THE ANTI-INFLAMMATORY SUCCESS PLAN

A Beginner's 28-Day Meal Plan, Strategies, and Self-Help Guide

STEPHEN WILLIAMS

TABLE OF CONTENTS

Anti-Inflammatory 28 Day meal plan	01-02
The Anti-Inflammatory Adventure Begins!	03
Week 1: Inflammation 101- Getting Started with the Basics	05
Day 1 Meal Plan	06-09
Flaxseeds: A Superstar in the Anti-Inflammatory Diet	10-11
Day 2 Meal Plan	12-15
Avocados, A Delicious Brain Food	16-17
Day 3 Meal Plan	18-21
Focus: Turmeric - The Golden Spice of Health	22-23
Day 4 Meal Plan	24-27
Cucumbers - The Cool Crusader	28-29
Day 5 Meal Plan	30-33
Papaya - The Tropical Anti-Inflammatory Star	34-35
Day 6 Meal Plan	36-39
Whole-Grain Toast - A Wholesome Foundation	40-41
Day 7 Meal Plan	42-45
Spinach - The Leafy Green Powerhouse	46-47
Completion of Week 1: A Thank You Note	48-52
Week 2: Flavorful Foods Fiesta	53-54
Day 8 Meal Plan	55-58
Cauliflower - The Cruciferous Marvel	59-60
Day 9 Meal Plan	61-64
Chickpeas - The Versatile Legume Powerhouse	65-66
Day 10 Meal Plan	67-70
Green Beans - The Vibrant Veggie Ally	71-72
Day 11 Meal Plan	73-76
Peaches: The Sweet Ally in Anti-Inflammatory Eating	77-78
Day 12 Meal Plan	79-82
Goat Cheese - The Tangy and Nutritious Delight	83-84
Day 13 Meal Plan	85-88
Sparkling Water - The Effervescent Hydrator	89-90
Day 14 Meal Plan	91-94
Blueberries - The Brain-Boosting, Anti-Inflammatory Superfruit	95-96
Completion of Week 2: A Gratitude Message	97-101

Day 15 Meal Plan	**102-105**
Chia Seeds - The Tiny Titans of Nutrition	**106-107**
Day 16 Meal Plan	**108-111**
Zucchini - The Versatile Vegetable for Health	**112-113**
Day 17 Meal Plan	**114-117**
Kiwi - The Tangy Vitamin Powerhouse	**118-119**
Day 18 Meal Plan	**120-123**
Trout - The Nutrient-Rich, Lean Protein	**124-125**
Day 19 Meal Plan	**126-129**
Mixed Nuts - The Heart-Healthy, Nutrient-Dense Snack	**130-131**
Day 20 Meal Plan	**132-135**
Tuna - The Lean Protein with Omega-3 Benefits	**136-137**
Day 21 Meal Plan	**138-141**
Asparagus - The Elegant and Nutritious Vegetable	**142-143**
Completion of Week 3: A Note of Thanks	**144-148**
Day 22 Meal Plan	**149-152**
Sweet Potato Fries vs. Regular Fries: A Nutritional Comparison	**153-154**
Day 23 Meal Plan	**155-158**
Olives - The Flavorful and Nutrient-Rich Fruit	**159-160**
Day 24 Meal Plan	**161-164**
Dark Chocolate - The Delicious Antioxidant Treat	**165-166**
Day 25 Meal Plan	**167-170**
Granola - The Crunchy, Wholesome Staple	**171-172**
Day 26 Meal Plan	**173-176**
Kale - The Leafy Green Superfood	**177-178**
Day 27 Meal Plan	**179-182**
Mango - The Tropical Nutrient Treasure	**183-184**
Day 28 Meal Plan	**185-188**
Completion of Week 4: A Message of Congratulations	**189-190**
How to Interpret Your Progress	**191**
Beyond the 28 Days: Sustaining an Anti-Inflammatory Lifestyle	**200**
Enhancing Your Anti-Inflammatory Journey Through Mindful Practices	**201**
Food to Avoid or minimize	**202**
F*** Ultra Processed Food	**205**
Integrating Anti-Inflammatory Choices in a Fast-Paced World	**208**
Acknowledgments and Further Learning Resources	**210**
	211

ANTI-INFLAMMATORY 28 DAY MEAL PLAN

Ready to turn down the heat on inflammation and turn up the dial on health and happiness?

Hey there, brave health explorer! Ready to embark on a 28-day adventure to calm the flames of inflammation? You're in the right place! This journey is all about transforming the way you eat to transform the way you feel.

Welcome to Your Personalized Path to Wellness

This book is designed to guide you through a transformative 28-day journey, focused on understanding and managing inflammation through a progressive meal plan, educational insights, and reflective practices.

Week-by-Week Inflammation Education

- Gradual Learning: Each week, we delve into different aspects of inflammation, starting with the basics and gradually building up to more complex concepts. This approach ensures you're not overwhelmed and can effectively integrate new information.
- Relevant Focus: The content is tailored to correspond with the weekly meal plans, providing context and deepening your understanding of how diet influences inflammation.

Progressive 28-Day Meal Plan

- Structured for Success: The meal plan is carefully structured to progress from simple, foundational meals in Week 1 to more diverse and adventurous meals in the following weeks. This progression is key in gently introducing your body to anti-inflammatory foods and habits.
- Variety and Exploration: As the weeks advance, you'll explore a wider range of anti-inflammatory foods, learning about their specific benefits and how they contribute to reducing inflammation and improving overall health.

Weekly Reflections Leading to Comprehensive Review

- Tracking Your Journey: At the end of each week, you'll have the opportunity to reflect on your experiences, feelings, and physical responses to the diet. This regular reflection helps in tracking your progress and tuning into your body's needs.
- Comprehensive Reflection Table: The book includes a detailed table for you to fill in at the back, providing a holistic view of your progress over the four weeks. This comprehensive reflection allows you to see patterns and overall improvements in various aspects of your health.

Deepening Knowledge with Spotlight on Foods

- Educational Insights: Throughout the book, we take a closer look at specific foods included in your meal plans. These spotlights provide deeper insights into why these foods were chosen, their health benefits, and how they combat inflammation.
- Informed Choices: Understanding the properties and benefits of these foods empowers you to make informed choices about your diet beyond the 28 days.

Equipping You with Tools for Lifelong Health

- Beyond the Diet: The book goes beyond just meal plans. It equips you with knowledge, strategies, and tools to continue managing inflammation through diet and lifestyle choices long after the 28 days are over.
- Empowerment Through Education: By the end of this journey, you'll have a comprehensive understanding of inflammation, how to manage it through diet, and how to incorporate mindful eating and stress reduction techniques into your daily life.

THE ANTI-INFLAMMATORY ADVENTURE BEGINS!, BUT WHAT IS IT ?

THE LOWDOWN ON CHRONIC INFLAMMATION

Imagine your body as a superhero, and inflammation is its trusty sidekick, jumping in when there's an injury or infection. But what happens when this sidekick starts overdoing it, causing more chaos than calm? That's chronic inflammation for you – a sneaky villain in disguise, linked to a whole host of health issues like arthritis, heart disease, and even some mood disorders.

Food: Your Secret Weapon Against Inflammation

Now, here's the exciting part: your kitchen is your secret lair, and your diet is one of the most powerful tools in your anti-inflammatory arsenal. Picture this: every bite you take is either fanning the flames of inflammation or dousing them with a big ol' bucket of water. This book is your map to choosing the water bucket every time!
Your 28-Day Anti-Inflammatory Blueprint
Over the next 28 days, we're goi
ng on a culinary quest filled with foods that love your body back. We're talking vibrant veggies, fantastic fruits, glorious grains, and other mouth-watering, inflammation-busting goodies. Each week, you'll get a new plan packed with great recipes and we'll help to improve knowledge and understanding of food in relation to inflammation.

FOODS TO AVOID

In the back of the book on page 205, you'll find a detailed list of foods, and substances, that are best avoided or minimized in an anti-inflammatory diet. Each food is scored on a scale of 1 to 5 based on its potential to exacerbate inflammation (with 1 being least problematic and 5 being most problematic).

F*** ULTRA PROCESSED FOOD

The Problem at a Glance:

- Health Risks: Ultra-processed foods are often laden with unhealthy ingredients that can exacerbate inflammation and lead to various health issues.
- Balance and Awareness: Learning how to identify and moderate the consumption of these foods is key to maintaining a healthy, anti-inflammatory diet.

In-Depth Exploration:

For a comprehensive guide on navigating the world of ultra-processed foods, refer to Page 208.

WHAT'S THE PLAN, STAN?

Week 1: Inflammation 101 - The Foundation Begins

In our initial week, we lay the groundwork for your anti-inflammatory journey. We start with the basics, introducing key concepts of inflammation, its impacts on health, and the principles of an anti-inflammatory lifestyle. This week is about setting a solid foundation, with simple yet effective meal plans that ease you into new eating habits. Expect to learn how everyday foods can either contribute to or reduce inflammation, and how to make choices that benefit your body.

Week 2: Flavorful Foods Fiesta - A Culinary Adventure

As you step into the second week, get ready for a culinary celebration! This week is all about exploring the vibrant world of anti-inflammatory foods. You'll discover a spectrum of flavors, colors, and textures, each bringing its unique health benefits. From colorful veggies to aromatic herbs and spices, your meals will be a delightful adventure. This week is designed to not only tantalize your taste buds but also show you the vast possibilities within a healthy diet.

Week 3: Mixin' It Up - Creativity in the Kitchen

Week three takes you deeper into the culinary journey. Here, we'll introduce a variety of new ingredients and cooking methods to add more excitement to your meals. It's all about creativity and experimentation, as you learn to mix and match different foods and flavors. This week encourages you to step out of your comfort zone and explore new dishes, showcasing how diverse and enjoyable an anti-inflammatory diet can be.

Week 4: Sustainable Swaps and Strategies - Building a Lasting Lifestyle

In our final week, we focus on sustainability. You'll learn how to make long-term changes to your diet and lifestyle that keep inflammation at bay. We'll cover practical tips for sustainable eating, how to make smart food swaps, and strategies to maintain your new eating habits. This week is about empowering you with the knowledge and tools to continue this healthful journey beyond the 28 days.

Reflect, Revisit, and Realize

At the end of each week, you'll have the opportunity to pause and reflect. Our dedicated reflection and notes pages are designed to help you gain insights into how the meal plans are influencing your health and wellbeing. These moments of introspection are vital for understanding your body's responses and the effectiveness of the diet. By regularly documenting your experiences, feelings, and any physical changes, you can track your progress and make adjustments as needed. These reflections not only provide a moment of pause in your busy week but are also a crucial component in realizing the full benefits of this transformative journey.

WEEK 1: INFLAMMATION 101- GETTING STARTED WITH THE BASICS

Ease into the anti-inflammatory lifestyle with simple, nourishing meals, complemented by healthy snacks and drinks.

UNDERSTANDING THE STRUCTURE OF WEEK 1

The Basics of Inflammation

- Acute vs. Chronic: In Week 1, we laid the groundwork by distinguishing between acute and chronic inflammation. Acute inflammation is your body's short-term response to injury or infection - think of it as a quick fix to a sudden problem. Chronic inflammation, however, is more like a slow burn that can lead to various health issues over time.
- Chronic Inflammation's Role: Chronic inflammation is linked to numerous diseases, including arthritis, heart disease, and even certain cancers. It's like having a low-level fire constantly burning in your body, which can eventually lead to significant damage.

The Science Behind Anti-Inflammatory Diets

- Food as Medicine: The meals in Week 1 were carefully chosen to introduce you to foods that are known for their anti-inflammatory properties. These foods, such as leafy greens, berries, nuts, and fatty fish, contain nutrients that help cool down inflammation.
- Gut Health Connection: There's a strong link between gut health and inflammation. The diet emphasizes foods that are not only anti-inflammatory but also gut-friendly, helping to restore and maintain a healthy gut microbiome.

DAY 1 MEAL PLAN

BREAKFAST: OATMEAL WITH BLUEBERRIES AND FLAXSEEDS
LUNCH: GRILLED CHICKEN SALAD WITH OLIVE OIL DRESSING
DINNER: BAKED SALMON WITH STEAMED BROCCOLI AND SWEET POTATO
SNACK: CARROT STICKS WITH HUMMUS
SNACK: ALMONDS
DRINK: GINGER TEA

BREAKFAST: OATMEAL WITH BLUEBERRIES AND FLAXSEEDS

INGREDIENTS

- ½ cup rolled oats
- 1 cup water or milk (dairy or almond milk)
- A handful of blueberries (fresh or frozen)
- 1 teaspoon ground flaxseeds

INSTRUCTIONS

- Measure and Mix: Add oats and liquid to the pot.
- Cook the Oatmeal: Heat on medium, bring to a gentle boil, then simmer for about 5 minutes.
- Check Consistency: Ensure oats are soft, adjusting cooking time if necessary.
- Add Toppings: Off heat, add blueberries and flaxseeds.
- Serve: Allow to cool briefly, then serve. Optionally, sweeten with honey or maple syrup.

KITCHEN TOOLS NEEDED
- Small pot
- Stirring spoon
- Serving bowl
- Measuring cup and spoon

LUNCH: GRILLED CHICKEN SALAD WITH OLIVE OIL DRESSING

INGREDIENTS

- 1 small chicken breast (3-4 oz)
- 2 cups mixed salad greens
- ¼ cup cherry tomatoes, halved
- ¼ cucumber, sliced
- 1 tablespoon olive oil
- ½ tablespoon lemon juice or vinegar
- Salt and pepper to taste
- Optional: red onion slices, avocado, nuts

INSTRUCTIONS

- Prepare Chicken: Season and grill the chicken, then slice it.
- Prepare Salad: Combine greens, tomatoes, and cucumber.
- Make Dressing: Mix olive oil, lemon juice/vinegar, salt, and pepper.
- Assemble Salad: Add dressing to greens, top with chicken.
- Serve: Enjoy your nutritious salad.

KITCHEN TOOLS NEEDED
- Grill pan or skillet
- Mixing bowl
- Knife and cutting board
- Measuring spoons
- Salad tongs or mixing spoons

DINNER: BAKED SALMON WITH STEAMED BROCCOLI AND SWEET POTATO

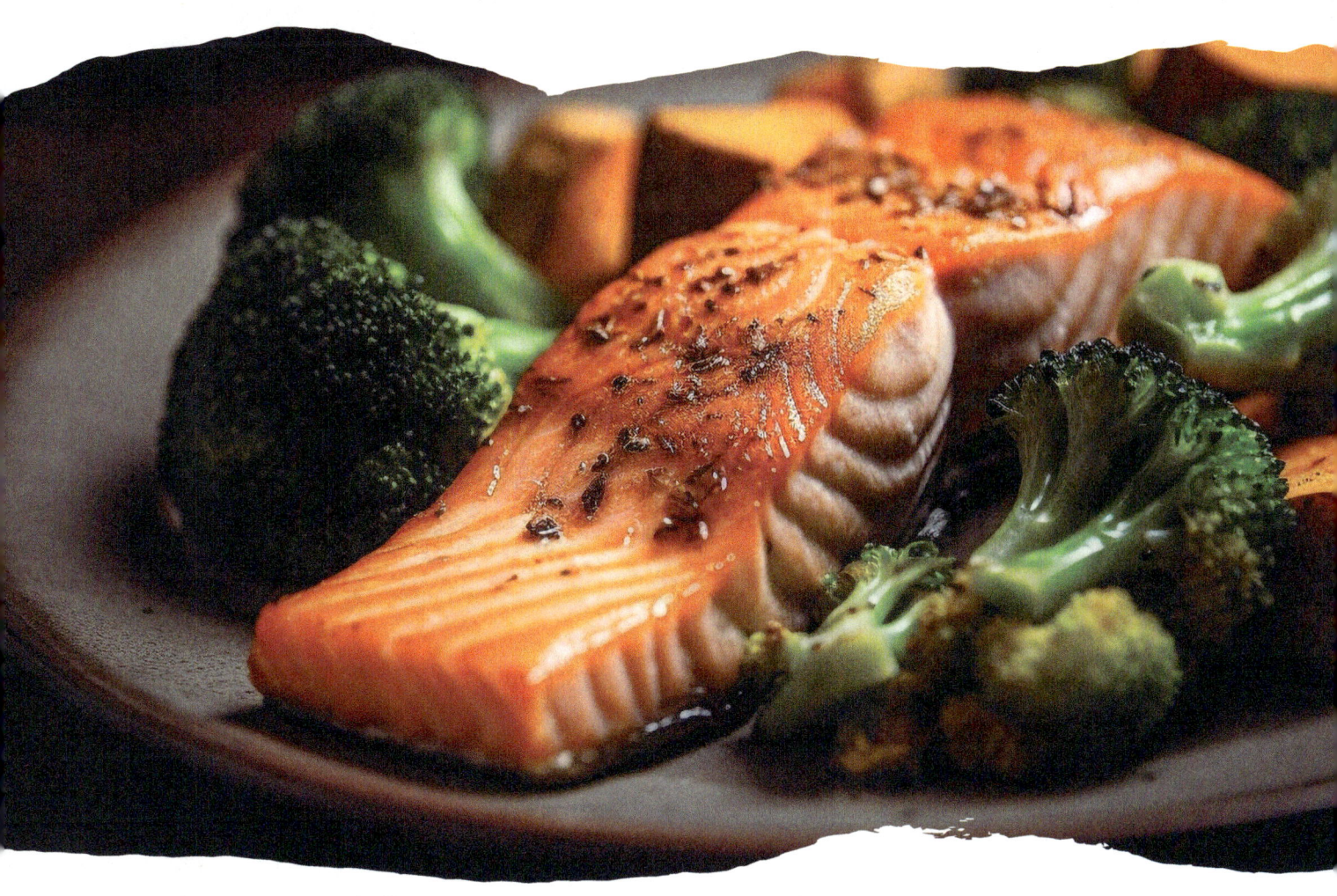

INGREDIENTS

- 1 salmon fillet (4-6 oz)
- 1 medium sweet potato
- 1 cup broccoli florets
- Olive oil
- Salt and pepper to taste
- Optional: herbs like dill or parsley

INSTRUCTIONS

- Prepare Sweet Potato: Peel, slice, season with oil and salt, and bake.
- Prepare Salmon: Season and wrap in foil, then bake with sweet potato.
- Steam Broccoli: Steam in a pot or microwave.
- Check and Serve: Ensure everything is cooked through, serve together.

KITCHEN TOOLS NEEDED

- Oven and baking sheet
- Steamer basket and pot or microwave-safe dish
- Knife and cutting board
- Aluminum foil
- Measuring spoons

DRINK: GINGER TEA

INGREDIENTS
- 1-inch piece of fresh ginger
- 1 cup water

PREPARATION TIME: ~15 MINUTES
- Boil water, add ginger, simmer, strain, and serve warm.

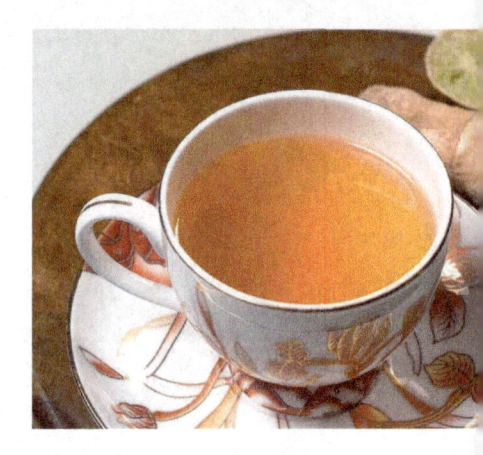

SNACK: CARROT STICKS WITH HUMMUS

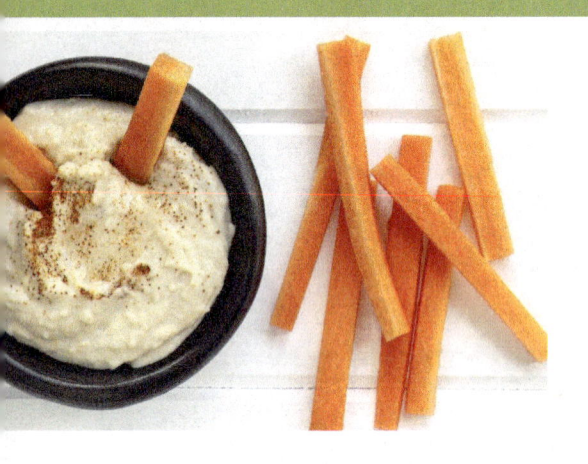

INGREDIENTS
- 1 large carrot
- 2 tablespoons hummus

PREPARATION TIME: ~5 MINUTES
- Peel and cut the carrot into sticks.
- Serve with hummus for dipping.

SNACK: ALMONDS

INGREDIENTS
- 10-15 raw or dry-roasted almonds

PREPARATION TIME: NONE, READY TO EAT.

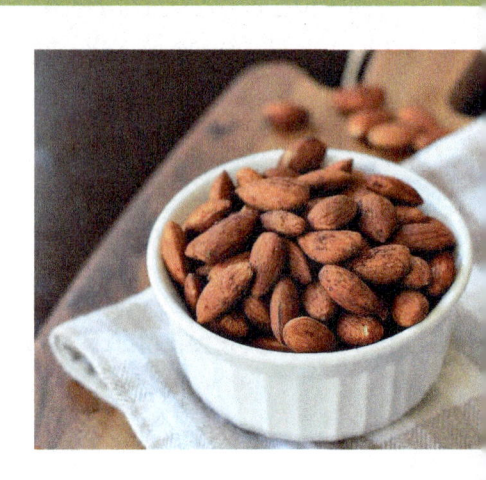

FLAXSEEDS: A SUPERSTAR IN THE ANTI-INFLAMMATORY DIET

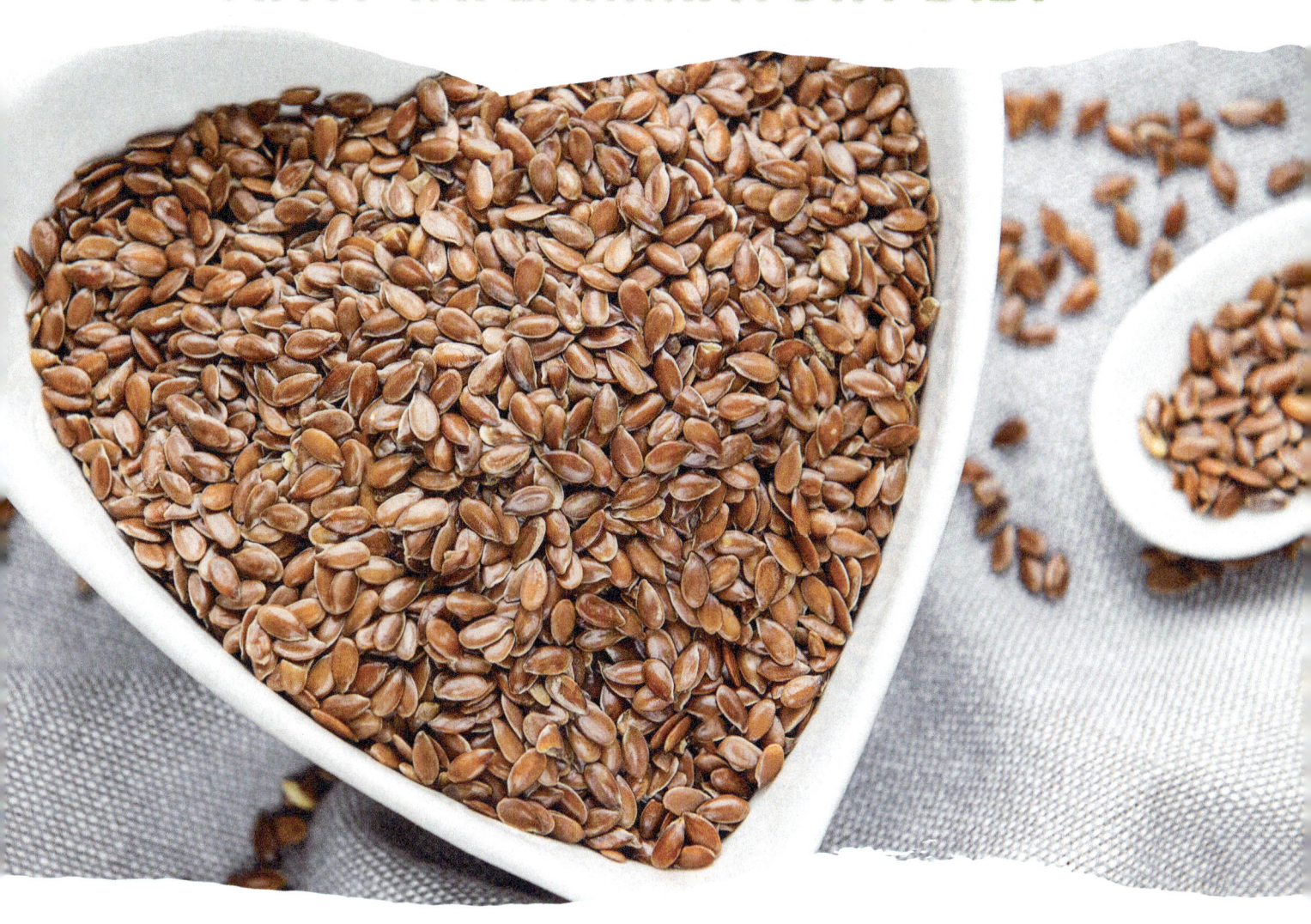

Flaxseeds on Day 1: A Thoughtful Introduction

Let's zoom in on why we kicked off our 28-Day Anti-Inflammatory Meal Plan with flaxseeds on Day 1. These little seeds are more than just a crunchy addition to your morning oatmeal; they're a powerhouse of anti-inflammatory benefits.

THE BENEFITS OF FLAXSEEDS

- Rich in Omega-3 Fatty Acids: Flaxseeds are loaded with alpha-linolenic acid (ALA), a type of omega-3 fatty acid, which is known for its anti-inflammatory properties. Starting your day with a dose of omega-3s helps set a positive, inflammation-reducing tone for the rest of your meals.
- High in Fiber: The fiber in flaxseeds aids digestion and helps maintain a healthy gut, which is crucial in managing inflammation. A healthy gut means less room for inflammation to wreak havoc.
- Lignans for Antioxidant Support: Flaxseeds contain lignans, which have antioxidant properties. Antioxidants combat free radicals in the body, reducing oxidative stress and inflammation.

COMPLEMENTING OTHER FOODS

- Synergy with Oatmeal and Blueberries: On Day 1, flaxseeds were paired with oatmeal and blueberries. This combination works beautifully as the fiber from oatmeal and antioxidants from blueberries complement the flaxseeds, enhancing their anti-inflammatory effects.
- Versatility: The beauty of flaxseeds lies in their versatility. They can be sprinkled over salads, blended into smoothies, or even used as an egg substitute in baking, making them an easy addition to various meals throughout the day.

A FOUNDATION FOR THE REST OF THE WEEK

- Building a Healthy Habit: By introducing flaxseeds on Day 1, we're setting up a healthy habit that can be carried forward. Their subtle taste and easy integration into meals make them a sustainable choice for long-term dietary planning.
- Prepping for Week 2's Diversity: As we gear up for Week 2's "Flavorful Foods Fiesta," flaxseeds serve as a foundational ingredient that can easily adapt to the introduction of more diverse flavors and foods.

Incorporating flaxseeds into your diet right from the start is a strategic move to harness their anti-inflammatory benefits. As you progress through the meal plan, you'll find that these tiny seeds are not only nutritious but also a versatile ally in your journey towards reducing inflammation and promoting overall health.

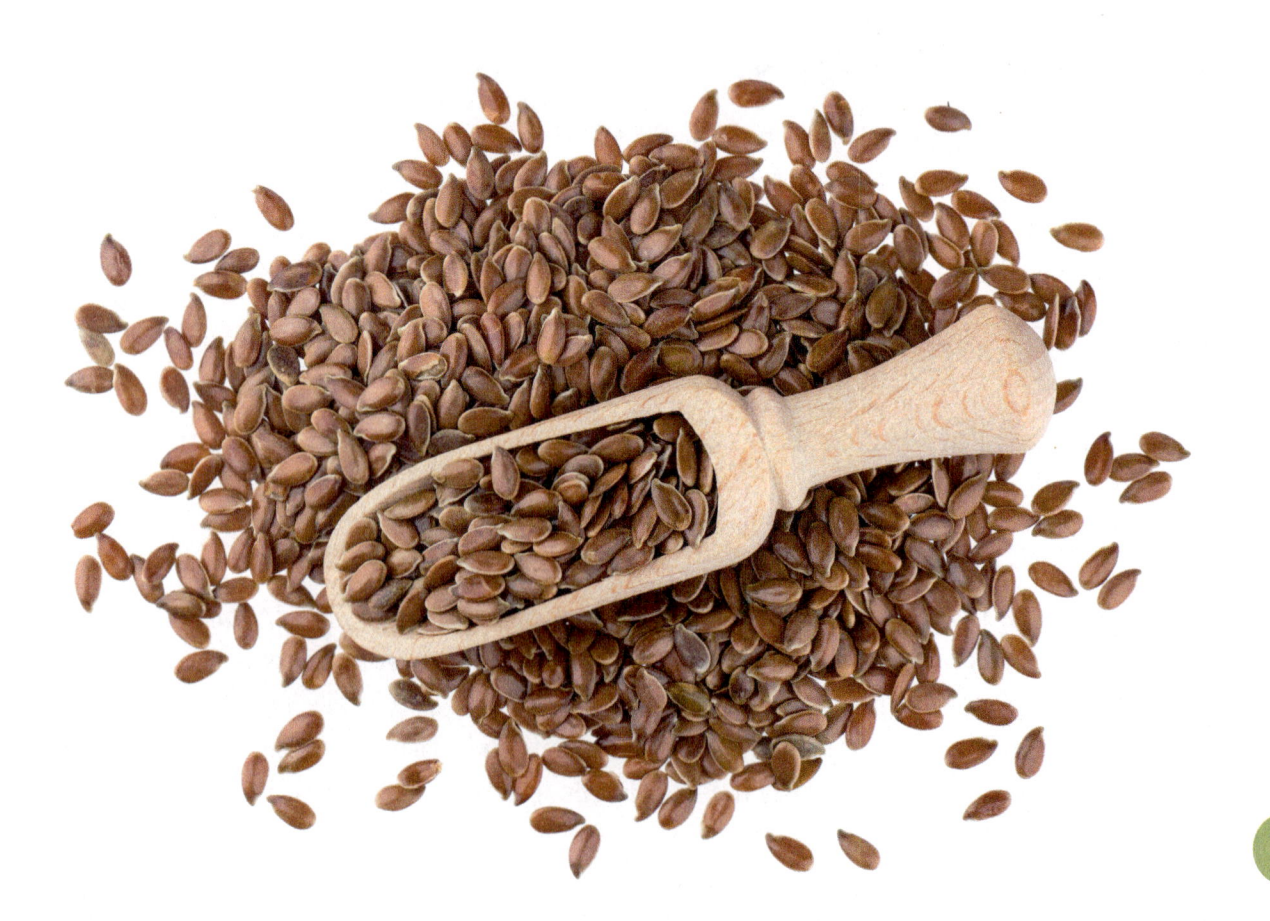

DAY 2 MEAL PLAN

BREAKFAST: GREEK YOGURT WITH HONEY AND WALNUTS
LUNCH: LENTIL SOUP WITH WHOLE-GRAIN BREAD
DINNER: GRILLED TURKEY BURGER WITH AVOCADO AND SIDE SALAD
SNACK: PINEAPPLE
SNACK: APPLE SLICES WITH ALMOND BUTTER
DRINK: CHAMOMILE TEA

BREAKFAST: GREEK YOGURT WITH HONEY AND WALNUTS

INGREDIENTS

- 1 cup Greek yogurt (plain or unsweetened)
- 1 tablespoon honey
- A handful of walnuts

INSTRUCTIONS

- Serve Yogurt: Scoop the Greek yogurt into a bowl.
- Add Toppings: Drizzle honey over the yogurt.
- Sprinkle Walnuts: Add a handful of walnuts on top.
- Stir and Enjoy: Mix slightly if desired and enjoy!

KITCHEN TOOLS NEEDED
- Spoon
- Serving bowl

LUNCH: LENTIL SOUP WITH WHOLE-GRAIN BREAD

INGREDIENTS

- Ingredients:
- 1 serving of pre-made or canned lentil soup
- 1 slice of whole-grain bread

INSTRUCTIONS

- Heat Soup: Warm the lentil soup in a pot over the stove or in a microwave-safe bowl.
- Prepare Bread: Toast the whole-grain bread if desired.
- Serve Together: Enjoy the soup with a side of whole-grain bread.

KITCHEN TOOLS NEEDED
- Pot or microwave-safe bowl
- Soup spoon

SNACK: APPLE SLICES WITH ALMOND BUTTER

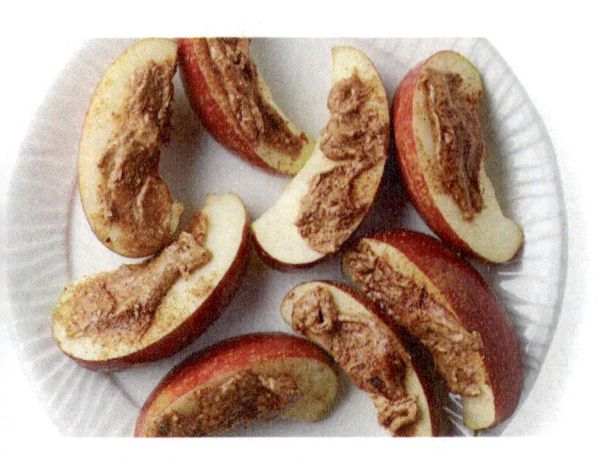

INGREDIENTS

- 1 apple
- 2 tablespoons almond butter

INSTRUCTIONS

- Slice Apple: Cut the apple into slices.
- Serve with Almond Butter: Place apple slices on a plate with a small spoonful of almond butter for dipping.

KITCHEN TOOLS NEEDED
- Knife and cutting board
- Small spoon

DINNER: GRILLED TURKEY BURGER WITH AVOCADO AND SIDE SALAD

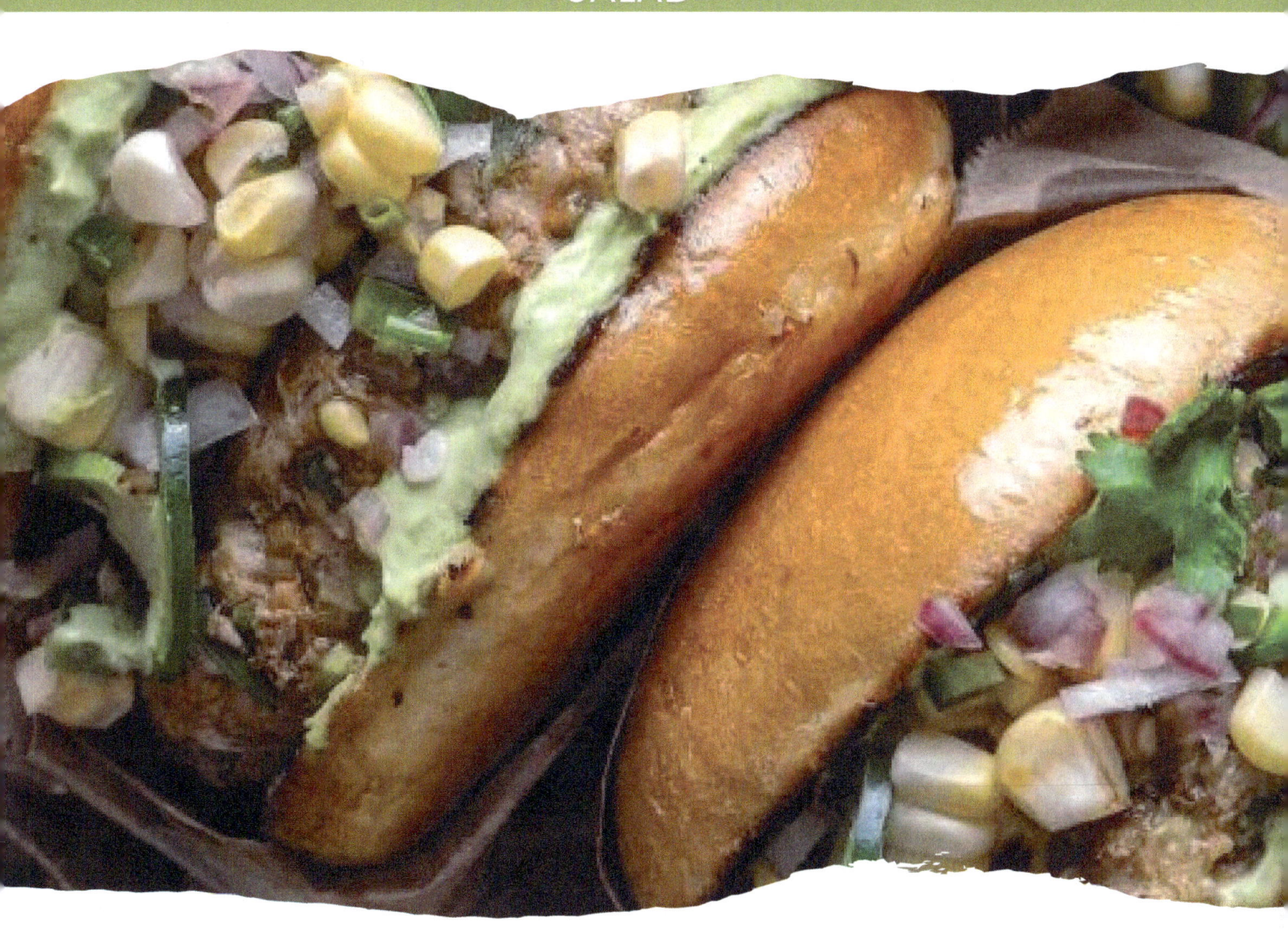

INGREDIENTS

- 1 turkey burger patty
- 1 whole-wheat burger bun
- 1/2 ripe avocado
- Lettuce, tomato, and other desired salad ingredients
- Olive oil and vinegar for dressing

INSTRUCTIONS

- Cook Turkey Burger: Grill the turkey patty until fully cooked.
- Prepare Avocado: Slice the avocado.
- Assemble Burger: Place the cooked turkey patty on the bun, add avocado slices.
- Make Side Salad: Toss together salad ingredients, drizzle with dressing.
- Serve: Enjoy the burger with the side salad.

KITCHEN TOOLS NEEDED
- Grill pan or skillet
- Knife and cutting board

DRINK: CHAMOMILE TEA

INGREDIENTS

- 1 chamomile tea bag
- 1 cup water

INSTRUCTIONS

- Boil Water: Heat water.
- Steep Tea: Place the tea bag in a mug, pour hot water over it.

KITCHEN TOOLS NEEDED

- Kettle or pot for boiling water
- Mug

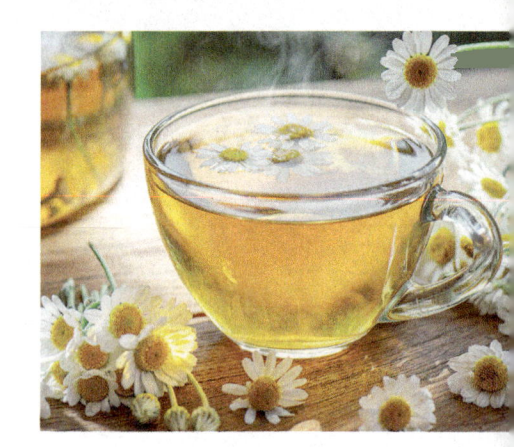

SNACK: PINEAPPLE

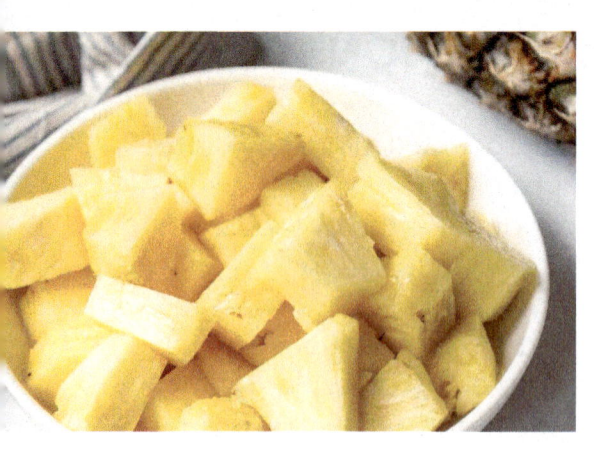

INGREDIENTS

- A small serving of pineapple (fresh or canned in juice)

INSTRUCTIONS

- Prepare Pineapple: If fresh, peel and cut the pineapple into chunks. If canned, drain the juice.

KITCHEN TOOLS NEEDED

- Knife and cutting board (if using fresh pineapple)

AVOCADOS, A DELICIOUS BRAIN FOOD

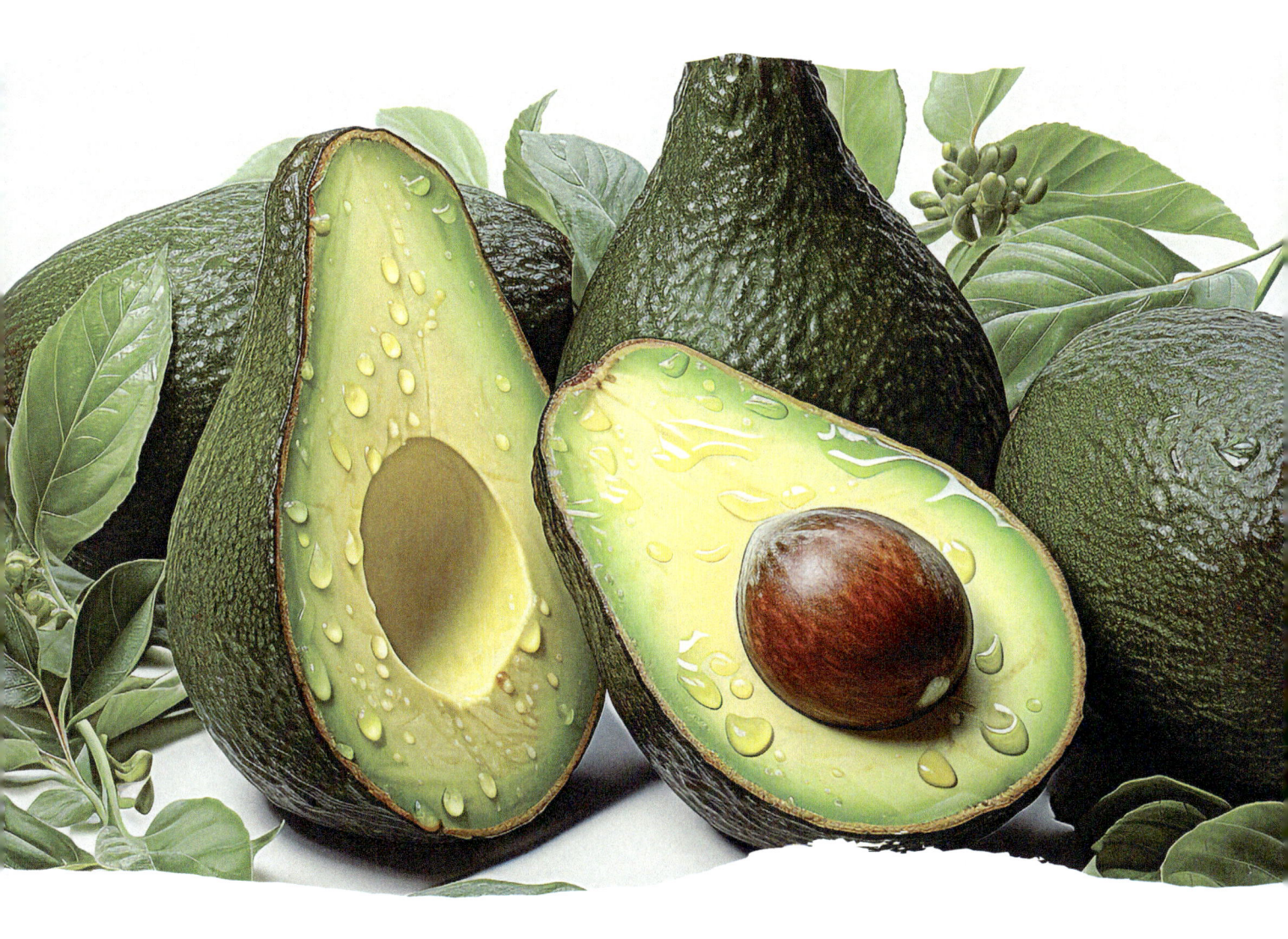

On Day 2 of our Anti-Inflammatory Meal Plan, avocados take the stage, especially in your dinner with that scrumptious grilled turkey burger. Avocados aren't just tasty and versatile; they're a brain food and a powerful ally in your anti-inflammatory arsenal.

THE BENEFITS OF AVOCADOS

- Packed with Healthy Fats: Avocados are rich in monounsaturated fats, which are great for heart health and brain function. These fats help reduce inflammation and are essential for a healthy nervous system, supporting brain health and cognitive function.
- Loaded with Fiber and Nutrients: They're also high in fiber, contributing to gut health, and packed with nutrients like potassium and vitamins E, C, and B-6, all of which play a role in reducing inflammation and supporting overall well-being.
- Brain Health Champion: The healthy fats in avocados are particularly beneficial for the brain. They contribute to the health of the nerve cells in the brain, aiding in the processes that support memory, learning, and overall cognitive function.

COMPLEMENTING THE DAY'S MEALS

- With the Turkey Burger: In your dinner, the avocado adds a creamy texture and a richness that complements the lean protein of the turkey burger. This combination ensures a satisfying meal that's both brain-friendly and anti-inflammatory.
- Throughout the Day: The versatile nature of avocados means they can be easily incorporated into various meals, whether it's as a spread on whole-grain toast for breakfast or added to a salad for lunch.

PREPARING FOR A NUTRIENT-RICH WEEK

- A Daily Dose of Brain Health: By incorporating avocados early in the week, we're emphasizing the importance of brain health in conjunction with anti-inflammatory eating. It's about looking after your body as a whole, brain included.
- Setting Up for a Flavorful Journey: As we move towards the "Flavorful Foods Fiesta" in Week 2, avocados serve as a reminder of the richness and diversity of flavors that can be enjoyed within an anti-inflammatory diet.

In short, avocados are much more than just a delicious addition to your meal; they're a nutrient-rich, brain-boosting food that plays a significant role in reducing inflammation and supporting overall health. As you continue on this 28-day journey, consider avocados your creamy companion in achieving both delicious and healthful meals.

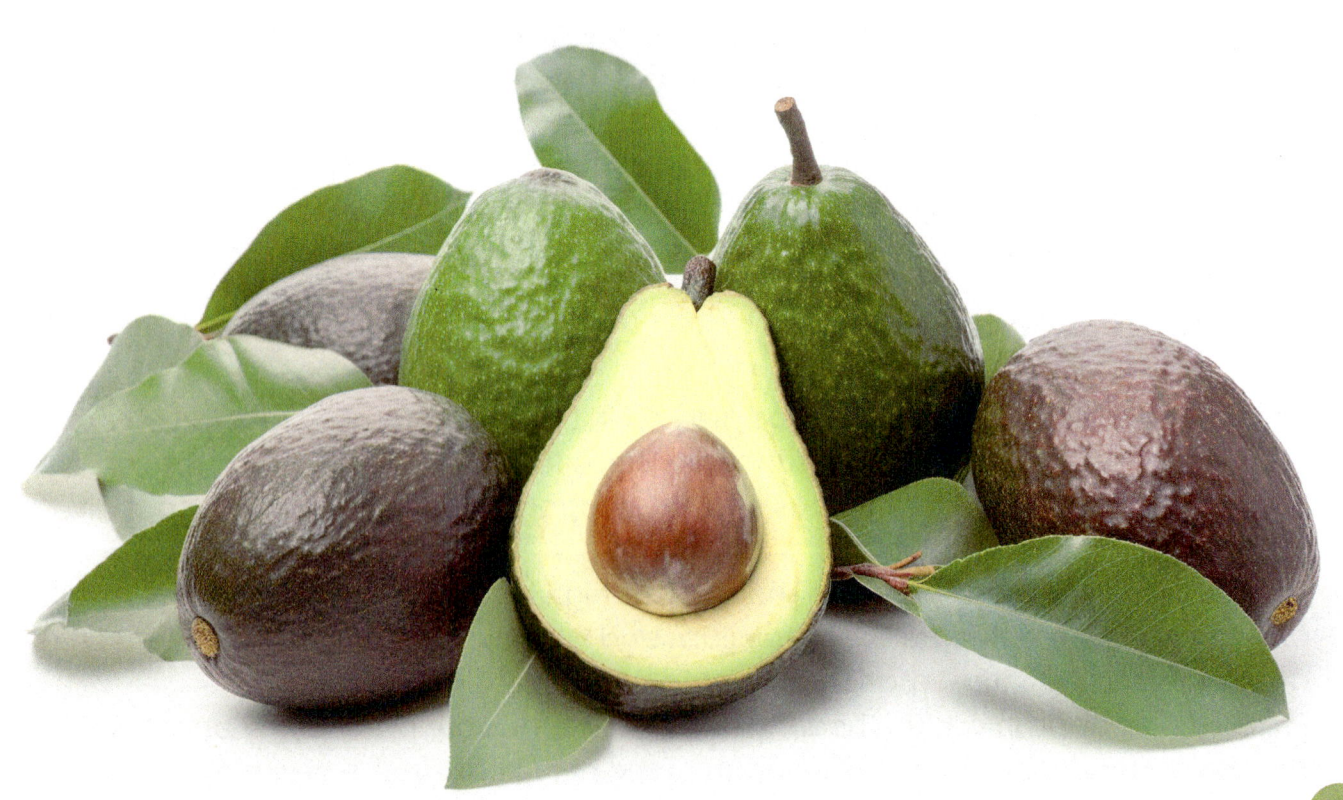

DAY 3 MEAL PLAN

BREAKFAST: SCRAMBLED EGGS WITH SPINACH AND TOMATOES
LUNCH: QUINOA BOWL WITH MIXED VEGGIES AND LEMON-TAHINI DRESSING
DINNER: BAKED COD WITH ASPARAGUS AND BROWN RICE
SNACK: A SMALL ORANGE
SNACK: CUCUMBER SLICES WITH GUACAMOLE
DRINK: TURMERIC AND LEMON WATER

BREAKFAST: SCRAMBLED EGGS WITH SPINACH AND TOMATOES

INGREDIENTS

- 2 eggs
- A handful of fresh spinach
- 1 small tomato, chopped
- Olive oil or butter for cooking
- Salt and pepper to taste

INSTRUCTIONS

- Prep Ingredients: Wash spinach and chop tomato.
- Cook Eggs: Beat the eggs in a bowl. Heat oil or butter in a skillet, pour in the eggs.
- Add Vegetables: Add spinach and tomato to the skillet.
- Scramble: Cook while stirring until eggs are set. Season with salt and pepper.
- Serve: Enjoy your healthy scrambled eggs.

KITCHEN TOOLS NEEDED
- Spoon
- Skillet
- Spatula
- Knife and cutting board

LUNCH: QUINOA BOWL WITH MIXED VEGGIES AND LEMON-TAHINI DRESSING

INGREDIENTS

- ½ cup cooked quinoa
- A mix of your favorite veggies (like bell peppers, carrots, and broccoli)
- 1 tablespoon tahini
- Juice of ½ lemon
- Salt and pepper to taste

INSTRUCTIONS

- Prepare Veggies: Chop the veggies into bite-sized pieces.
- Make Dressing: Whisk together tahini, lemon juice, salt, and pepper.
- Assemble Bowl: Place quinoa in a bowl, top with veggies.
- Add Dressing: Drizzle the lemon-tahini dressing over the top.
- Serve: Mix everything together and enjoy.

KITCHEN TOOLS NEEDED
- Bowl
- Knife and cutting board
- Small whisk or spoon

DINNER: BAKED COD WITH ASPARAGUS AND BROWN RICE

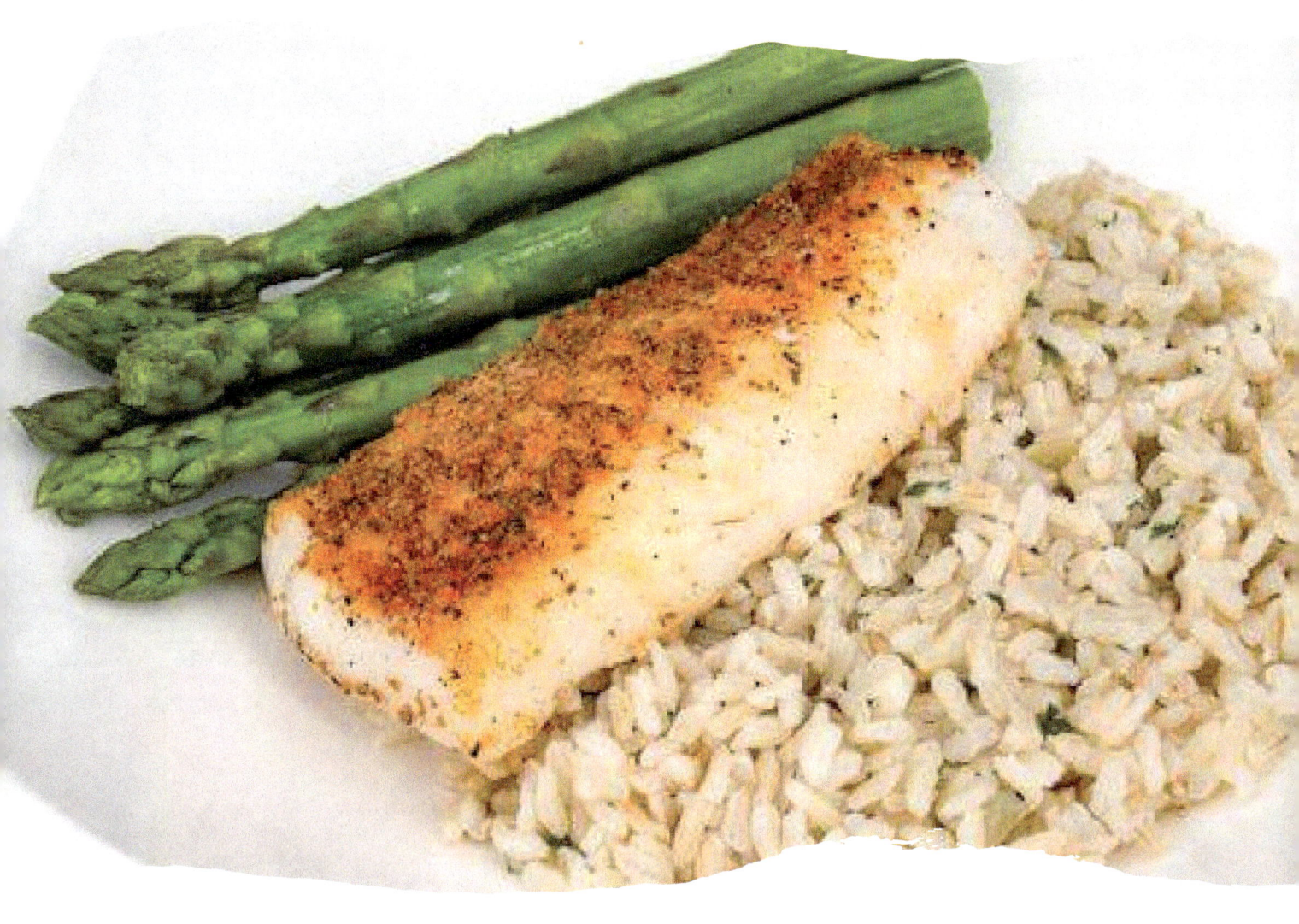

INGREDIENTS

- 1 cod fillet (about 4-6 oz)
- A bunch of asparagus
- ½ cup brown rice
- Olive oil
- Salt and pepper to taste

INSTRUCTIONS

- Cook Rice: Cook brown rice according to package instructions.
- Prepare Cod and Asparagus: Preheat oven to 400ºF (200ºC). Season cod with salt and pepper. Trim asparagus ends and toss with olive oil.
- Bake: Place cod and asparagus on a baking sheet. Bake for about 12-15 minutes.
- Check and Serve: Ensure cod is cooked through and asparagus is tender. Serve alongside the cooked brown rice.

KITCHEN TOOLS NEEDED
- Oven and baking sheet
- Pot for rice
- Knife and cutting board

DRINK: TURMERIC AND LEMON WATER

INGREDIENTS

- 1 cup water
- ½ teaspoon turmeric powder
- Juice of ½ lemon

INSTRUCTIONS

- Boil Water: Heat water in a kettle or pot.
- Mix Ingredients: Add turmeric and lemon juice to a mug.
- Combine: Pour hot water into the mug, stir well.
- Serve: Drink while warm, stirring occasionally as turmeric may settle.

KITCHEN TOOLS NEEDED

- Kettle or pot for boiling water
- Mug
- Spoon

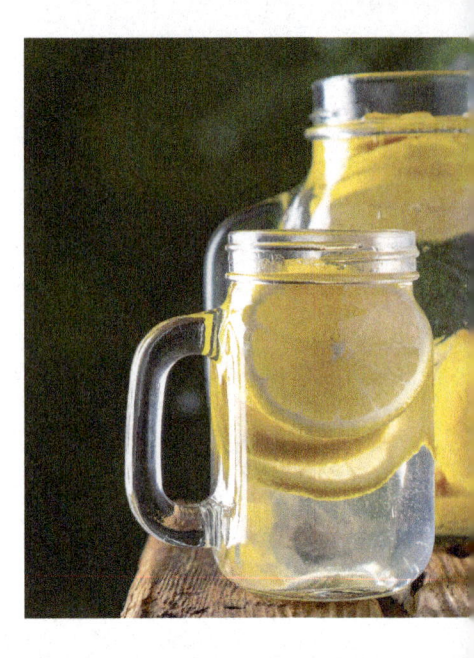

SNACK: CUCUMBER SLICES WITH GUACAMOLE

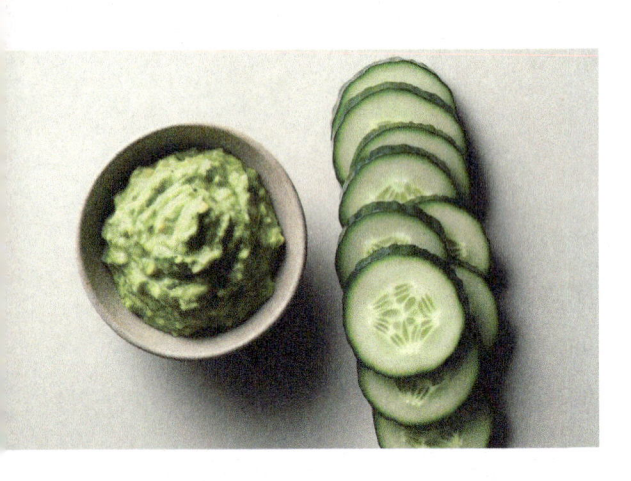

INGREDIENTS

- 1 small cucumber
- 2 tablespoons guacamole

INSTRUCTIONS

- Slice Cucumber: Cut the cucumber into slices.
- Serve with Guacamole: Enjoy the cucumber slices with a side of guacamole for dipping.

KITCHEN TOOLS NEEDED

- Knife and cutting board

SNACK: A SMALL ORANGE

INGREDIENTS

- 1 small orange

PREPARATION TIME: NONE, READY TO EAT.

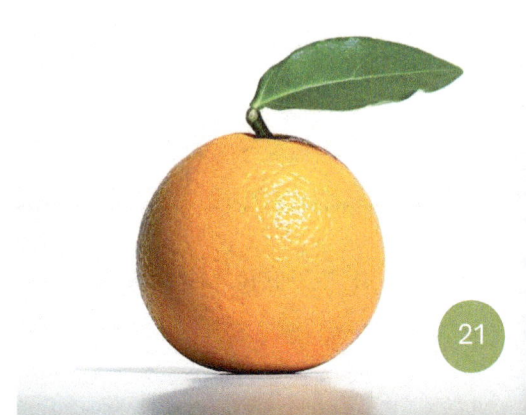

TURMERIC – THE GOLDEN SPICE OF HEALTH

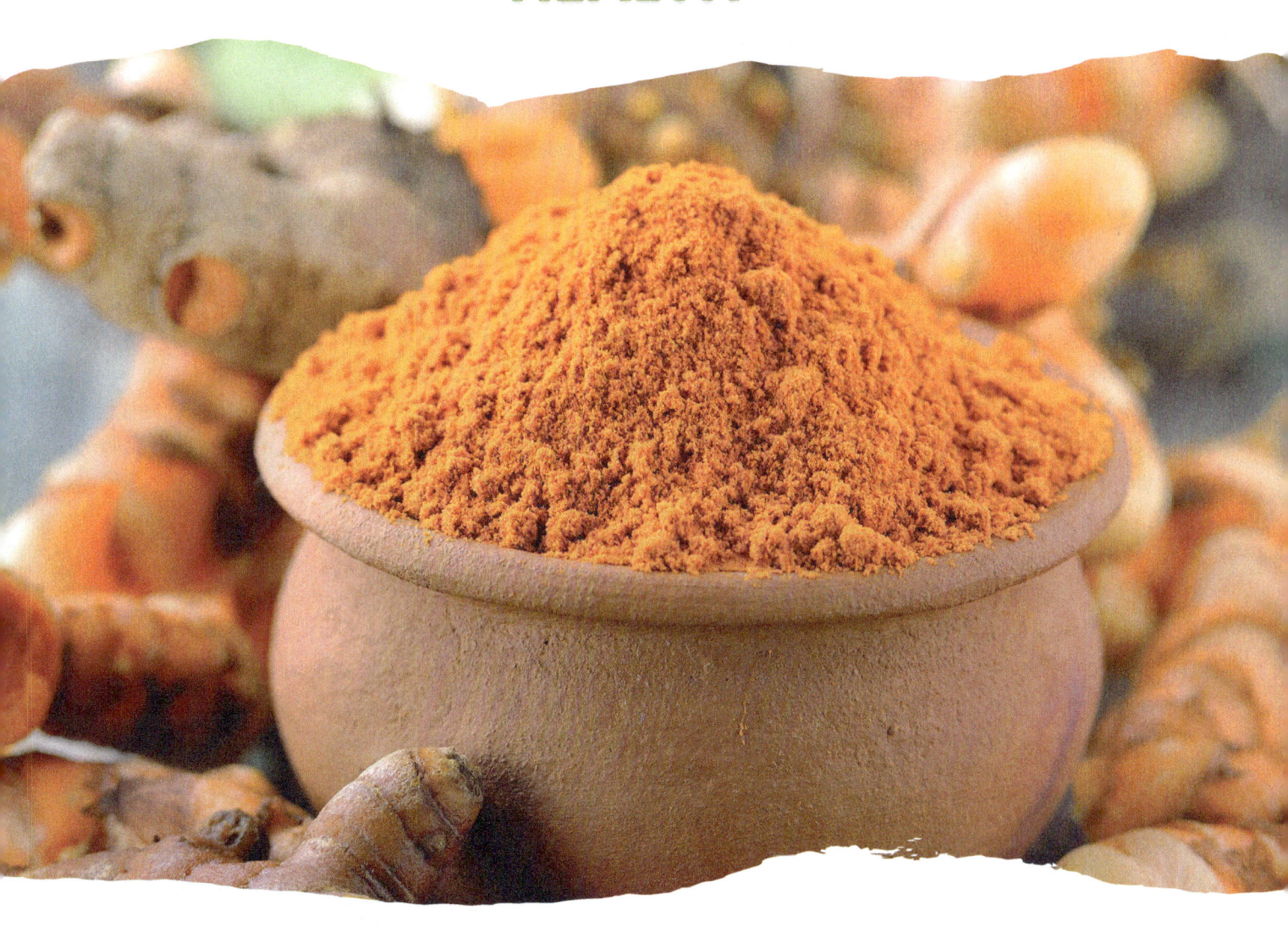

Turmeric in Day 3: A Spice That Does More Than Just Flavor
On Day 3 of our Anti-Inflammatory Meal Plan, we introduce turmeric, notably in your turmeric and lemon water. This golden spice is renowned not just for its ability to add flavor and color but also for its impressive health benefits.

The Wonders of Turmeric

- Anti-Inflammatory Powerhouse: The active compound in turmeric, curcumin, is a potent anti-inflammatory agent. It helps in reducing inflammation throughout the body, making it a valuable addition to an anti-inflammatory diet.
- Boosts Brain Health: Curcumin in turmeric is also linked to improved brain function. It can increase levels of brain-derived neurotrophic factor (BDNF), a protein that plays a vital role in the health of nerve cells, aiding in memory and learning.
- Antioxidant Abilities: Turmeric is a powerful antioxidant that can neutralize free radicals, protecting cells from damage and reducing oxidative stress, which is often a contributor to chronic inflammation.

COMPLEMENTING THE DAY'S MEALS

- With the Dinner: The inclusion of turmeric in the drink complements the baked cod and asparagus dinner, adding an extra layer of anti-inflammatory benefits to an already nutritious meal.
- Throughout the Day: Turmeric can be sprinkled on various foods, from scrambled eggs to quinoa bowls, enhancing flavor while boosting health benefits.

PREPARING FOR A VIBRANT WEEK

- A Daily Dose of Wellness: Introducing turmeric early in the week sets the tone for a diet rich in anti-inflammatory ingredients. It's about more than just reducing inflammation; it's about enhancing overall health and vitality.
- Setting the Stage for Week 2's Fiesta: As we approach the "Flavorful Foods Fiesta," turmeric serves as a reminder of the diverse and vibrant flavors that can be part of an anti-inflammatory diet, each with its unique health benefits.

In essence, turmeric is a multifaceted spice, playing a significant role in reducing inflammation, boosting brain health, and fighting oxidative stress. Its inclusion in the meal plan is a testament to the fact that powerful health benefits can come from the most unassuming of spices. As you move forward in this 28-day journey, let turmeric be a golden thread, adding both color and health to your meals.

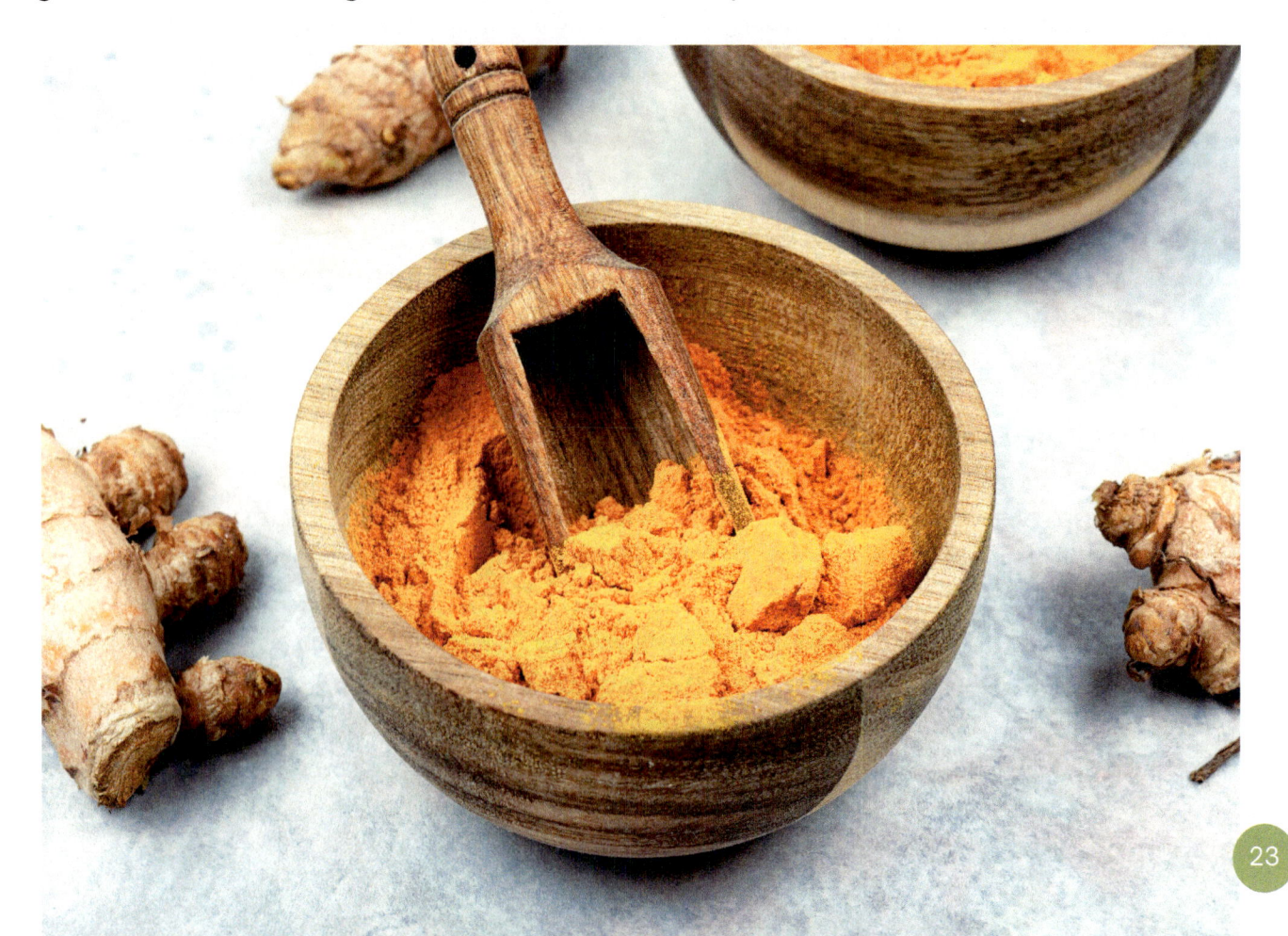

DAY 4 MEAL PLAN

BREAKFAST: SPINACH, BANANA, AND ALMOND MILK SMOOTHIE
LUNCH: TURKEY AND HUMMUS WRAP WITH CUCUMBER AND BELL PEPPER
DINNER: CHICKEN STIR-FRY WITH BROCCOLI AND CARROTS ON QUINOA
SNACK: MIXED BERRIES
SNACK: CELERY STICKS WITH PEANUT BUTTER
DRINK: GREEN TEA

BREAKFAST: SPINACH, BANANA, AND ALMOND MILK SMOOTHIE

INGREDIENTS

- 1 cup fresh spinach
- 1 ripe banana
- 1 cup almond milk
- Optional: a scoop of protein powder or a tablespoon of honey for sweetness

INSTRUCTIONS

- Combine Ingredients: Place spinach, banana, and almond milk in the blender. Add protein powder or honey if using.
- Blend: Blend on high until smooth.
- Serve: Pour into a glass and enjoy your refreshing smoothie.

KITCHEN TOOLS NEEDED
- Blender
- Measuring cup

LUNCH: TURKEY AND HUMMUS WRAP WITH CUCUMBER AND BELL PEPPER

INGREDIENTS

- 1 whole-grain wrap or tortilla
- 2-3 slices of turkey breast
- 2 tablespoons hummus
- Sliced cucumber
- Sliced bell pepper

INSTRUCTIONS

- Prepare Veggies: Slice cucumber and bell pepper.
- Assemble Wrap: Spread hummus on the wrap. Add turkey slices, cucumber, and bell pepper.
- Roll and Serve: Roll the wrap tightly, cut in half, and enjoy.

KITCHEN TOOLS NEEDED
- Knife and cutting board

DINNER: CHICKEN STIR-FRY WITH BROCCOLI AND CARROTS ON QUINOA

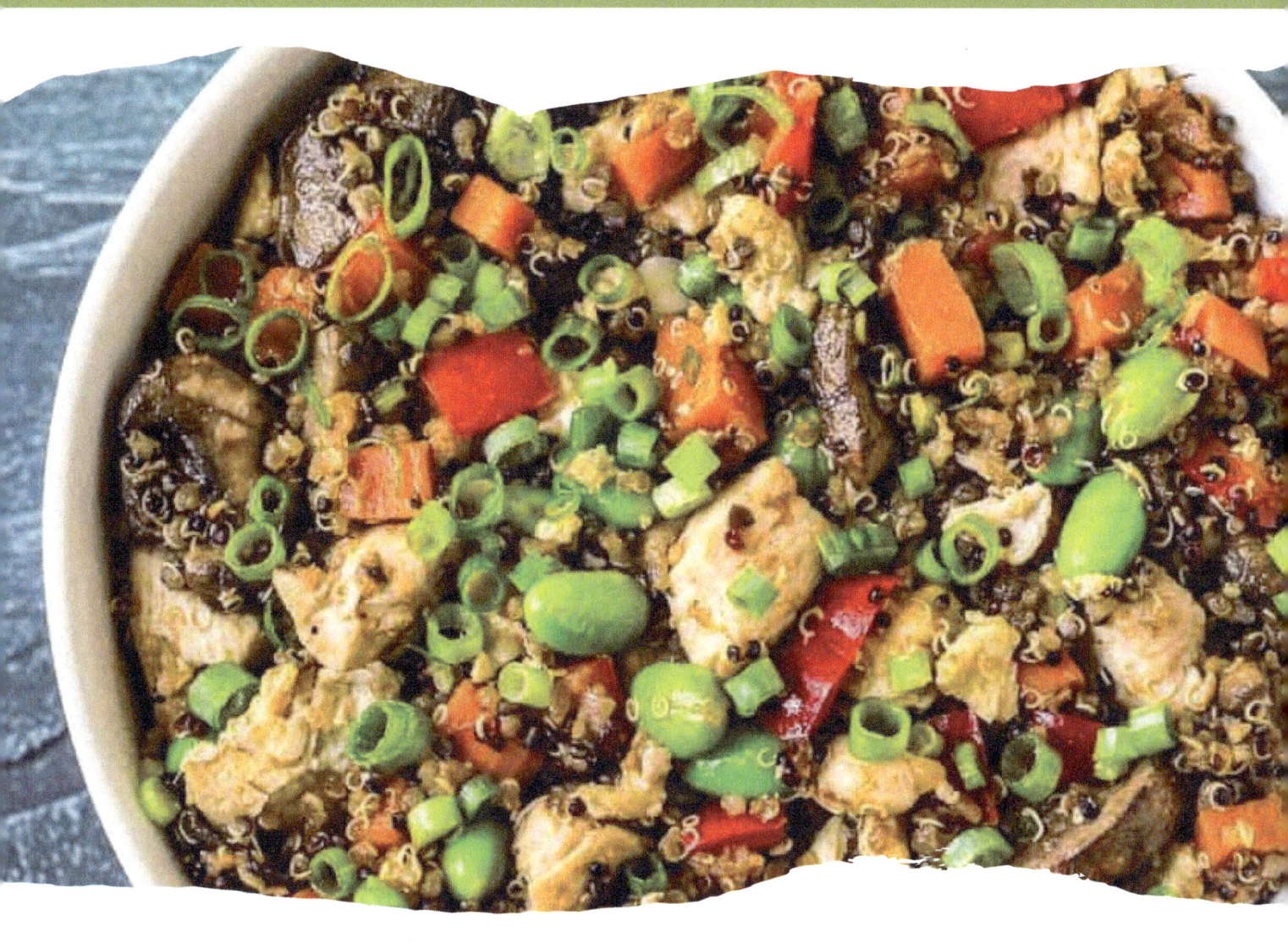

INGREDIENTS

- 1 chicken breast, cut into bite-sized pieces
- 1 cup broccoli florets
- 1 carrot, sliced
- ½ cup quinoa
- Soy sauce or a stir-fry sauce
- Olive oil or sesame oil

INSTRUCTIONS

- Cook Quinoa: Cook quinoa according to package instructions.
- Prepare Stir-Fry: Heat oil in a skillet or wok. Add chicken pieces and cook until browned.
- Add Vegetables: Add broccoli and carrots, stir-fry until vegetables are tender.
- Season: Add soy sauce or stir-fry sauce, mix well.
- Serve: Place cooked quinoa on a plate, top with the chicken and vegetable stir-fry.

KITCHEN TOOLS NEEDED
- Skillet or wok
- Pot for quinoa
- Knife and cutting board

DRINK: GREEN TEA

INGREDIENTS
- 1 green tea bag
- 1 cup water

INSTRUCTIONS
- Boil Water: Heat water in a kettle or pot.
- Steep Tea: Place the tea bag in a mug, pour hot water over it.
- Wait and Enjoy: Let the tea steep for about 3-5 minutes before drinking.

KITCHEN TOOLS NEEDED
- Kettle or pot for boiling water
- Mug

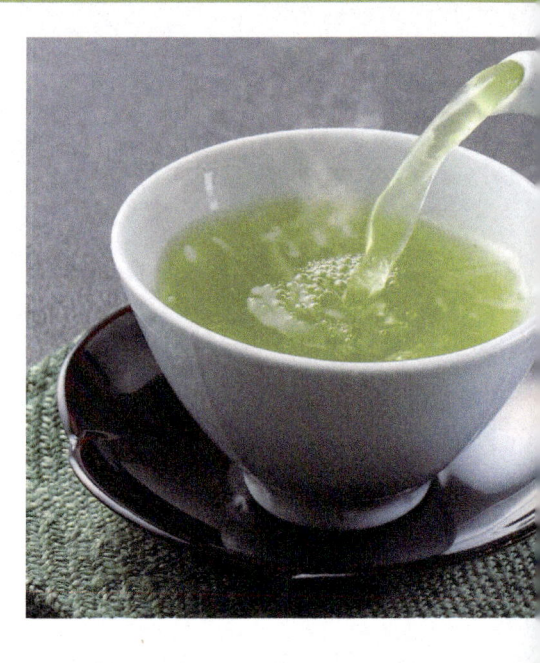

SNACK: CELERY STICKS WITH PEANUT BUTTER

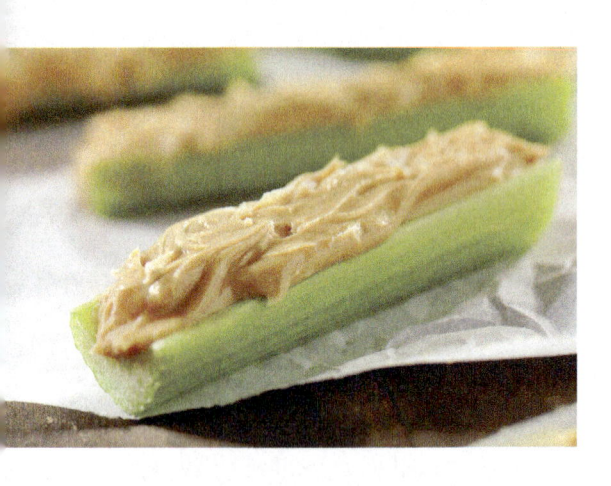

INGREDIENTS
- 2-3 celery stalks
- 2 tablespoons peanut butter

INSTRUCTIONS
- Prepare Celery: Wash and cut the celery into sticks.
- Serve with Peanut Butter: Enjoy celery sticks with peanut butter for dipping.

KITCHEN TOOLS NEEDED
- Knife and cutting board

SNACK: MIXED BERRIES

INGREDIENTS
- A cup of mixed berries (like strawberries, blueberries, and raspberries)

PREPARATION TIME: NONE, READY TO EAT.

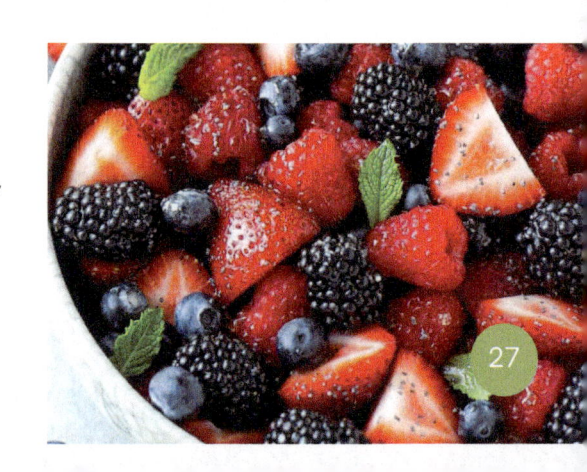

CUCUMBERS - THE COOL CRUSADER

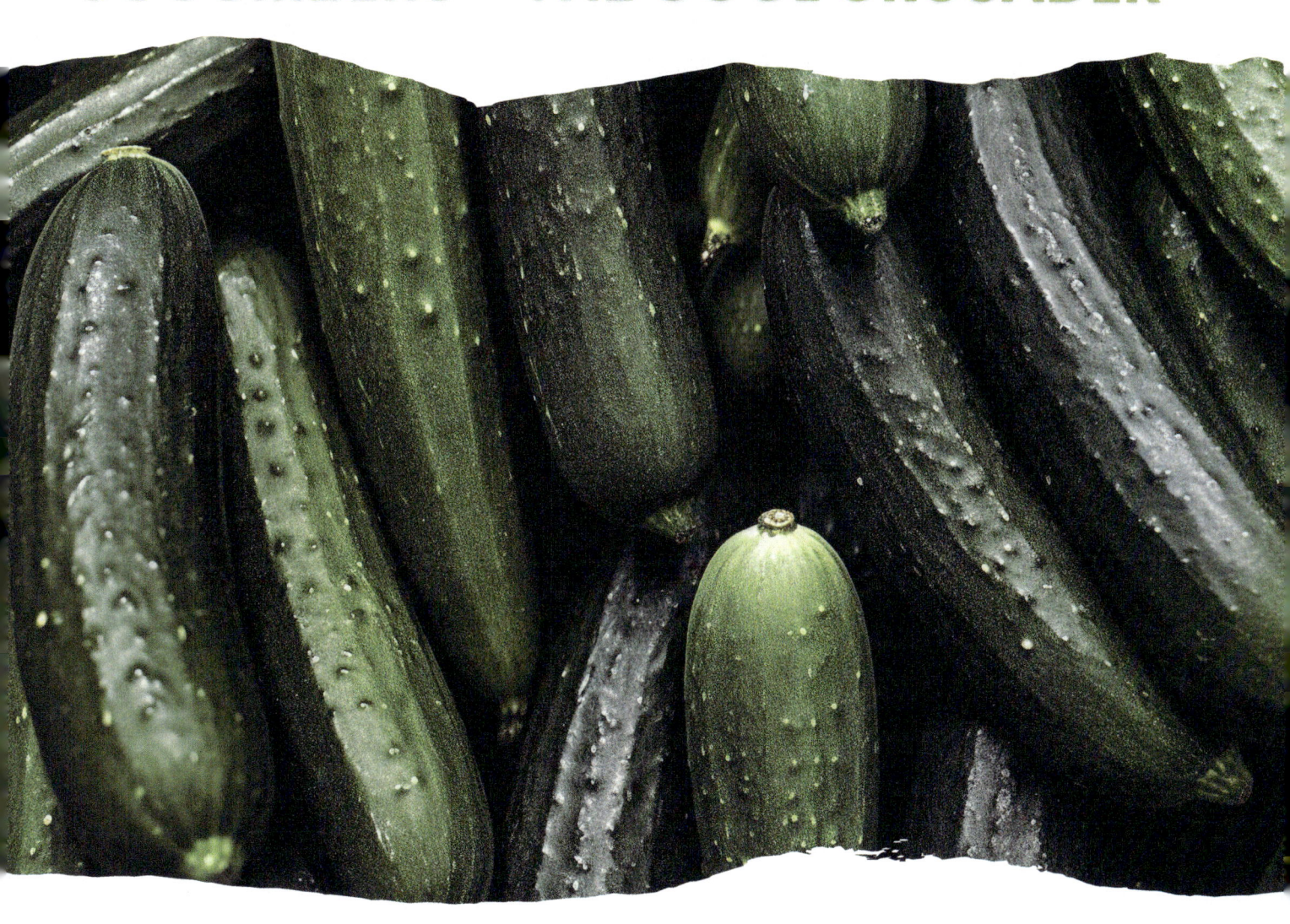

Cucumbers on Day 4: More Than Just a Crunch
On Day 4 of our Anti-Inflammatory Meal Plan, cucumbers make a refreshing appearance, especially in your turkey and hummus wrap. This crisp, cool veggie is often underrated, but it's packed with benefits that go beyond its satisfying crunch.

The Refreshing Benefits of Cucumbers

- Hydration Hero: Cucumbers are incredibly hydrating, composed of about 95% water. This high water content helps in flushing out toxins and maintaining healthy hydration levels, crucial for reducing inflammation.
- Rich in Nutrients, Low in Calories: Despite their high water content, cucumbers are a good source of several vitamins and minerals, including vitamin K, potassium, and magnesium, all while being low in calories.
- Skin and Digestive Health: The silica in cucumbers promotes healthy skin, while their fiber content aids digestion. A healthy digestive system is key in managing inflammation.

Complementing the Day's Meals

- With the Lunch Wrap: In your turkey and hummus wrap, cucumbers add not just a crunch but also a freshness that balances the richness of the hummus and the protein from the turkey, creating a meal that's light yet satisfying.
- Snack Time: As a snack, cucumbers can be a refreshing palate cleanser, perfect for pairing with a creamy and rich peanut butter.

Setting the Stage for the Rest of the Week

- A Daily Dose of Freshness: Incorporating cucumbers early in the week emphasizes the importance of hydration and fresh, nutrient-rich foods in an anti-inflammatory diet. It's about creating meals that are as rejuvenating as they are delicious.
- Prepping for Week 2's Flavor Fiesta: As we move towards more diverse flavors, cucumbers serve as a reminder of the simple yet powerful impact that even the most basic vegetables can have on our overall health.

In summary, cucumbers are a fantastic addition to your anti-inflammatory arsenal. They're not just a sidekick to salads but a versatile, hydrating, and nutrient-packed vegetable that can elevate any meal. As you continue through this 28-day journey, let cucumbers be a staple in your diet, offering a burst of freshness and a host of health benefits.

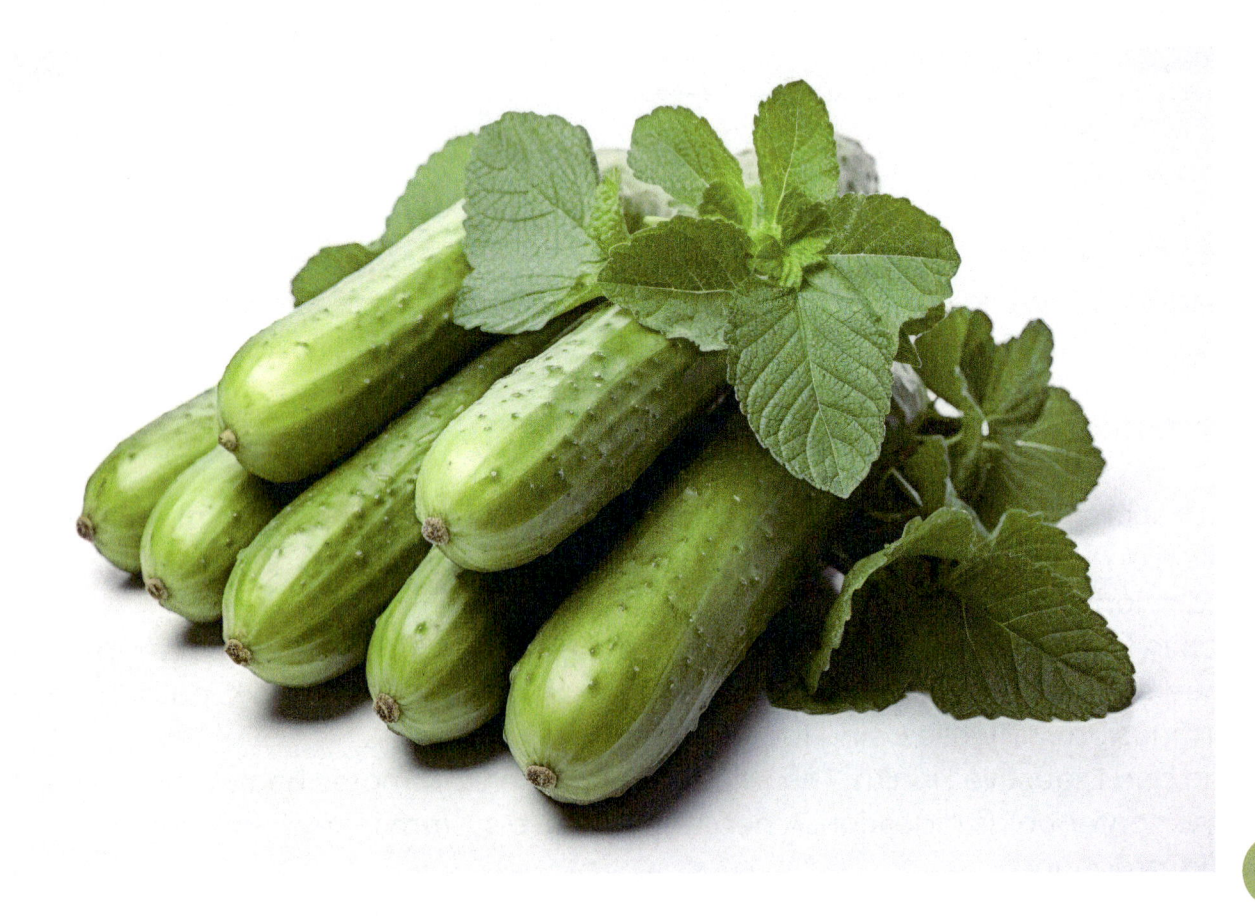

DAY 5 MEAL PLAN

BREAKFAST: CHIA PUDDING WITH MIXED BERRIES AND ALMONDS
LUNCH: KALE SALAD WITH GRILLED CHICKEN, AVOCADO, AND BALSAMIC VINAIGRETTE
DINNER: GRILLED SHRIMP WITH GARLIC, LEMON, AND SAUTÉED GREENS
SNACK: A SMALL PEAR
SNACK: SLICES OF PAPAYA
DRINK: HERBAL TEA WITH A HINT OF MINT

BREAKFAST: CHIA PUDDING WITH MIXED BERRIES AND ALMONDS

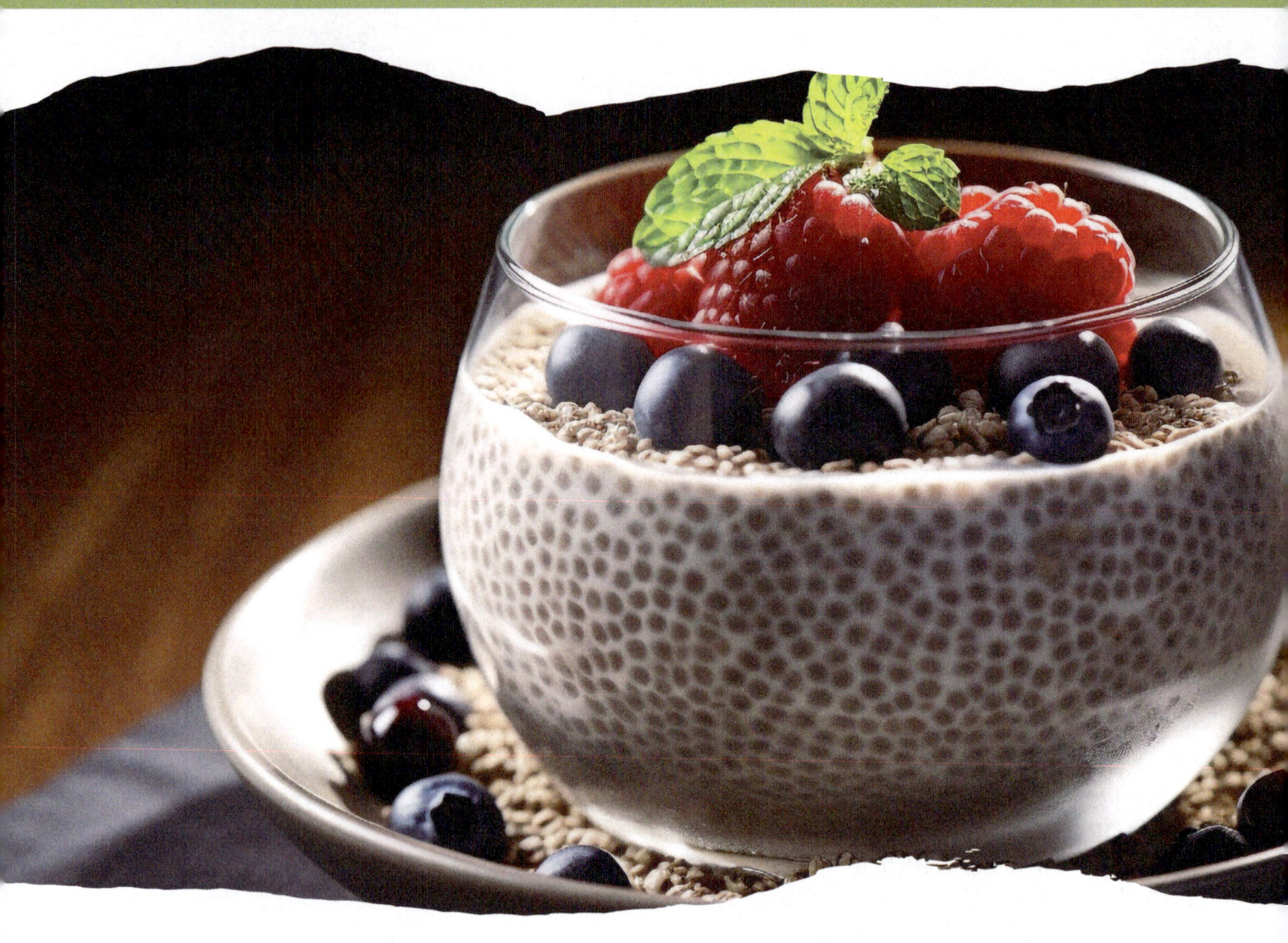

INGREDIENTS

- 3 tablespoons chia seeds
- 1 cup almond milk (or any milk of your choice)
- A handful of mixed berries (fresh or frozen)
- A handful of almonds, chopped
- Optional: honey or maple syrup for sweetness

INSTRUCTIONS

- Prepare Chia Pudding: Mix chia seeds with almond milk in a bowl or jar. Let it sit for a few minutes, then stir again to prevent clumping.
- Refrigerate: Cover and refrigerate for at least 2 hours or overnight.
- Add Toppings: Before serving, top with mixed berries and chopped almonds. Sweeten if desired.

KITCHEN TOOLS NEEDED
- Bowl or jar
- Spoon
- Measuring cups and spoons

LUNCH: KALE SALAD WITH GRILLED CHICKEN, AVOCADO, AND BALSAMIC VINAIGRETTE

INGREDIENTS

- 2 cups kale, chopped
- 1 small chicken breast, grilled and sliced
- ½ avocado, sliced
- 1 tablespoon balsamic vinegar
- 2 tablespoons olive oil
- Salt and pepper to taste

INSTRUCTIONS

- Prepare Chicken: Season and grill the chicken, then let it rest and slice.
- Prepare Salad: Place chopped kale in a bowl.
- Make Dressing: Whisk together balsamic vinegar, olive oil, salt, and pepper.
- Assemble Salad: Add avocado and grilled chicken to kale. Drizzle with dressing.
- Serve: Toss everything together and enjoy.

KITCHEN TOOLS NEEDED

- Grill pan or skillet
- Mixing bowl
- Knife and cutting board
- Whisk or fork

DINNER: GRILLED SHRIMP WITH GARLIC, LEMON, AND SAUTÉED GREENS

INGREDIENTS

- 6-8 large shrimp, peeled and deveined
- 1 garlic clove, minced
- Juice of ½ lemon
- 2 cups mixed greens (like spinach and Swiss chard)
- Olive oil
- Salt and pepper to taste

INSTRUCTIONS

- Prepare Shrimp: Marinate shrimp with garlic, lemon juice, salt, and pepper.
- Grill Shrimp: Cook shrimp in a grill pan or skillet until pink and opaque.
- Sauté Greens: In another skillet, sauté greens in olive oil until wilted.
- Serve: Plate shrimp with sautéed greens on the side.

KITCHEN TOOLS NEEDED

- Grill pan or skillet
- Another skillet for greens
- Knife and cutting board
- Measuring spoons

DRINK: HERBAL TEA WITH A HINT OF MINT

INGREDIENTS
- 1 herbal tea bag (any flavor)
- A few fresh mint leaves
- 1 cup boiling water

INSTRUCTIONS
- Boil Water: Heat water in a kettle or pot.
- Steep Tea: Place the tea bag and mint leaves in a mug. Pour hot water over them.
- Serve: Let the tea steep for about 5 minutes before drinking.

KITCHEN TOOLS NEEDED
- Kettle or pot for boiling water
- Mug

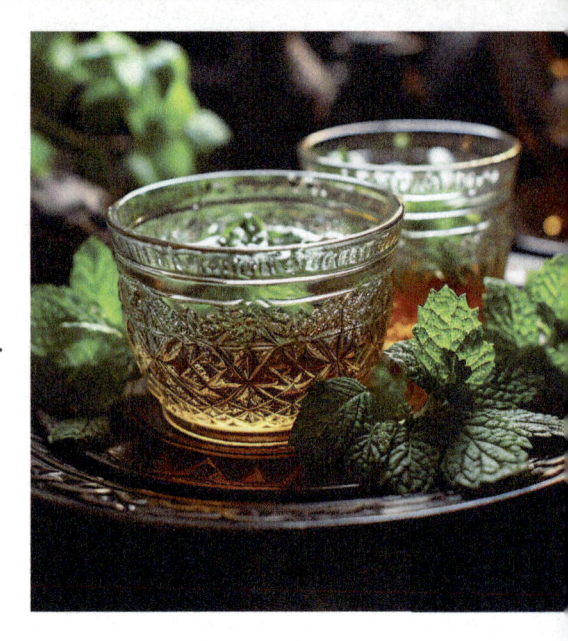

SNACK: SLICES OF PAPAYA

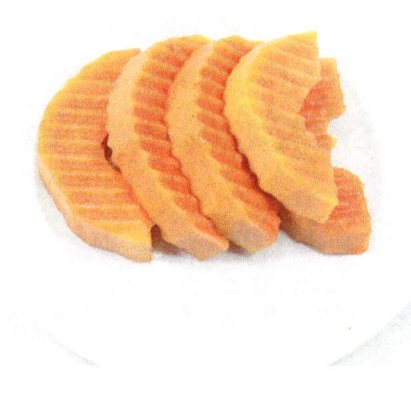

INGREDIENTS
- A few slices of papaya

PREPARATION TIME: ~5 MINUTES
- Peel and slice the papaya.

SNACK: A SMALL PEAR

INGREDIENTS
- 1 small pear

PREPARATION TIME: NONE, READY TO EAT.

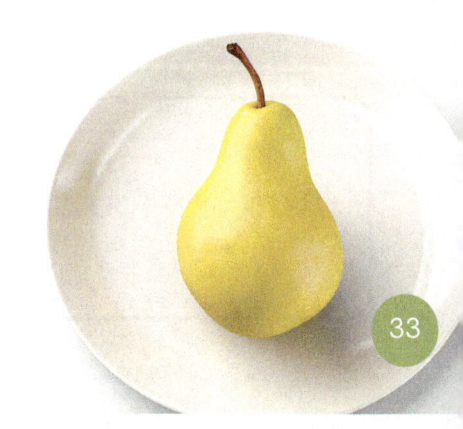

PAPAYA – THE TROPICAL ANTI-INFLAMMATORY STAR

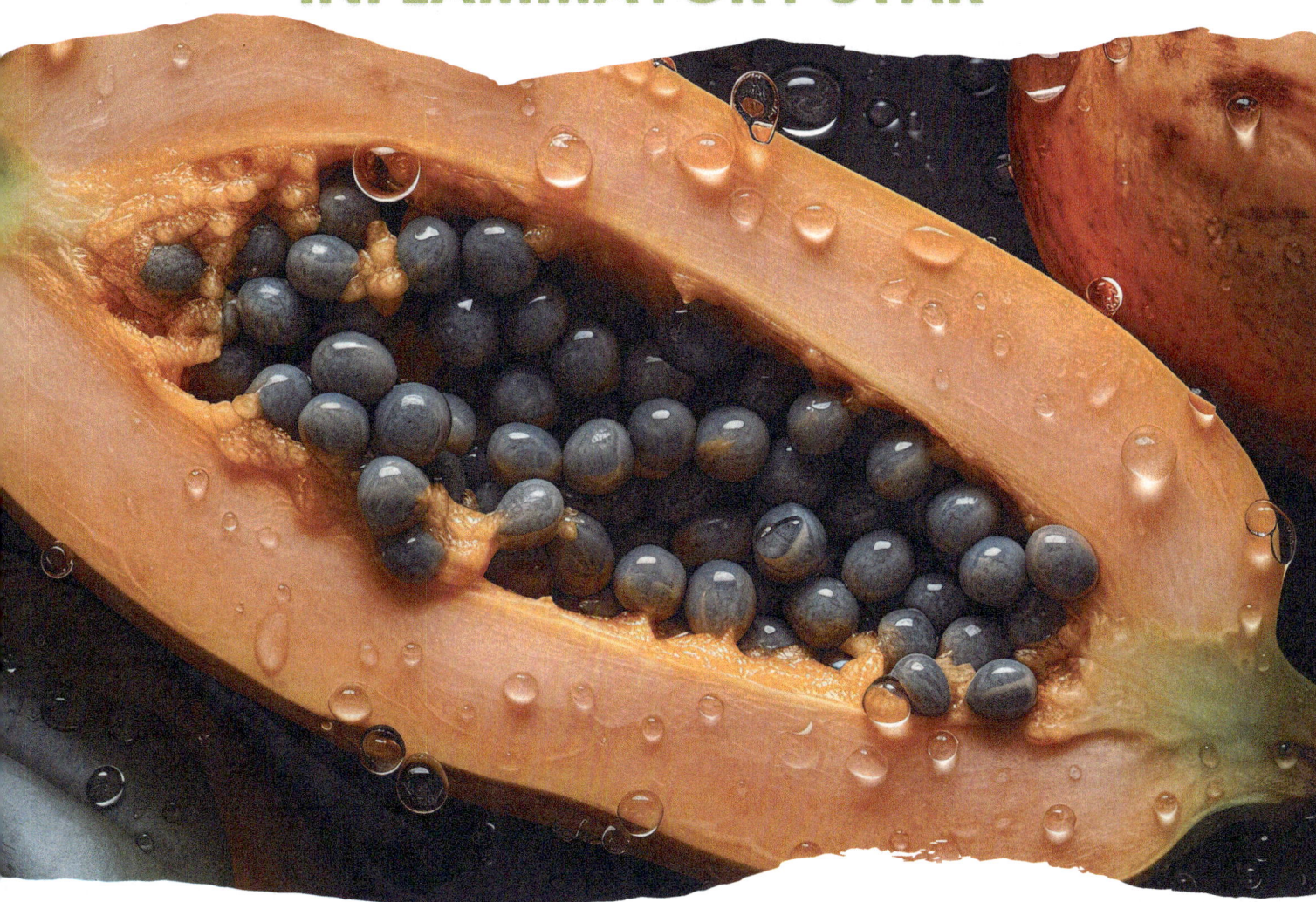

Papaya on Day 5: A Sweet Boost to Your Diet
Day 5 of our Anti-Inflammatory Meal Plan introduces the tropical delight, papaya, as a snack. This fruit is not just a sweet treat; it's loaded with health benefits that align perfectly with our anti-inflammatory goals.

The Sweet Benefits of Papaya

- Digestive Health Ally: Papaya contains an enzyme called papain, which aids in digestion by breaking down proteins. This makes it an excellent choice for promoting gut health, an essential aspect of controlling inflammation.
- Rich in Antioxidants: Papaya is packed with antioxidants like carotenoids that help fight free radicals in the body. This reduces oxidative stress, which can lead to inflammation.
- Immune System Booster: High in vitamins C and A, papaya supports the immune system, helping your body to combat inflammation more effectively.

Complementing the Day's Meals

- As a Snack: The sweet, refreshing flavor of papaya offers a delightful contrast to the savory notes of your lunch and dinner, making it a perfect midday snack. It's a great way to satisfy your sweet tooth naturally while reaping health benefits.
- With Dinner: The light, digestive-friendly nature of papaya makes it a great follow-up to your dinner of grilled shrimp and sautéed greens, helping in winding down the day with a soothing, tropical touch.

Preparing for a Nutrient-Rich Finish

- A Daily Dose of Tropical Wellness: By incorporating papaya into your diet, we emphasize the importance of including a variety of fruits, each with its unique health properties. It's about enjoying the diversity of nature's bounty in your quest to reduce inflammation.
- Setting Up for Week 2's Flavorful Journey: As we move towards more diverse and vibrant flavors, papaya serves as a reminder of the exciting and delicious possibilities that lie within an anti-inflammatory diet. It's a testament to how a diet aimed at reducing inflammation can also be full of delightful and exotic flavors.

In short, papaya is more than just a tropical indulgence; it's a fruit packed with digestive health benefits, antioxidants, and immune-boosting nutrients. As you continue through this 28-day journey, let papaya be a reminder of the joy and health benefits that come from incorporating a variety of fruits into your diet.

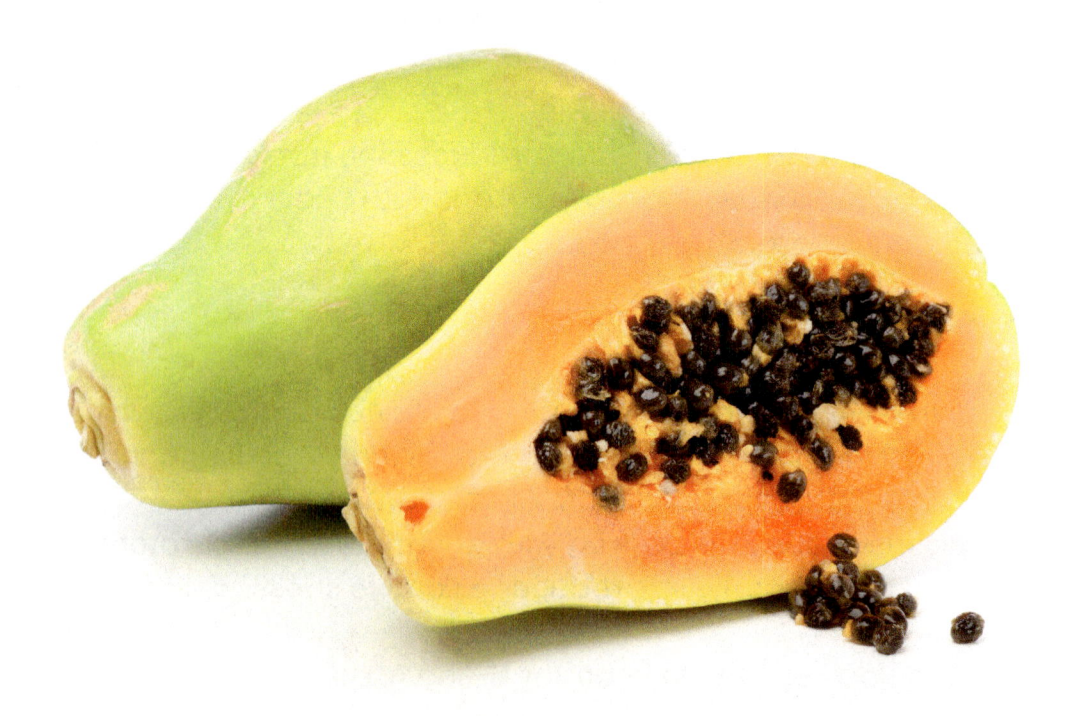

DAY 6 MEAL PLAN

BREAKFAST: WHOLE-GRAIN TOAST WITH ALMOND BUTTER AND SLICED BANANA
LUNCH: VEGGIE AND HUMMUS PLATTER
DINNER: BEEF STEW WITH ROOT VEGETABLES
SNACK: A SMALL HANDFUL OF CASHEWS
SNACK: A FEW CHERRY TOMATOES
DRINK: INFUSED WATER WITH CUCUMBER AND LEMON

BREAKFAST: WHOLE-GRAIN TOAST WITH ALMOND BUTTER AND SLICED BANANA

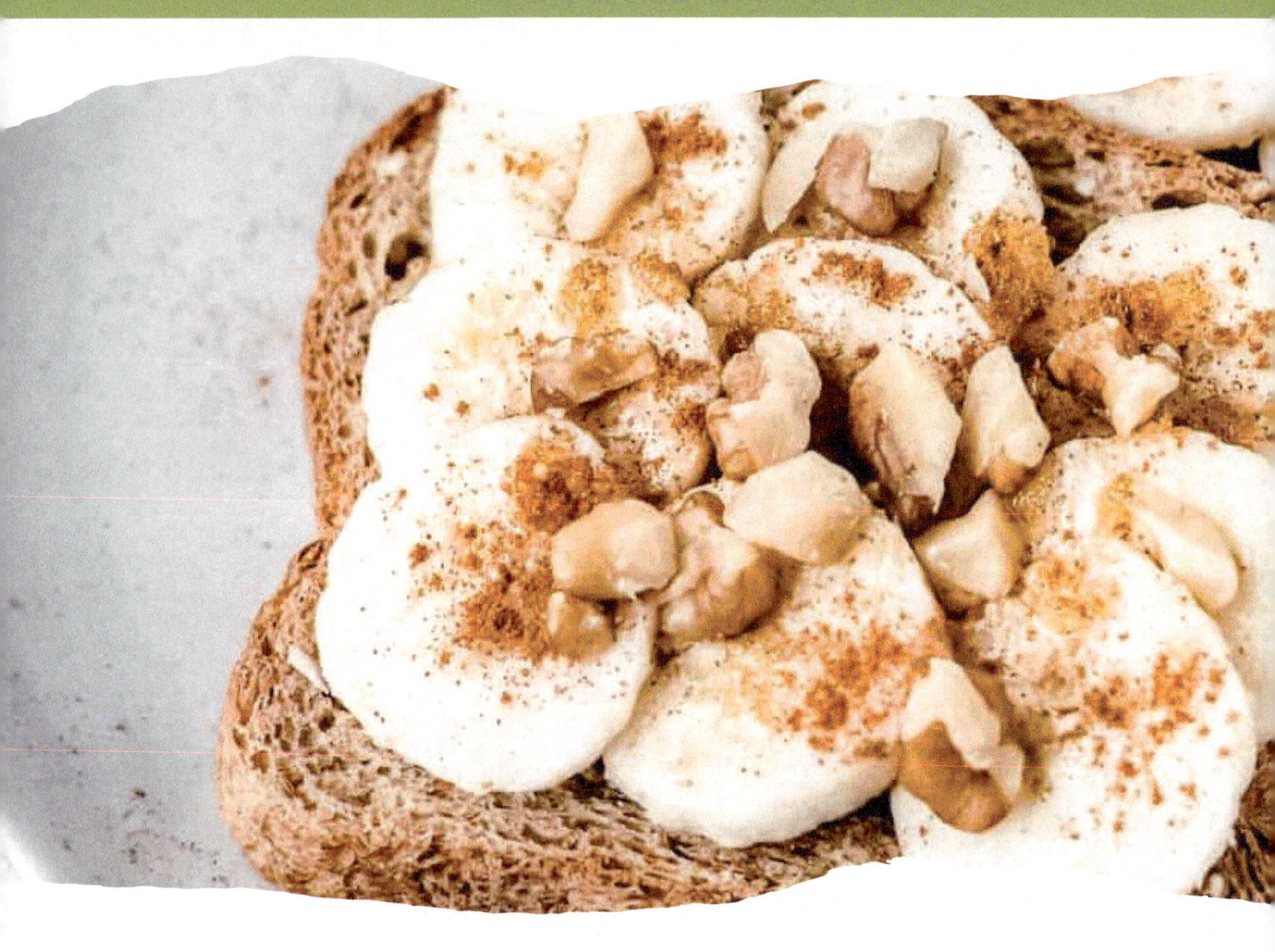

INGREDIENTS

- 1 slice whole-grain bread
- 2 tablespoons almond butter
- 1 banana, sliced

INSTRUCTIONS

- Toast Bread: Toast the whole-grain bread to your liking.
- Spread Almond Butter: Spread almond butter evenly over the toast.
- Add Banana: Top with sliced banana.
- Serve: Enjoy this nutritious and filling breakfast.

KITCHEN TOOLS NEEDED
- Toaster
- Knife and cutting board
- Butter knife or spreader

LUNCH: VEGGIE AND HUMMUS PLATTER

INGREDIENTS

- A variety of veggies (like carrots, cucumbers, bell peppers, and celery), cut into sticks
- ¼ cup hummus

INSTRUCTIONS

- Prepare Veggies: Cut the vegetables into stick or bite-sized pieces.
- Arrange Platter: Place hummus in a small bowl or on a plate, surround with veggie sticks.
- Serve: Dip veggies in hummus and enjoy.

KITCHEN TOOLS NEEDED
- Knife and cutting board

DINNER: BEEF STEW WITH ROOT VEGETABLES

INGREDIENTS

- ½ lb beef stew meat, cut into cubes
- 1 carrot, chopped
- 1 potato, chopped
- 1 parsnip, chopped
- 1 onion, chopped
- 2 cups beef broth
- Salt, pepper, and herbs to taste

INSTRUCTIONS

- Prepare Ingredients: Chop all vegetables and meat.
- Cook Stew: In a pot or slow cooker, combine meat, vegetables, broth, and seasonings. Cook until meat is tender and vegetables are cooked through.
- Serve: Enjoy a hearty and comforting dinner.

KITCHEN TOOLS NEEDED
- Pot or slow cooker
- Knife and cutting board
- Measuring cups

DRINK: INFUSED WATER WITH CUCUMBER AND LEMON

INGREDIENTS
- A few slices of cucumber
- A few slices of lemon
- 1 liter of water

INSTRUCTIONS
- Prepare Ingredients: Slice cucumber and lemon.
- Infuse Water: Add cucumber and lemon slices to water in a pitcher or bottle.
- Chill: Refrigerate for an hour or more to infuse flavors.
- Serve: Enjoy refreshing and hydrating infused water.

KITCHEN TOOLS NEEDED
- Pitcher or large bottle
- Knife and cutting board

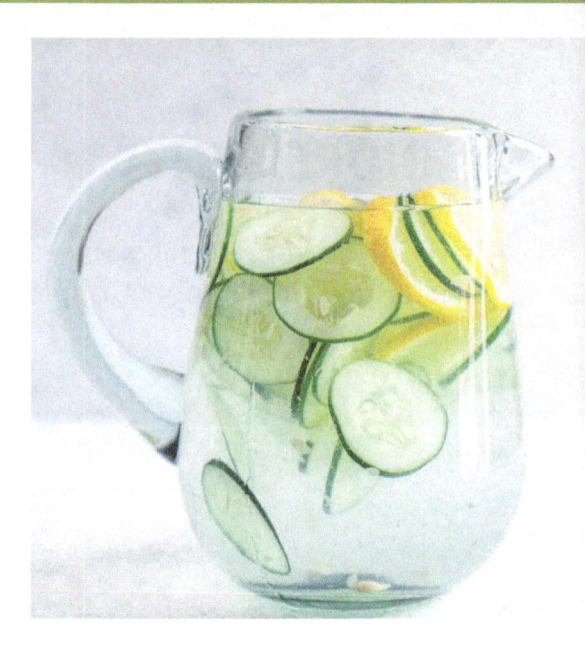

SNACK: A FEW CHERRY TOMATOES

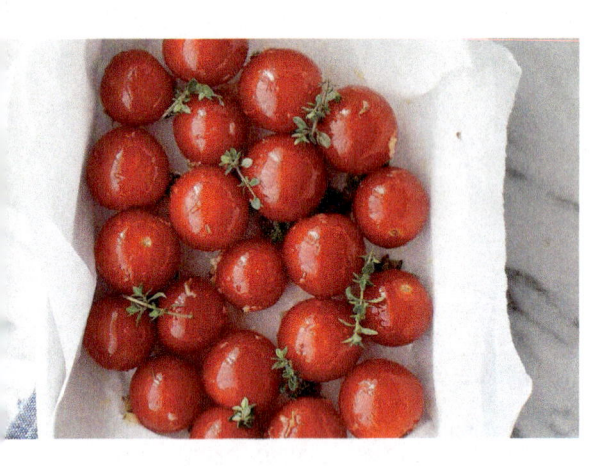

INGREDIENTS
- A handful of cherry tomatoes

PREPARATION TIME: NONE, READY TO EAT.

SNACK: A SMALL HANDFUL OF CASHEWS

INGREDIENTS
- A small handful of cashews (about 10-15 nuts)

PREPARATION TIME: NONE, READY TO EAT.

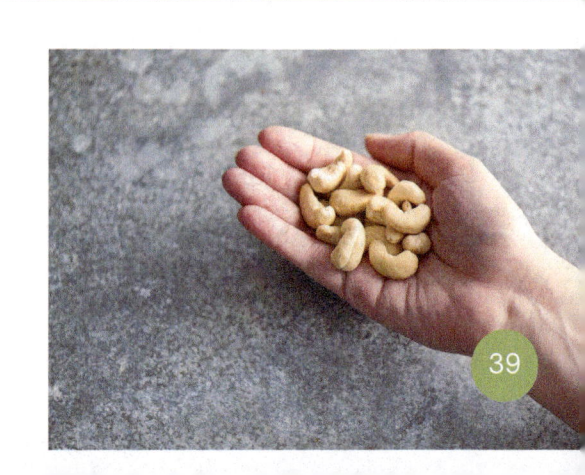

WHOLE-GRAIN TOAST - A WHOLESOME FOUNDATION

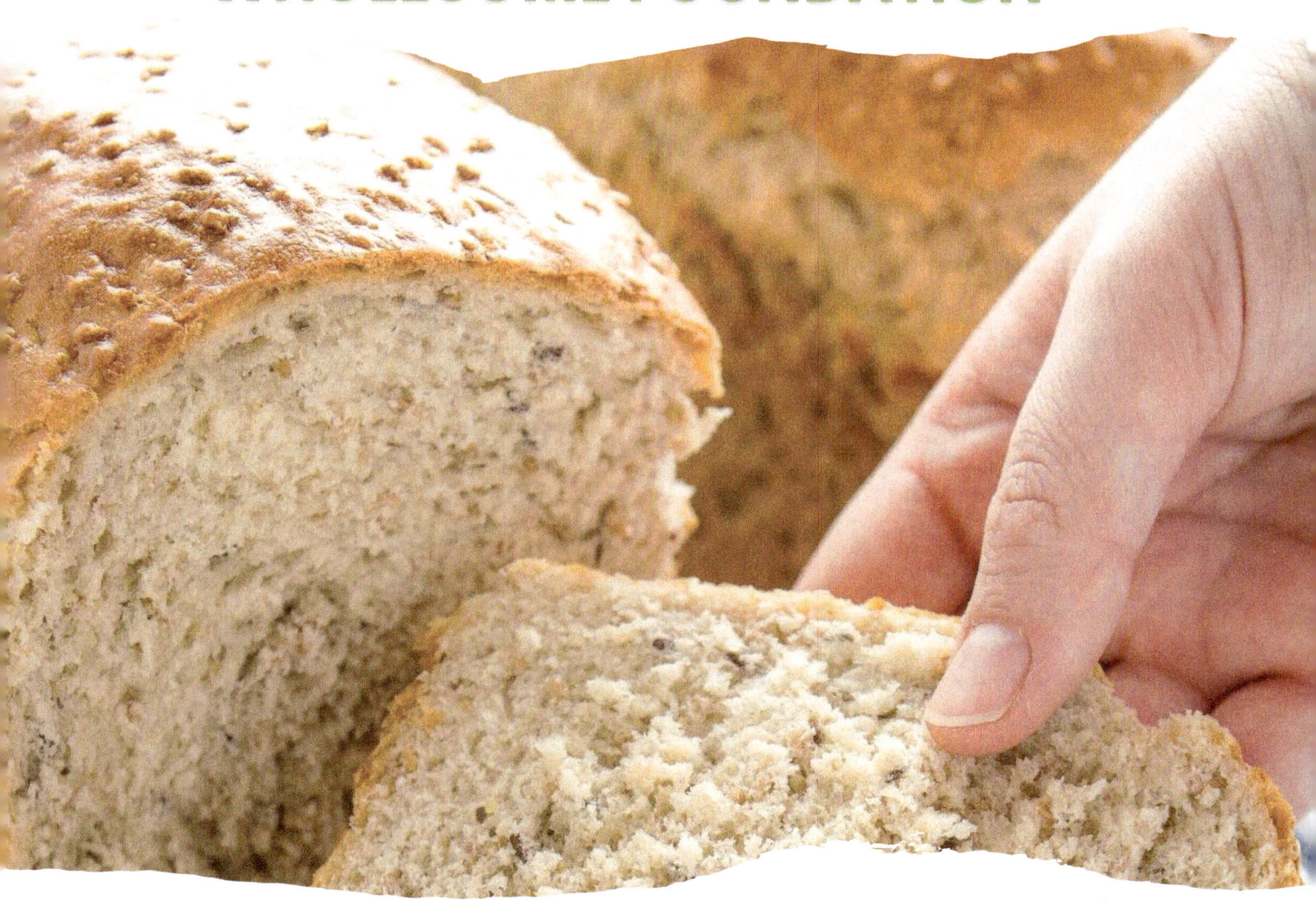

Whole-Grain Toast on Day 6: More Than Just a Base for Toppings
On Day 6 of our Anti-Inflammatory Meal Plan, we start the day with whole-grain toast. This isn't just your regular toast; it's a nutritional powerhouse that lays a solid foundation for a day filled with anti-inflammatory eating.

The Whole-Grain Advantage

- Nutrient-Dense Choice: Whole grains are rich in essential nutrients like fiber, B vitamins, antioxidants, and trace minerals (iron, zinc, copper, and magnesium). Unlike white bread, whole-grain toast retains all parts of the grain, ensuring you get all these benefits.
- Gut Health and Beyond: The fiber in whole grains promotes healthy digestion and gut health, which is crucial in managing inflammation. A healthy gut is less likely to contribute to systemic inflammation.
- Steady Energy Release: Whole grains have a lower glycemic index compared to white bread. This means they provide a more gradual release of energy, preventing spikes in blood sugar levels that can lead to inflammation.

Complementing the Day's Meals

- With Breakfast: Paired with almond butter and banana, whole-grain toast offers a balance of complex carbs, healthy fats, and proteins. This combination provides sustained energy and a range of anti-inflammatory benefits.
- Throughout the Day: The fiber and nutrients in whole-grain toast also help keep you full, reducing the temptation for less healthy snacks and supporting a consistent, anti-inflammatory diet throughout the day.

Setting the Stage for a Nourishing End to the Week

- A Foundation for Daily Wellness: By incorporating whole-grain toast at the start of the day, we emphasize the importance of choosing nutrient-dense, whole foods that support long-term health and inflammation management.
- Preparing for Week 2's Diverse Flavors: As we continue to explore a variety of foods in Week 2, whole-grain toast serves as a versatile base that can be adapted to many flavors and toppings, showcasing the flexibility and deliciousness of an anti-inflammatory diet.

In essence, whole-grain toast is much more than a simple breakfast item; it's a nutritious, versatile, and satisfying food that supports your anti-inflammatory goals. As you enjoy its wholesome goodness, remember that every bite is a step towards a healthier, more balanced lifestyle.

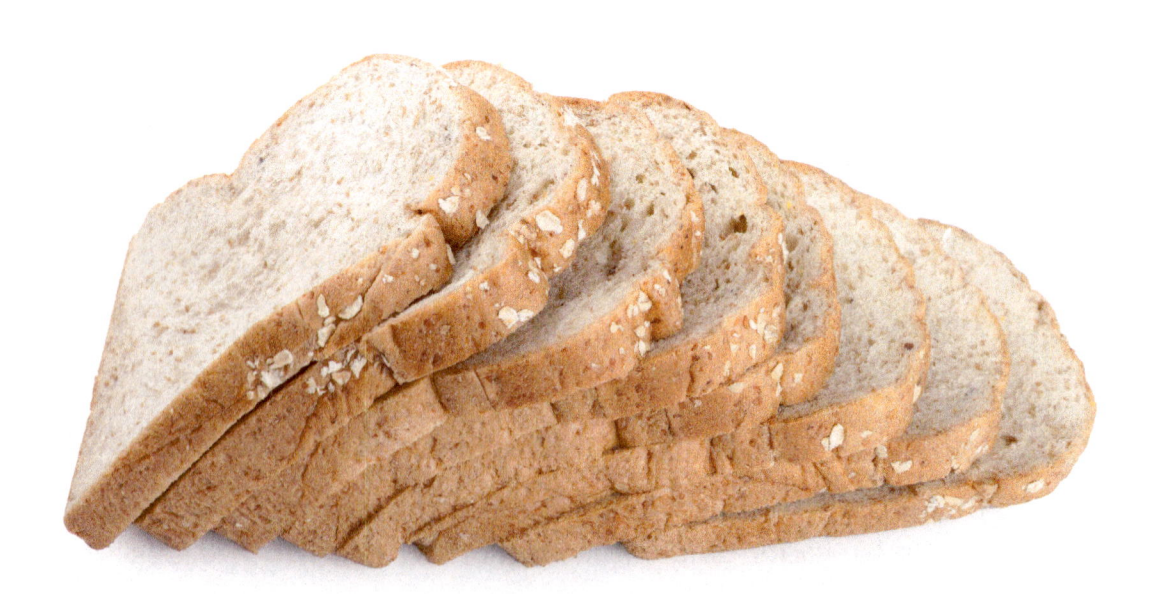

DAY 7 MEAL PLAN

BREAKFAST: OVERNIGHT OATS WITH CHIA SEEDS, APPLE SLICES, AND CINNAMON
LUNCH: SPINACH AND GOAT CHEESE SALAD WITH GRILLED SALMON
DINNER: ROASTED CHICKEN WITH BRUSSELS SPROUTS AND QUINOA
SNACK: A KIWI
SNACK: BELL PEPPER STRIPS WITH TZATZIKI
DRINK: CHAMOMILE TEA WITH A SLICE OF LEMON

BREAKFAST: OVERNIGHT OATS WITH CHIA SEEDS, APPLE SLICES, AND CINNAMON

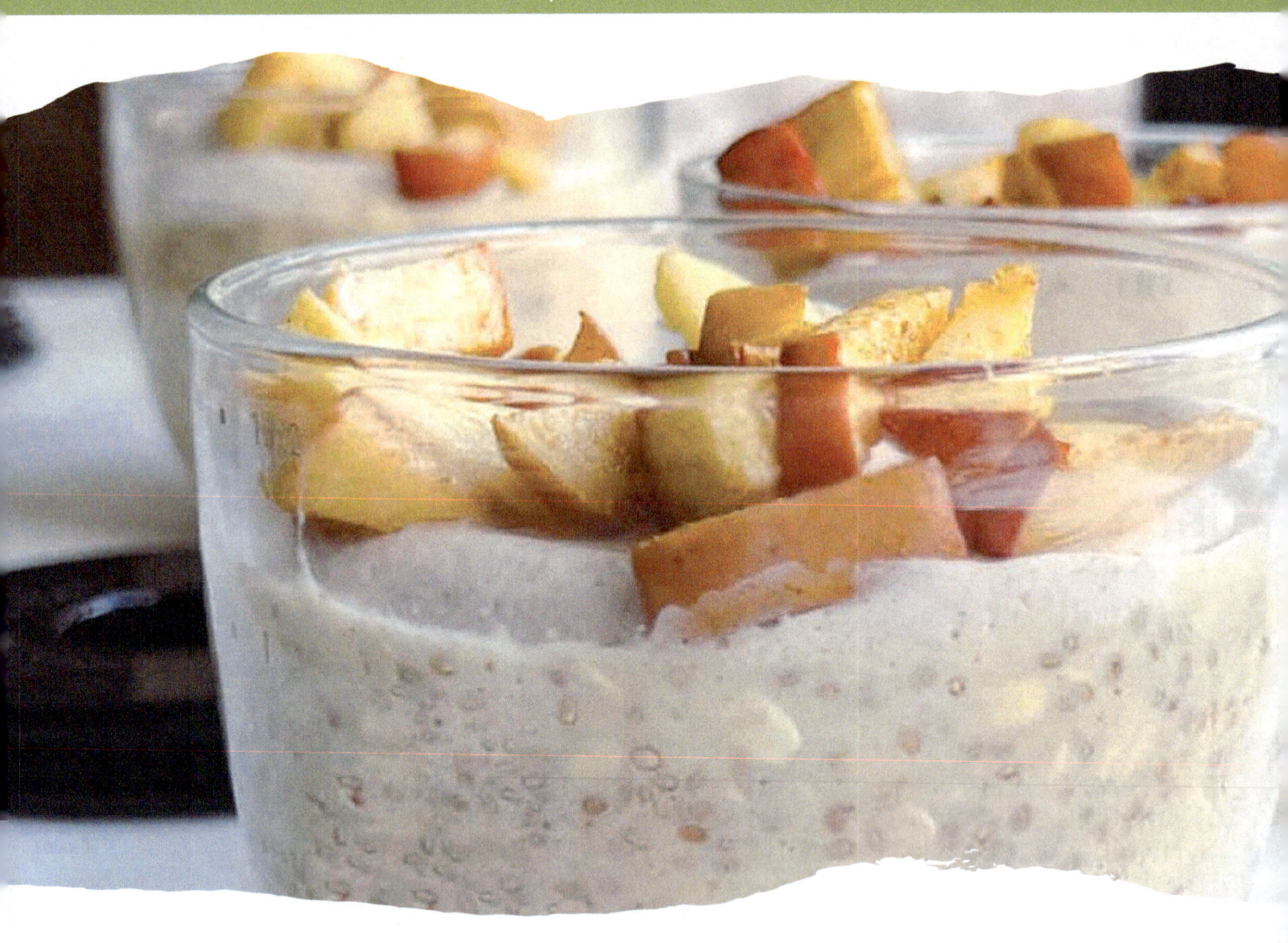

INGREDIENTS

- ½ cup rolled oats
- 1 tablespoon chia seeds
- ¾ cup almond milk or milk of choice
- 1 apple, sliced
- ½ teaspoon cinnamon

INSTRUCTIONS

- Prepare Oats: In a jar or bowl, mix oats, chia seeds, and almond milk.
- Refrigerate: Seal and refrigerate overnight.
- Add Toppings: In the morning, add apple slices and sprinkle with cinnamon.
- Serve: Stir and enjoy a healthy, ready-to-eat breakfast.

KITCHEN TOOLS NEEDED

- Jar or bowl with a lid
- Knife and cutting board

LUNCH: SPINACH AND GOAT CHEESE SALAD WITH GRILLED SALMON

INGREDIENTS

- 2 cups fresh spinach
- 2-3 oz goat cheese, crumbled
- 1 salmon fillet (about 4-6 oz)
- Olive oil
- Salt and pepper
- Balsamic vinaigrette or dressing of choice

INSTRUCTIONS

- Prepare Salmon: Season salmon with salt and pepper, grill until cooked through.
- Assemble Salad: Place spinach in a bowl, top with crumbled goat cheese.
- Add Salmon: Once cooked, place the salmon on the salad.
- Dress and Serve: Drizzle with vinaigrette and serve.

KITCHEN TOOLS NEEDED
- Grill pan or skillet
- Mixing bowl
- Knife and cutting board

DINNER: ROASTED CHICKEN WITH BRUSSELS SPROUTS AND QUINOA

INGREDIENTS

- 1 chicken breast
- 1 cup Brussels sprouts, halved
- ½ cup quinoa
- Olive oil
- Salt and pepper

INSTRUCTIONS

- Cook Quinoa: Prepare quinoa according to package instructions.
- Prepare and Roast Chicken and Brussels Sprouts: Season chicken and Brussels sprouts with oil, salt, and pepper. Roast in the oven until chicken is cooked and Brussels sprouts are tender.
- Serve: Plate chicken with quinoa and Brussels sprouts.

KITCHEN TOOLS NEEDED
- Oven and baking tray
- Pot for quinoa
- Knife and cutting board

DRINK: CHAMOMILE TEA WITH A SLICE OF LEMON

INGREDIENTS
- 1 chamomile tea bag
- 1 slice of lemon
- 1 cup water

INSTRUCTIONS
- Boil Water: Heat water in a kettle or pot.
- Steep Tea: Place the tea bag and lemon slice in a mug, add hot water.
- Serve: Let the tea steep for about 5 minutes before enjoying.

KITCHEN TOOLS NEEDED
- Kettle or pot for boiling water
- Mug

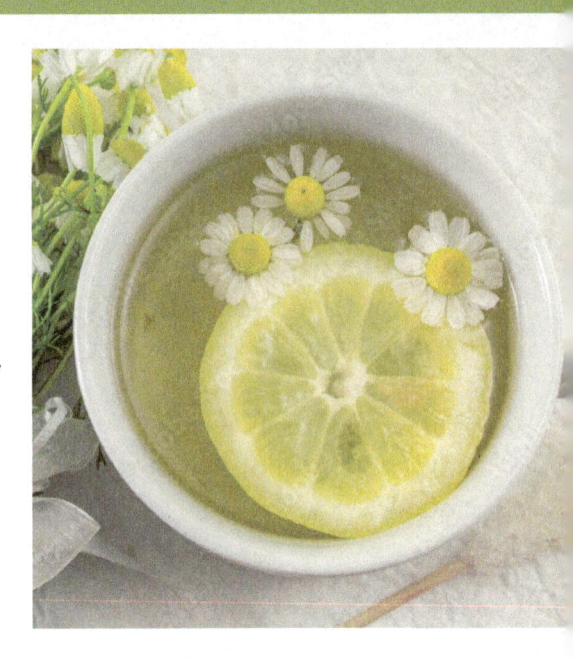

SNACK: BELL PEPPER STRIPS WITH TZATZIKI

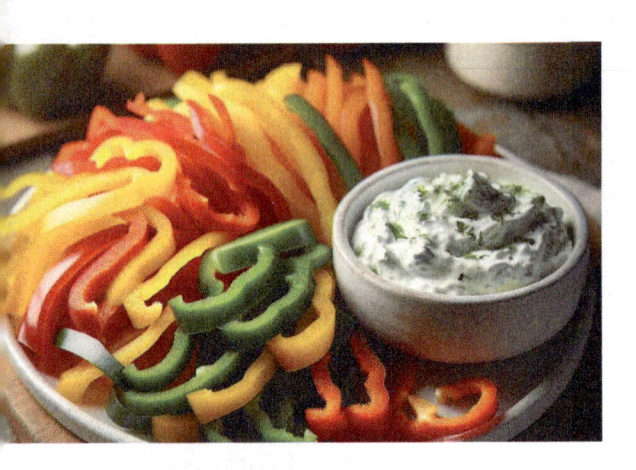

INGREDIENTS
- 1 bell pepper, sliced into strips
- ¼ cup tzatziki sauce

INSTRUCTIONS
- Prepare Bell Pepper: Slice the bell pepper into strips.
- Serve: Enjoy the pepper strips with a side of tzatziki for dipping.

KITCHEN TOOLS NEEDED
- Knife and cutting board

SNACK: A KIWI

INGREDIENTS
- 1 kiwi

PREPARATION TIME: NONE, READY TO EAT AFTER PEELING.

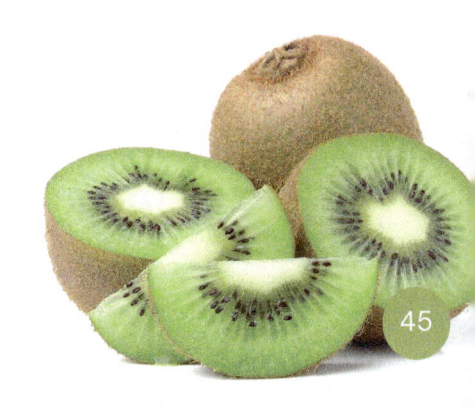

SPINACH – THE LEAFY GREEN POWERHOUSE

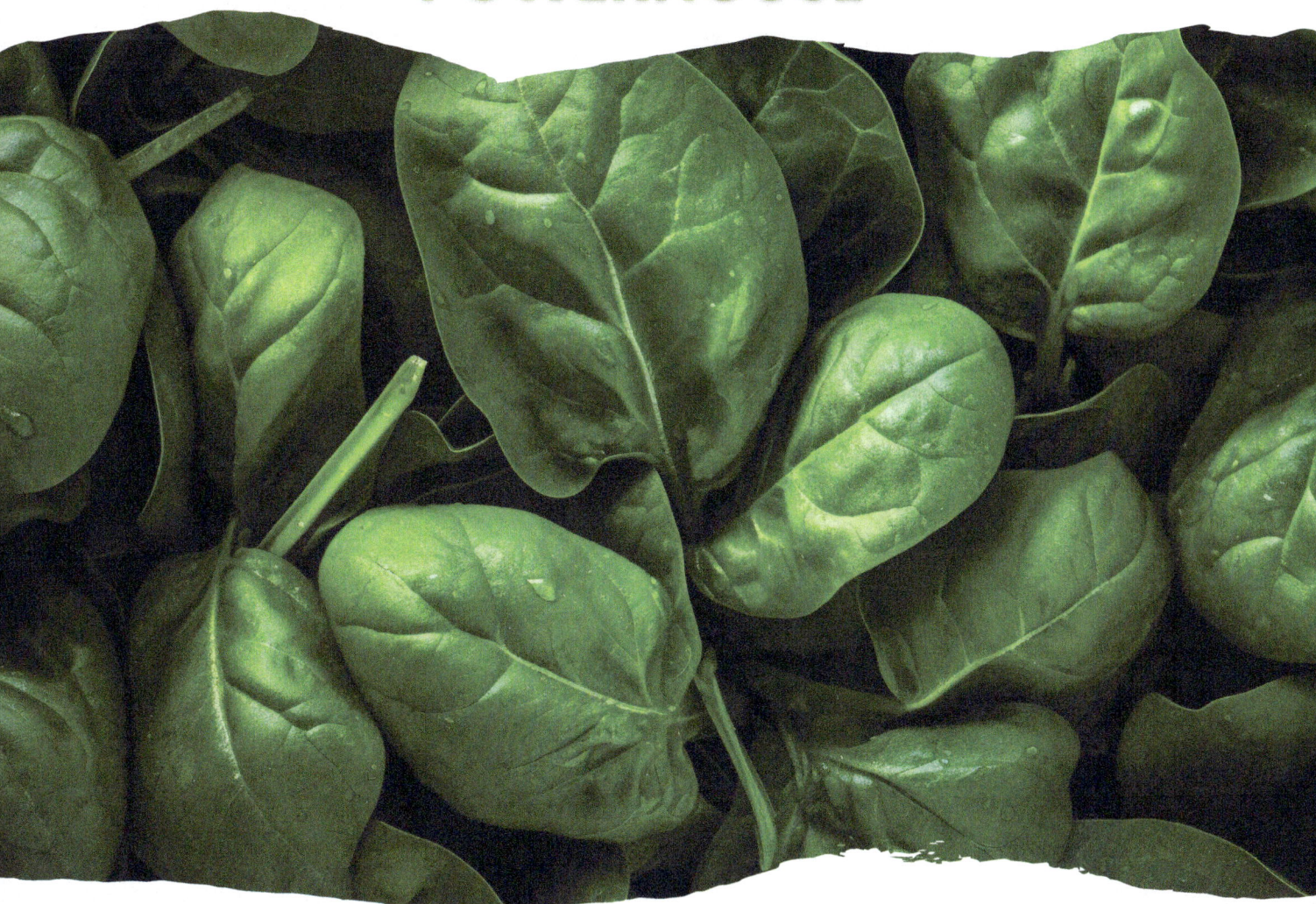

Spinach on Day 7: A Vital Ingredient for Vibrant Health
As we round off the week in our Anti-Inflammatory Meal Plan, let's zoom in on spinach, featured in your lunch salad. This leafy green is not just for Popeye; it's a nutritional superhero for anyone looking to combat inflammation and boost overall health.

The Super Benefits of Spinach

- Nutrient-Rich: Spinach is packed with vitamins and minerals, including high levels of vitamin K, vitamin A, manganese, folate, and iron. These nutrients play a crucial role in reducing inflammation and supporting overall bodily functions.
- Antioxidant Haven: Rich in antioxidants like lutein and zeaxanthin, spinach helps combat oxidative stress in the body, a key contributor to inflammation. These antioxidants are also great for eye health.
- Bone Health and Beyond: The vitamin K in spinach is crucial for bone health. It works with calcium to improve bone density, reducing the risk of fractures and osteoporosis.

Complementing the Day's Meals

- In the Lunch Salad: Paired with goat cheese and grilled salmon, spinach forms a powerhouse of anti-inflammatory nutrients, creating a meal that's not only satisfying but also packed with health benefits.
- Versatile Ingredient: Spinach's versatility makes it easy to include in various meals throughout the day, whether it's a green smoothie for breakfast, a leafy salad for lunch, or sautéed as a side for dinner.

Setting the Stage for Ongoing Wellness

- A Leafy Foundation for Health: Incorporating spinach into your diet, as seen on Day 7, emphasizes the importance of including leafy greens for their dense nutritional profile and anti-inflammatory properties.
- Prepping for a Diverse Diet: As we move forward in our meal plan, spinach serves as a reminder of the importance of greens in an anti-inflammatory diet, offering a range of options to keep meals both healthful and flavorful.

In summary, spinach is a quintessential component of an anti-inflammatory diet. Its rich nutritional profile and versatility make it an ideal ingredient for a variety of meals, contributing significantly to reducing inflammation and promoting overall health. As you continue your dietary journey, let spinach be a staple in your quest for a balanced and vibrant lifestyle.

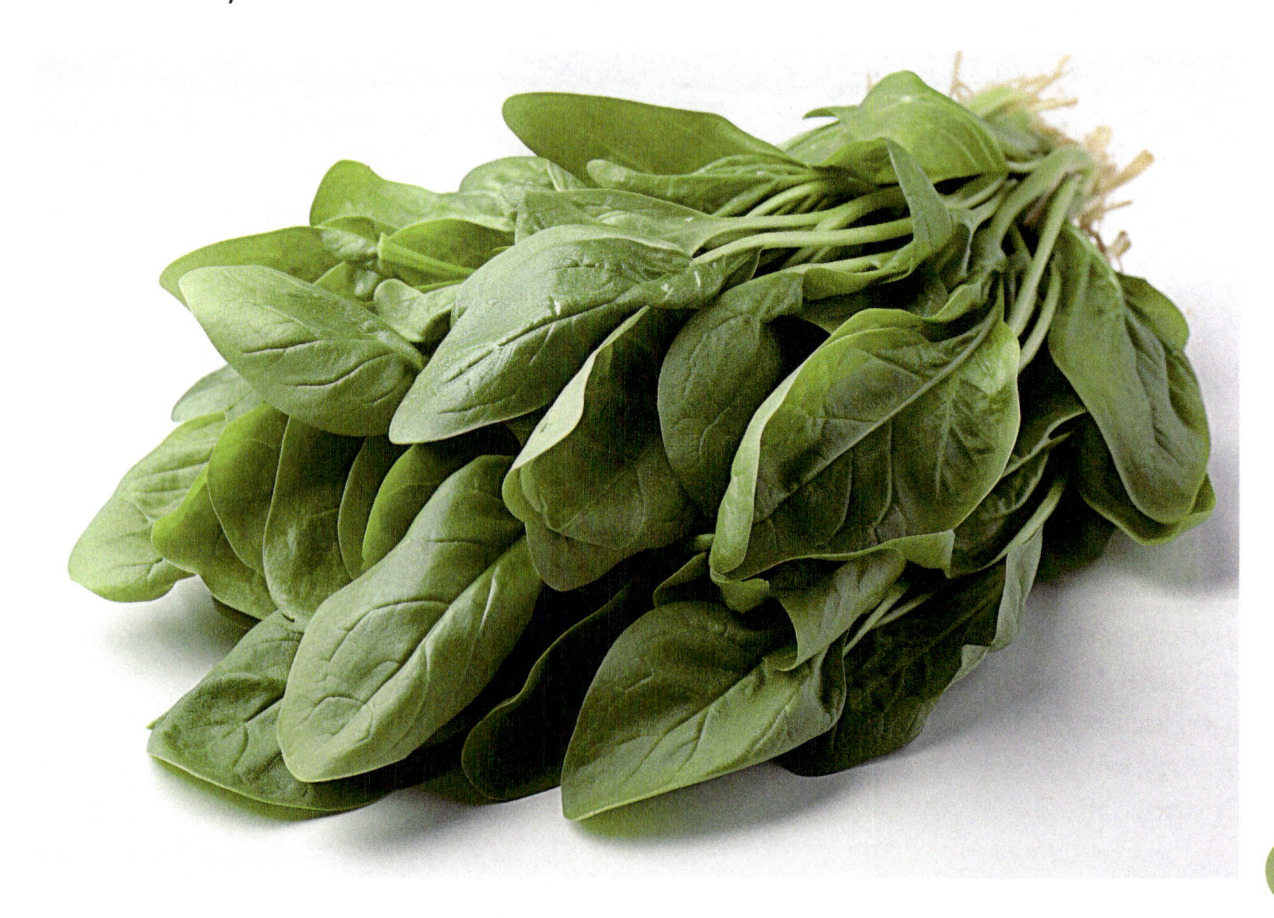

COMPLETION OF WEEK 1: A THANK YOU NOTE

Celebrating Your First Milestone

Congratulations on successfully completing Week 1 of the Anti-Inflammatory Meal Plan! As you embark on this journey towards better health and wellness, we want to extend a heartfelt thank you for joining us in this transformative endeavor.

Gratitude for Your Commitment

- Appreciation: We deeply appreciate your dedication and effort in embracing the changes this week. It's not just about following a diet; it's about taking a significant step towards a healthier lifestyle.
- Acknowledging Challenges: We recognize that adapting to new dietary habits can be challenging. Your willingness to explore and embrace these changes is commendable and a testament to your commitment to your health.

Encouragement for the Journey Ahead

- Continued Support: As you move forward in this journey, remember that each week is a building block towards achieving your health goals. We're here to support you every step of the way.
- Celebration of Progress: Each day you follow this plan, you're making a positive impact on your health. We encourage you to celebrate these small victories and the progress you've made.

As you reflect on your experiences from Week 1, we invite you to assess how your body and mind have responded to the diet. Please use the Body Awareness Scale on the following page to help gauge your progress and tune into your body's needs. Your feedback and reflections are invaluable as you continue on this path to wellness. Once again, thank you for being a part of this journey, and we look forward to continuing this adventure with you!

WEEK 1 REFLECTION

After completing Week 1 of the Anti-Inflammatory Meal Plan, it's important to reflect on how your body has responded to the dietary changes. Use the following scale to rate your experiences in various aspects of your health and well-being. Rate each category from 1 to 10 (where 1 is 'no improvement' and 10 is 'significant improvement').

1. Digestive Comfort

- Question: How would you rate the overall comfort of your digestive system this week?
- Rating (1-10): _ _ _ _ _

2. Energy Levels

- Question: How do you feel about your energy levels after following the meal plan for a week?
- Rating (1-10): _ _ _ _ _

3. Sleep Quality

- Question: Have you noticed any changes in the quality of your sleep?
- Rating (1-10): _ _ _ _ _

4. Mood and Mental Clarity

- Question: How has your mood and mental clarity been affected by the dietary changes?
- Rating (1-10): _ _ _ _ _

5. Physical Comfort and Pain Levels

- Question: If you previously experienced any physical discomfort or pain, have you noticed any changes in its intensity or frequency?
- Rating (1-10): _ _ _ _ _

6. Skin Health

- Question: Have there been any noticeable changes in your skin health/appearance?
- Rating (1-10): _ _ _ _ _

7. Cravings and Appetite Control

- Question: How would you rate your control over cravings and appetite this week?
- Rating (1-10): _ _ _ _ _

8. Overall Well-being

- Question: Considering all factors, how would you rate your overall well-being after Week 1?
- Rating (1-10): _ _ _ _ _

Notes

Notes

- Daily Observations: Note any specific reactions or feelings on a day-to-day basis. This can include changes in mood, energy levels, digestive reactions, or any other physical or mental responses you notice.

- Dietary Adaptations: If you made any modifications to the meal plan, such as substituting ingredients or altering meal times, document these changes. This can help you understand how different foods or eating patterns affect you.

- Challenges and Successes: Reflect on any challenges you faced, such as cravings or difficulty in meal preparation, and how you addressed them. Also, celebrate successes, like resisting a particular craving or noticing positive changes in your health.

- Physical and Emotional Well-being: Expand on the ratings you provided by describing in more detail how you feel physically and emotionally. This could include noting any reduction in pain, improvements in skin health, or changes in mental clarity and mood.

- Future Adjustments: Based on your week's experience, jot down any thoughts on what you might want to try differently in the upcoming week. This could be trying new recipes, adjusting portion sizes, or incorporating more of a particular type of food.

- Questions and Research: If you have questions or areas of curiosity that arose during the week, such as the effects of certain foods or why you experienced specific reactions, note these down. You can then research these topics or discuss them with a healthcare professional.

- Overall Reflection: Conclude with a general reflection on how the week went, what you learned about your body's response to the diet, and how you feel about continuing with the meal plan.

WEEK 2: FLAVORFUL FOODS FIESTA

Adding Color and Variety to Your Anti-Inflammatory Diet
This week, we're spicing things up with a diverse array of colorful, anti-inflammatory foods that are as tasty as they are beneficial.

ENHANCING UNDERSTANDING BEFORE TRANSITIONING TO WEEK 2

Unpacking the Anti-Inflammatory Diet

- Bioactive Compounds in Foods: Many foods included in Week 1, like blueberries and nuts, contain bioactive compounds (like flavonoids and omega-3 fatty acids) that actively reduce inflammation. These compounds inhibit inflammatory pathways in the body and promote healing.
- Synergy in Meals: The combination of foods in Week 1 was designed to create a synergy that amplifies their anti-inflammatory effects. For instance, the healthy fats in salmon enhance the absorption of fat-soluble nutrients from vegetables, maximizing their benefits.
- Importance of Dietary Fiber: High-fiber foods, such as leafy greens and whole grains, play a crucial role in maintaining gut health. A healthy gut microbiome is essential in managing systemic inflammation, as it helps regulate immune responses and reduce harmful bacterial overgrowth.

Preparing for Week 2: Expanding the Palette

Reinforcing Foundations at the End of Week 1
As we wrap up the first week of our Anti-Inflammatory Meal Plan, let's further bolster our understanding of how our diet can combat chronic inflammation. This deeper knowledge will not only enhance our appreciation of the foods we're eating but also prepare us for the exciting variety in Week 2.

The Science Behind Anti-Inflammatory Foods

- Understanding Inflammatory Pathways: Inflammation is the body's natural response to protect itself, but chronic inflammation can lead to various health problems. Certain foods contain compounds that help modulate these inflammatory pathways, reducing the risk of chronic diseases.
- Role of Antioxidants: Antioxidants in foods like blueberries and nuts combat oxidative stress, a key contributor to inflammation. They neutralize free radicals, preventing them from causing cellular damage.
- Omega-3 Fatty Acids: Found in foods like salmon, these fatty acids are crucial in reducing inflammation. They play a role in creating resolvins and protectins, which help terminate inflammation in the body.

Integrating Holistic Practices

- Holistic Dietary Approach: An anti-inflammatory diet isn't just about individual foods; it's about the overall pattern of eating. A balanced diet rich in whole foods, healthy fats, lean proteins, and a variety of fruits and vegetables is key.
- Hydration and Inflammation: Proper hydration is crucial in managing inflammation. Water helps flush out toxins and keeps cells functioning optimally.

Preparing for Week 2: Embracing Diversity

- Dietary Diversity: Week 2 will introduce a wider array of fruits, vegetables, grains, and proteins. Each of these foods brings unique anti-inflammatory compounds and health benefits.
- Culinary Exploration: We'll be exploring different culinary traditions and recipes that incorporate these principles, making the diet enjoyable and sustainable.

Mind and Body Connection

- Mindful Eating and Stress Reduction: Understanding the connection between the mind and inflammation is crucial. Techniques like mindful eating, meditation, and regular physical activity can significantly impact your body's inflammatory response. At the back of the book, Page x (INSERT PAGE NUMBER HERE LABRI ONCE COMPLETED, SO THE READER CAN GO TO THE PAGE PLEASE!) . we have detailed stress reduction techniques with mindful eating program).

As we move forward into Week 2, armed with a richer understanding and appreciation for the anti-inflammatory diet, we're well-prepared to enjoy and benefit from the varied and flavorful meals ahead. This journey is about nourishing not just the body but also the mind, creating a harmonious balance for long-term health and wellness. Let's step into the next week with enthusiasm for the new flavors and experiences that await!

DAY 8 MEAL PLAN

BREAKFAST: SPINACH AND MUSHROOM OMELET
LUNCH: QUINOA SALAD WITH CHERRY TOMATOES, CUCUMBER, AND FETA
DINNER: CHICKEN CURRY WITH TURMERIC, GINGER, AND CAULIFLOWER RICE
SNACK: SLICED RED BELL PEPPER WITH GUACAMOLE
SNACK: A HANDFUL OF GRAPES
DRINK: MATCHA GREEN TEA

BREAKFAST: SPINACH AND MUSHROOM OMELET

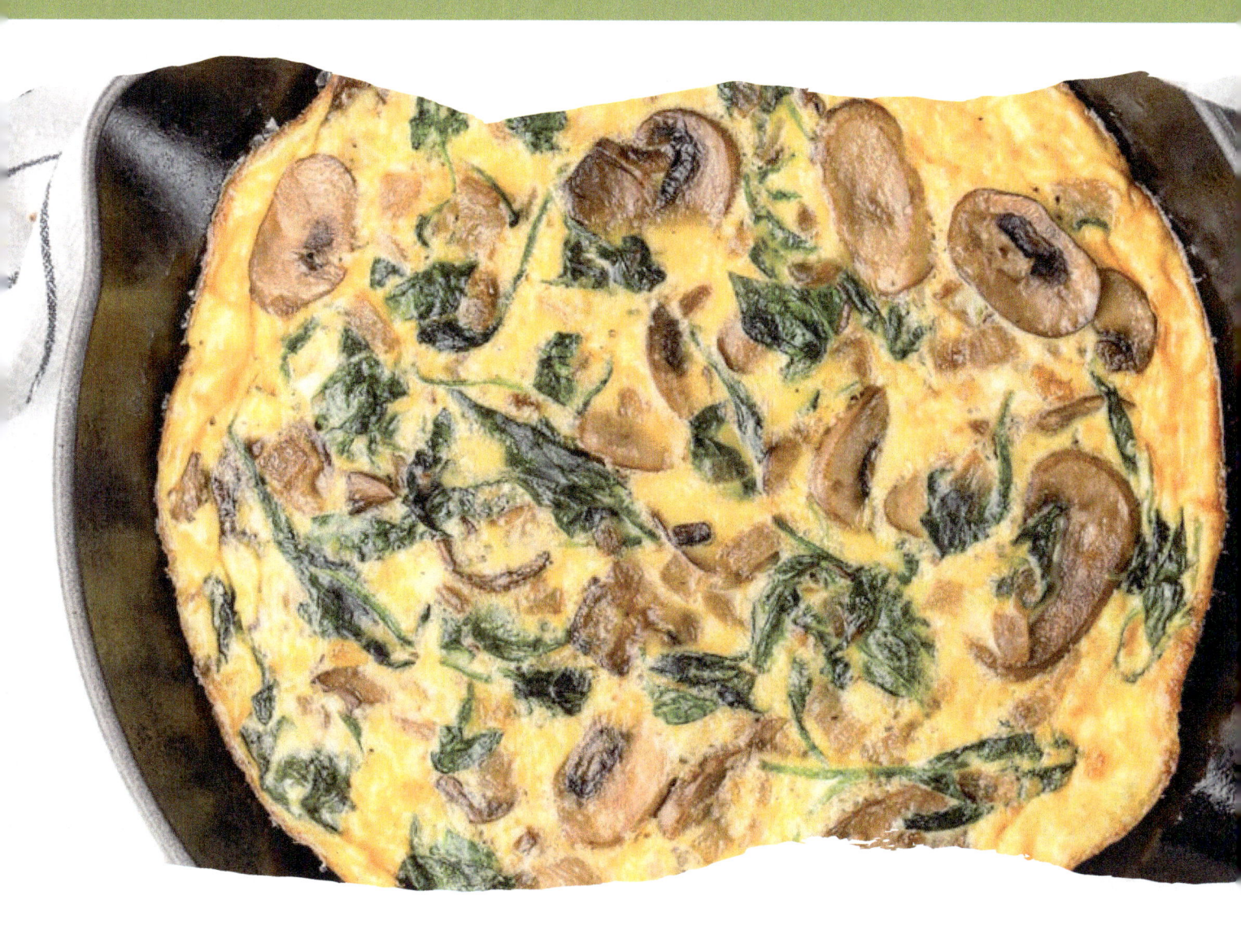

INGREDIENTS

- 2 eggs
- 1 cup fresh spinach, chopped
- ½ cup mushrooms, sliced
- Salt and pepper to taste
- Olive oil or butter for cooking

INSTRUCTIONS

- Prepare Ingredients: Chop spinach and slice mushrooms.
- Beat Eggs: Whisk eggs in a bowl, season with salt and pepper.
- Cook Omelet: In a pan, cook mushrooms, add spinach, then pour eggs over. Cook until set, fold over.

KITCHEN TOOLS NEEDED

- Frying pan
- Spatula
- Knife and cutting board
- Mixing bowl

LUNCH: QUINOA SALAD WITH CHERRY TOMATOES, CUCUMBER, AND FETA

INGREDIENTS

- 1 cup cooked quinoa
- ½ cup cherry tomatoes, halved
- ½ cucumber, diced
- ¼ cup feta cheese, crumbled
- Olive oil and lemon juice for dressing
- Salt and pepper to taste

INSTRUCTIONS

- Combine Salad Ingredients: In a bowl, mix quinoa, tomatoes, cucumber, and feta.
- Dress Salad: Drizzle with olive oil and lemon juice, season with salt and pepper.

KITCHEN TOOLS NEEDED

- Mixing bowl
- Knife and cutting board

DINNER: CHICKEN CURRY WITH TURMERIC, GINGER, AND CAULIFLOWER RICE

INGREDIENTS

- 1 chicken breast, cut into pieces
- 1 cup cauliflower rice
- 1 tablespoon curry powder (with turmeric and ginger)
- 1 cup coconut milk
- Olive oil for cooking
- Salt to taste

INSTRUCTIONS

- Cook Chicken: Sauté chicken with curry powder until browned.
- Add Coconut Milk: Pour in coconut milk, simmer until chicken is cooked.
- Prepare Cauliflower Rice: Cook cauliflower rice in a separate pan.
- Serve: Plate the chicken curry over cauliflower rice.

KITCHEN TOOLS NEEDED

- Skillet or saucepan
- Knife and cutting board

DRINK: MATCHA GREEN TEA

INGREDIENTS

- 1 teaspoon matcha green tea powder
- 1 cup hot water

INSTRUCTIONS

- Prepare Matcha: Whisk matcha powder with hot water until frothy.
- Serve: Enjoy the rich and energizing matcha tea.

KITCHEN TOOLS NEEDED

- Tea bowl or mug
- Whisk or spoon

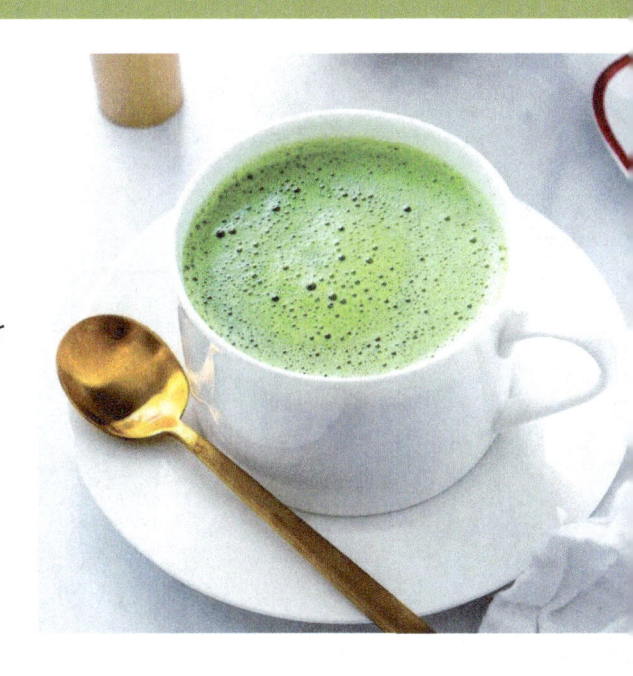

SNACK: SLICED RED BELL PEPPER WITH GUACAMOLE

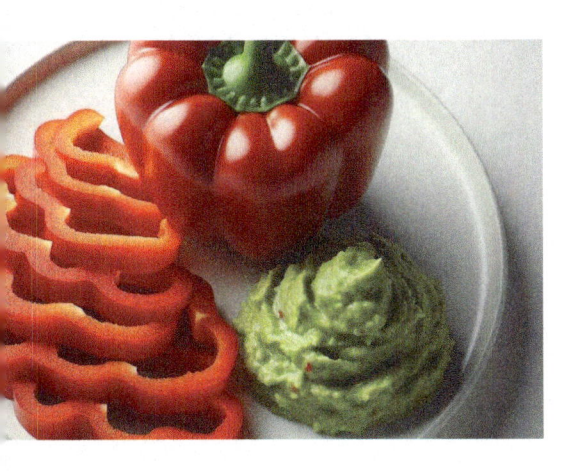

INGREDIENTS

- 1 red bell pepper
- ¼ cup guacamole

INSTRUCTIONS

- Slice Pepper: Cut the bell pepper into strips.
- Serve with Guacamole: Enjoy the pepper slices dipped in guacamole.

KITCHEN TOOLS NEEDED

- Knife and cutting board

SNACK: A HANDFUL OF GRAPES

INGREDIENTS

- A handful of grapes (any variety)

PREPARATION TIME: NONE, READY TO EAT.

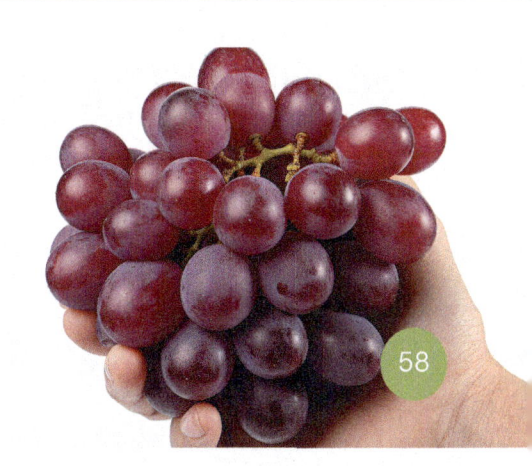

CAULIFLOWER - THE CRUCIFEROUS MARVEL

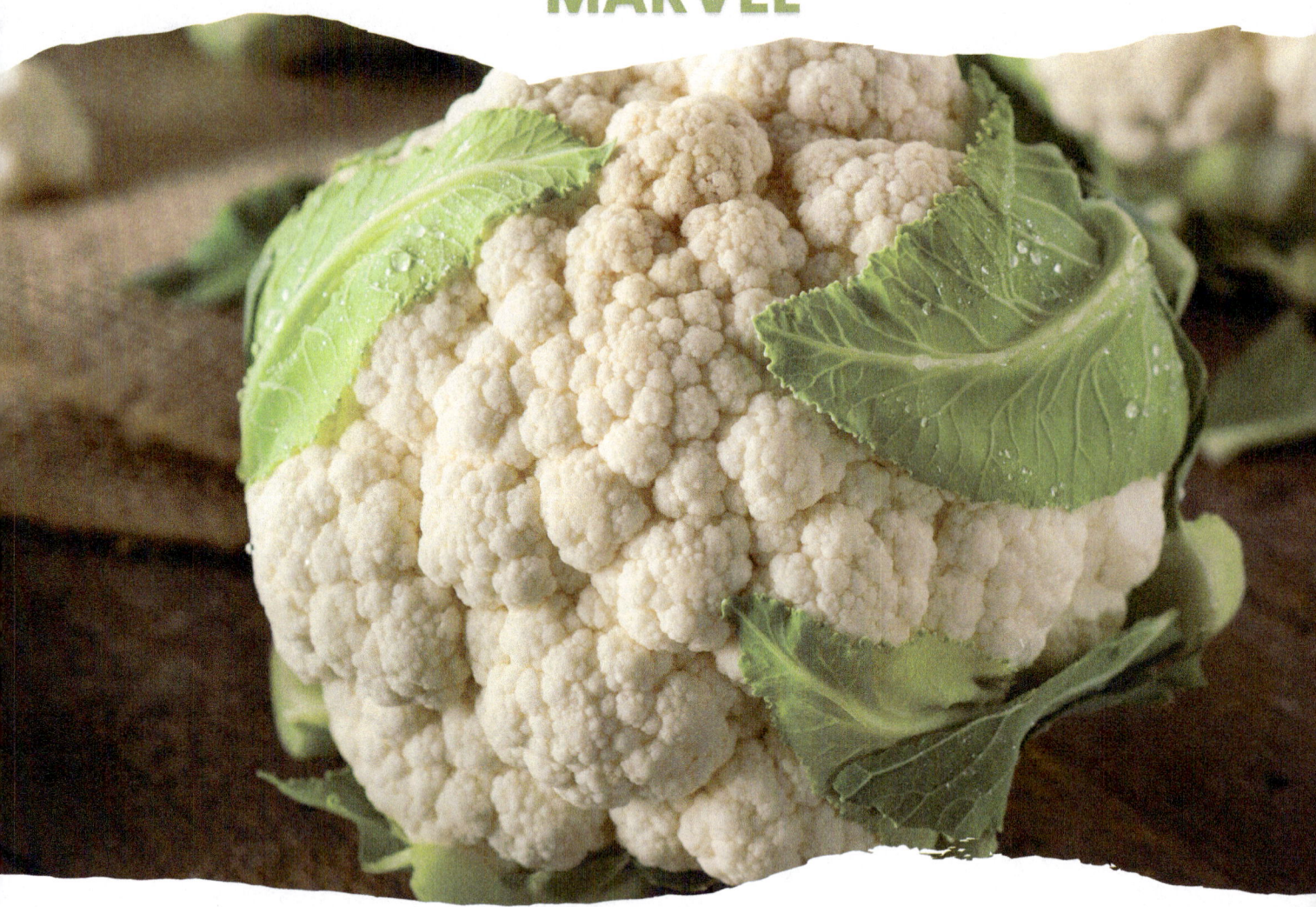

Cauliflower in Our Anti-Inflammatory Meal Plan
As we delve deeper into our Anti-Inflammatory Meal Plan, it's time to spotlight cauliflower, an unsung hero of the cruciferous family. This versatile vegetable is not only a culinary chameleon but also a powerhouse of nutrients and health benefits, making it an invaluable addition to our daily diet.

The Remarkable Benefits of Cauliflower

- Nutrient Density: Cauliflower is a treasure trove of vitamins and minerals. It's an excellent source of vitamins C and K, folate, and fiber, contributing to reduced inflammation and improved digestion.
- Rich in Antioxidants: Packed with antioxidants like glucosinolates and isothiocyanates, cauliflower helps in neutralizing harmful free radicals. This action is crucial in reducing oxidative stress and inflammation in the body.
- Supports Heart and Brain Health: Regular consumption of cauliflower has been linked to enhanced heart and brain health, thanks to its anti-inflammatory properties that help in reducing the risk of chronic diseases

Integrating Cauliflower into Daily Meals

- Adaptable in Various Recipes: Cauliflower's mild flavor and adaptability make it perfect for various culinary uses – from roasted cauliflower as a side dish to cauliflower rice or even as a pizza crust for a healthier alternative.
- Incorporation in Lunches and Dinners: It can be seamlessly added to salads, stews, and stir-fries, enhancing the meal's nutritional value without overpowering other flavors.

Paving the Way for a Health-Conscious Future

- A Versatile Vegetable for Every Diet: Cauliflower's low-calorie yet high-fiber content makes it ideal for various dietary needs, from weight management to diabetic diets.
- Inspiring Creative and Healthful Cooking: As we explore more recipes in our meal plan, cauliflower stands out as an ingredient that inspires creativity in the kitchen, allowing for healthful and delicious meal options.

In conclusion, cauliflower is a cornerstone in the realm of anti-inflammatory foods. Its impressive nutrient profile, coupled with its versatility in cooking, makes it an essential ingredient for anyone pursuing a health-focused diet. Incorporating cauliflower into your meals can significantly aid in reducing inflammation and promoting overall well-being. As your dietary adventure continues, let cauliflower be a key player in your diverse and nutritious culinary repertoire.

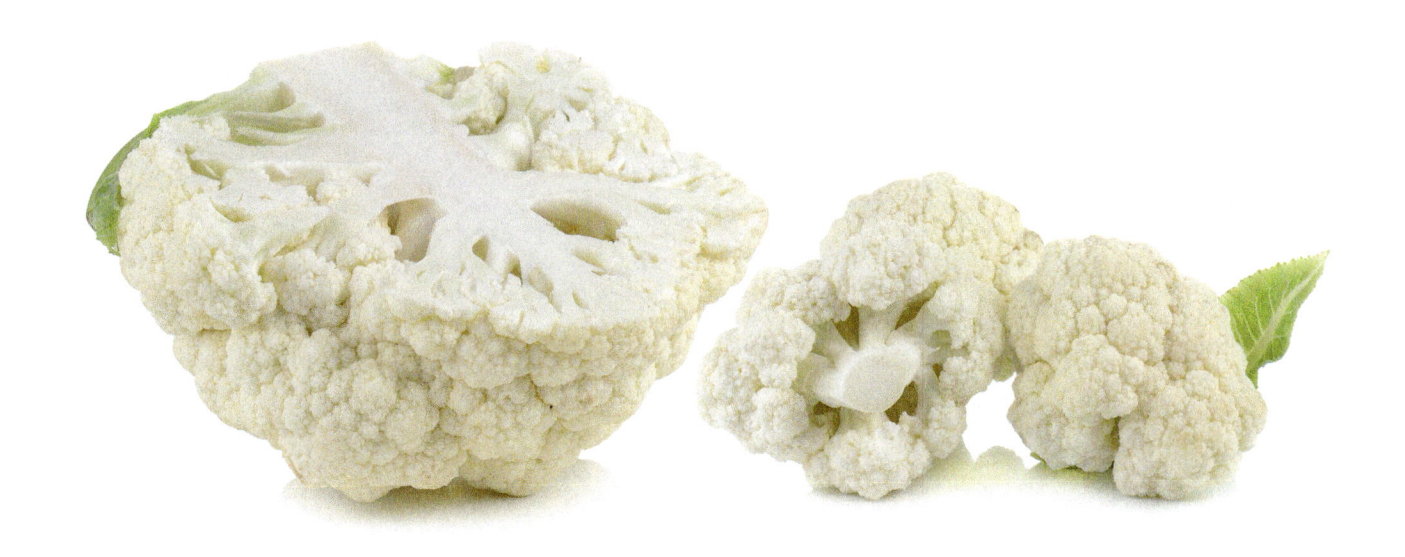

DAY 9 MEAL PLAN

BREAKFAST: WHOLE GRAIN PANCAKES WITH MIXED BERRIES AND GREEK YOGURT
LUNCH: MEDITERRANEAN CHICKPEA SALAD
DINNER: BAKED TROUT WITH ROASTED BRUSSELS SPROUTS AND BUTTERNUT SQUASH
SNACK: A MEDIUM-SIZED APPLE
SNACK: A SMALL HANDFUL OF PUMPKIN SEEDS
DRINK: ROOIBOS TEA

BREAKFAST: WHOLE GRAIN PANCAKES WITH MIXED BERRIES AND GREEK YOGURT

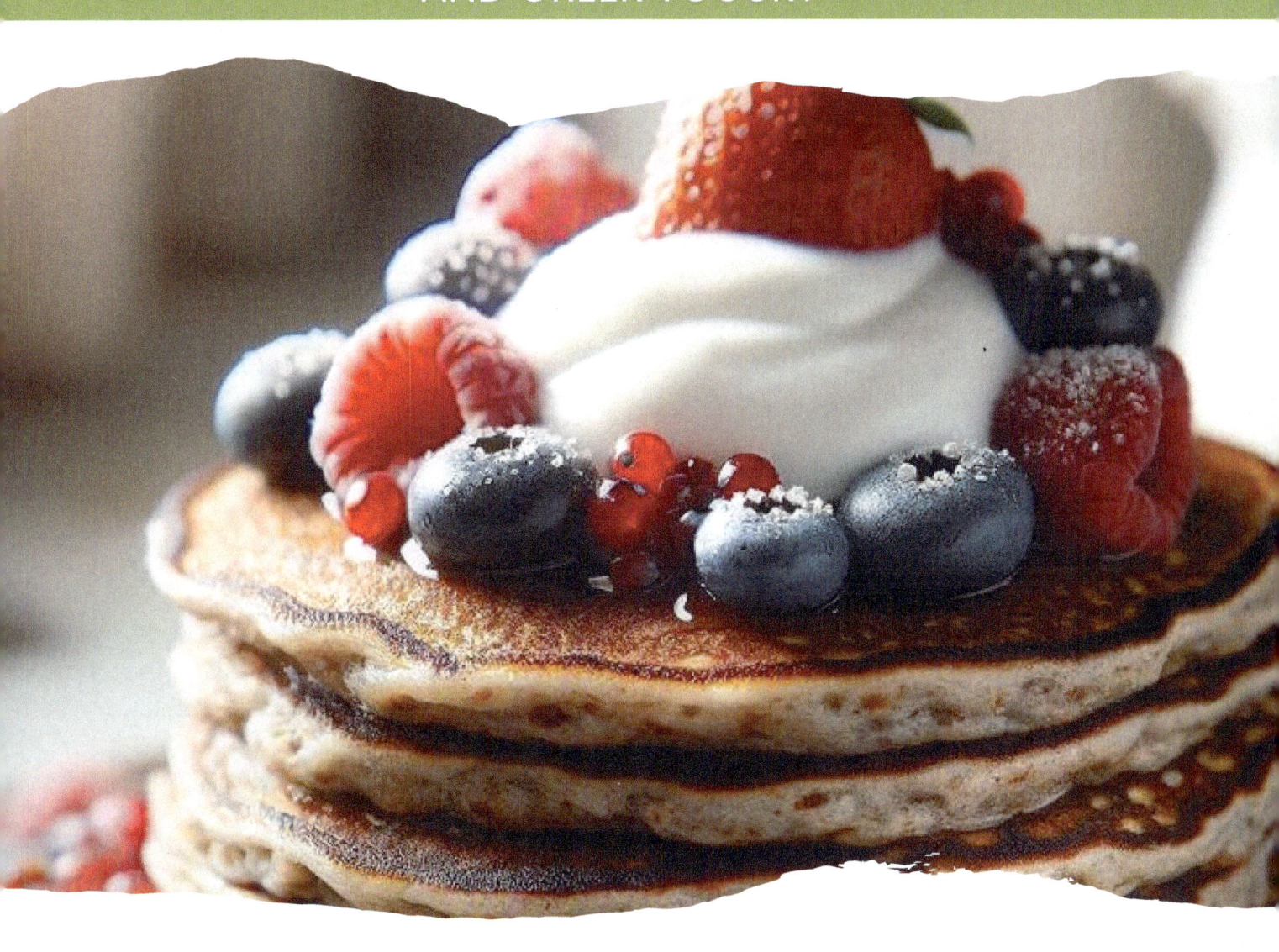

INGREDIENTS

- Whole grain pancake mix (as per package instructions)
- Mixed berries (strawberries, blueberries, raspberries)
- Greek yogurt for topping

INSTRUCTIONS

- Prepare Pancake Batter: Follow the instructions on the pancake mix package.
- Cook Pancakes: Pour batter onto a heated griddle, cook until golden brown on both sides.
- Top with Berries and Yogurt: Serve pancakes topped with a mix of berries and a dollop of Greek yogurt.

KITCHEN TOOLS NEEDED
- Griddle or frying pan
- Mixing bowl
- Spatula

LUNCH: MEDITERRANEAN CHICKPEA SALAD

INGREDIENTS

- 1 cup cooked chickpeas
- ½ cup olives, sliced
- ¼ red onion, finely chopped
- Tahini dressing (tahini, lemon juice, water, salt)
- Optional: cherry tomatoes, cucumber

INSTRUCTIONS

- Combine Salad Ingredients: In a bowl, mix chickpeas, olives, and red onion.
- Prepare Dressing: Whisk together tahini, lemon juice, water, and salt.
- Dress Salad: Toss the salad with the tahini dressing.

KITCHEN TOOLS NEEDED
- Mixing bowl
- Knife and cutting board

DINNER: BAKED TROUT WITH ROASTED BRUSSELS SPROUTS AND BUTTERNUT SQUASH

INGREDIENTS

- 1 trout fillet
- 1 cup Brussels sprouts, halved
- 1 cup butternut squash, cubed
- Olive oil, salt, and pepper for seasoning

INSTRUCTIONS

- Prepare Vegetables: Toss Brussels sprouts and butternut squash with olive oil, salt, and pepper. Roast in the oven until tender.
- Prepare Trout: Season the trout fillet and bake alongside the vegetables.
- Check and Serve: Ensure everything is cooked through, then serve together.

KITCHEN TOOLS NEEDED
- Oven and baking tray
- Knife and cutting board

DRINK: ROOIBOS TEA

INGREDIENTS

- 1 rooibos tea bag
- 1 cup boiling water

INSTRUCTIONS

- Boil Water: Heat the water.
- Steep Tea: Place the tea bag in a mug and pour hot water over it.

KITCHEN TOOLS NEEDED

- Kettle or pot for boiling water
- Mug

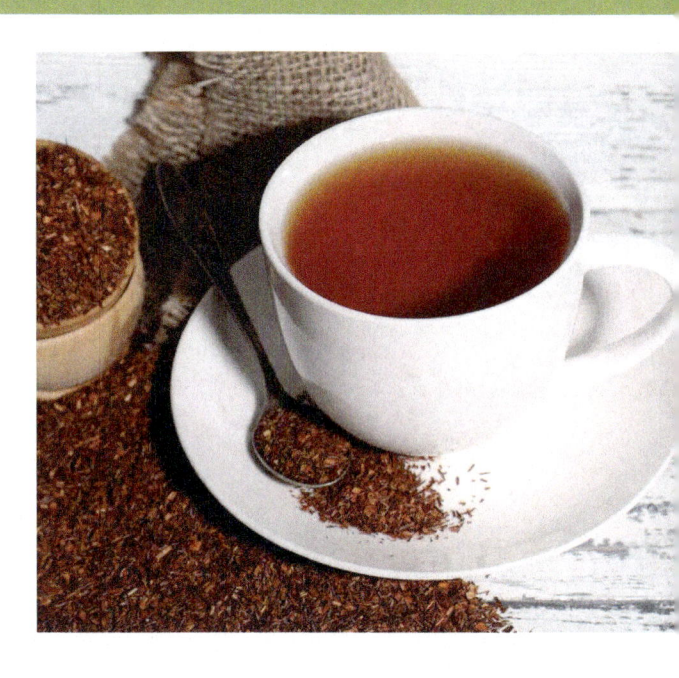

SNACK: A MEDIUM-SIZED APPLE

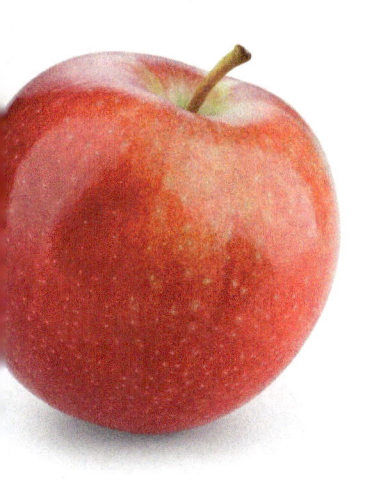

INGREDIENTS

- A Medium-sized Apple

PREPARATION TIME: NONE, READY TO EAT.

SNACK: A SMALL HANDFUL OF PUMPKIN SEEDS

INGREDIENTS

- A small handful of pumpkin seeds

PREPARATION TIME: NONE, READY TO EAT AFTER PEELING.

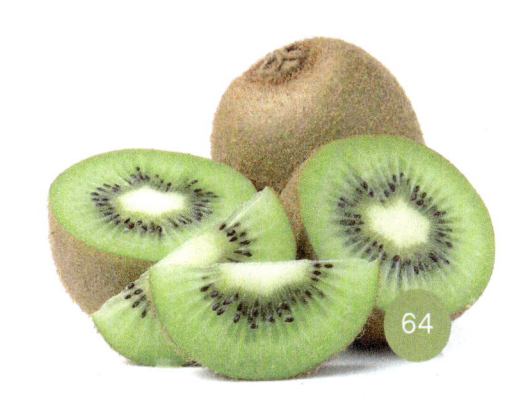

CHICKPEAS - THE VERSATILE LEGUME POWERHOUSE

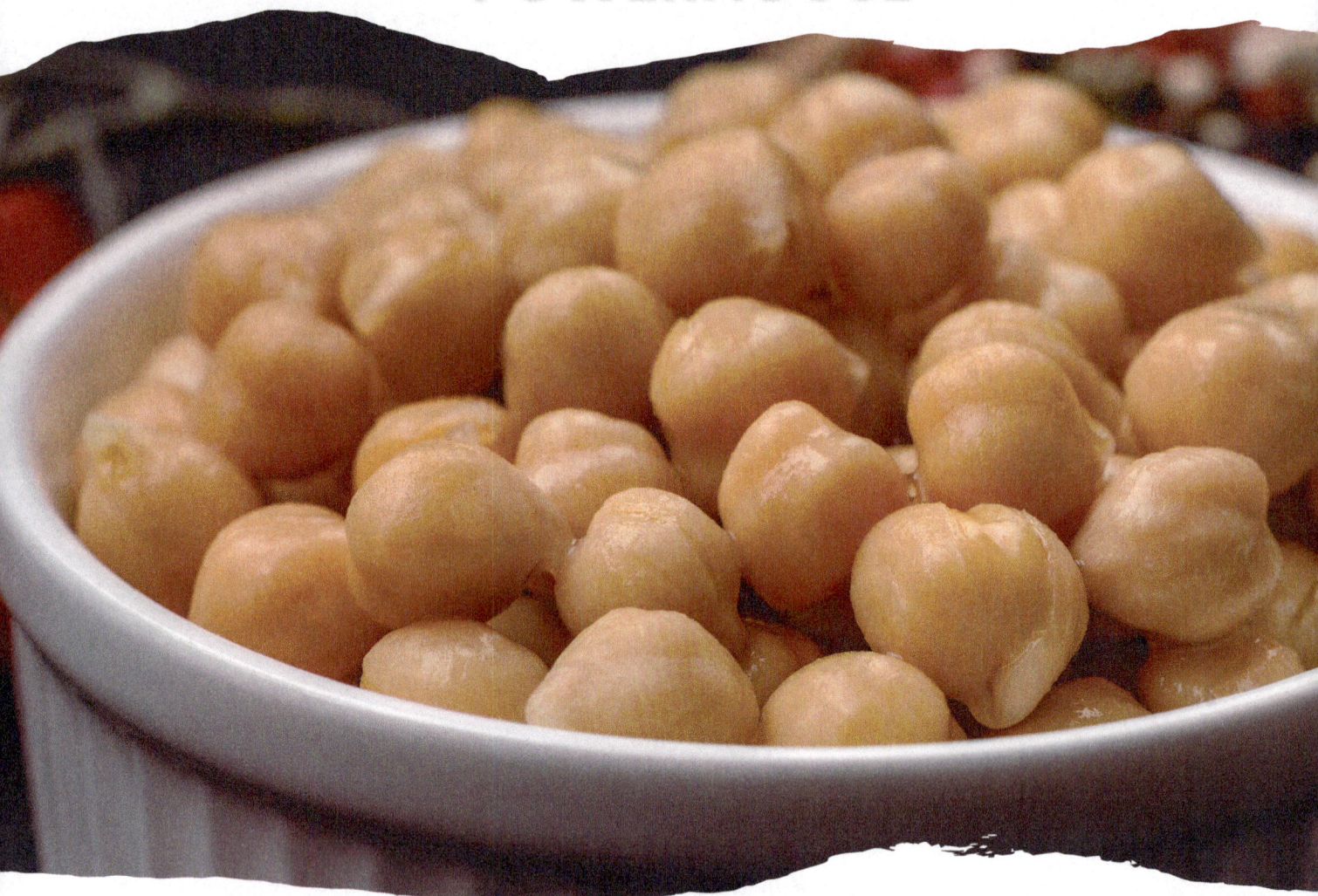

Continuing our exploration of beneficial foods in the Anti-Inflammatory Meal Plan, let's shine a light on chickpeas. Also known as garbanzo beans, these legumes are not only a staple in many cuisines worldwide but also a vital ingredient for anyone looking to boost their health and fight inflammation.

The Superlative Benefits of Chickpeas

- Nutrient-Rich: Chickpeas are a fantastic source of protein, especially important for those on plant-based diets. They also offer a wealth of other nutrients, including fiber, vitamins B6 and C, folate, and minerals like magnesium and potassium.
- Fights Inflammation: The high fiber content in chickpeas aids in digestion and gut health, while the protein and nutrients contribute to reducing inflammation throughout the body.
- Supports Heart Health: Regular consumption of chickpeas is linked to better heart health, thanks to their ability to lower cholesterol levels and improve blood pressure.

Incorporating Chickpeas into Daily Meals

- Versatility in Recipes: Chickpeas are incredibly versatile and can be included in a variety of dishes. They can be tossed into salads, blended into hummus, roasted for a crunchy snack, or added to soups and stews.
- A Star in Lunches and Dinners: They make a fantastic meat substitute in many dishes, adding heartiness and texture. Chickpeas can also be a star ingredient in vegetarian or vegan meals, providing essential protein.

Setting the Stage for Long-Term Health Benefits

- A Legume for All Diets: Their low glycemic index makes chickpeas a great option for those managing blood sugar levels, including diabetics.
- Encouraging Healthy Eating Habits: The presence of chickpeas in our meal plan underscores the importance of integrating legumes into our diet for their health benefits and their ability to make meals more satisfying and flavorful.

In summary, chickpeas are an invaluable component of an anti-inflammatory diet. Their rich nutritional profile and culinary flexibility make them a superb choice for a variety of dishes, contributing significantly to reducing inflammation and promoting overall health. As you continue your journey towards a balanced and healthful lifestyle, consider chickpeas as a staple in your dietary arsenal for both their health benefits and their delicious versatility.

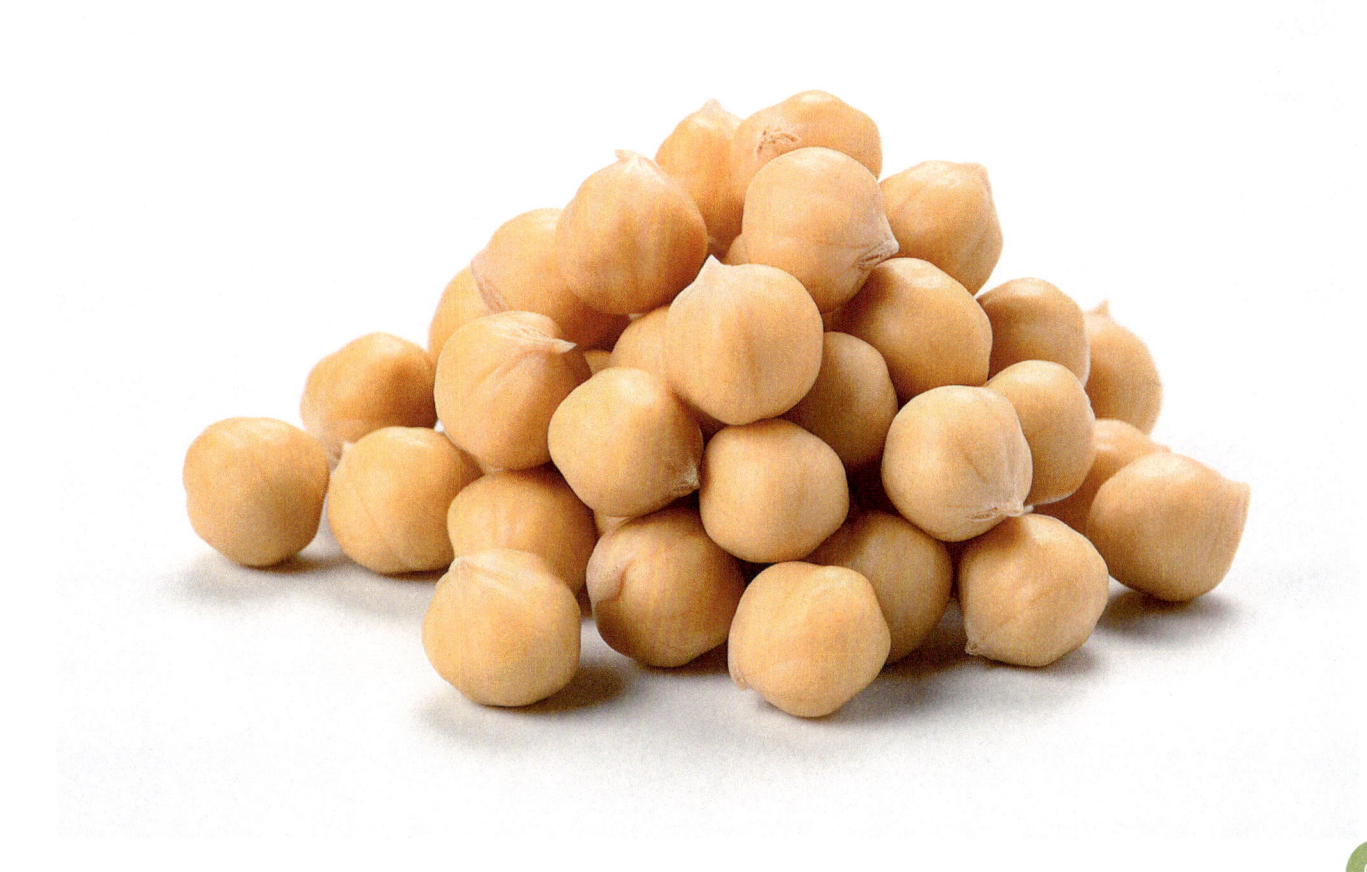

DAY 10 MEAL PLAN

BREAKFAST: BERRY AND BANANA SMOOTHIE
LUNCH: LENTIL SOUP WITH WHOLE-GRAIN BREAD
DINNER: GRILLED LAMB CHOPS WITH STEAMED GREEN BEANS AND QUINOA TABBOULEH
SNACK: CARROT STICKS WITH ALMOND BUTTER
SNACK: ORANGE SLICES
DRINK: LEMON AND GINGER WATER

BREAKFAST: BERRY AND BANANA SMOOTHIE

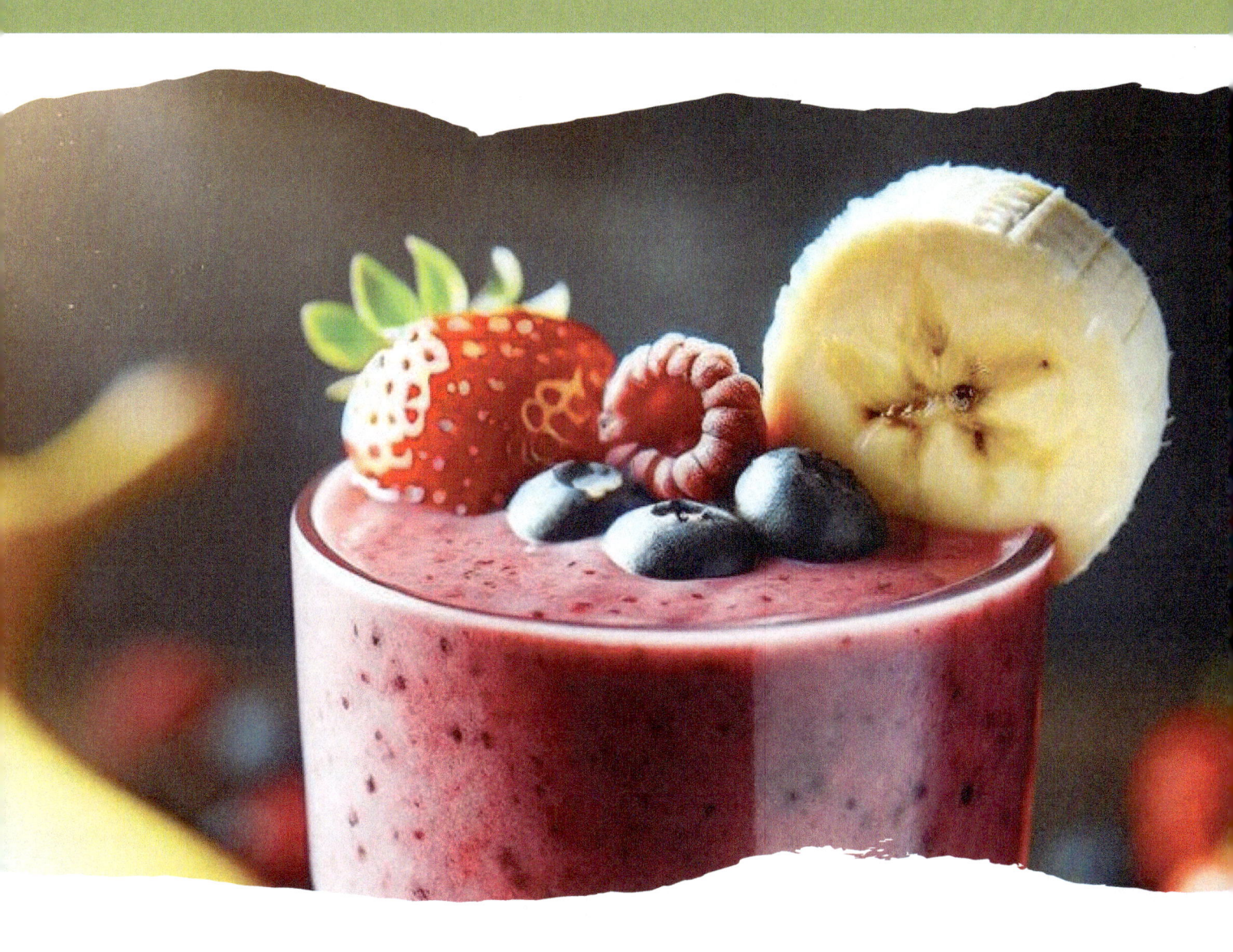

INGREDIENTS

- ½ cup mixed berries (fresh or frozen)
- 1 banana
- 1 cup almond milk
- 1 scoop protein powder (preferably vanilla or unflavored)

INSTRUCTIONS

- Blend Ingredients: Combine berries, banana, almond milk, and protein powder in the blender.
- Blend until Smooth: Blend until you get a smooth consistency.
- Serve: Pour into a glass and enjoy immediately.

KITCHEN TOOLS NEEDED
- Blender
- Measuring cup

LUNCH: LENTIL SOUP WITH WHOLE-GRAIN BREAD

INGREDIENTS

- 1 serving of pre-made or canned lentil soup
- 1 slice of whole-grain bread

INSTRUCTIONS

- Heat Soup: Warm the lentil soup in a pot on the stove or in a microwave-safe bowl.
- Prepare Bread: Toast the whole-grain bread if desired.
- Serve Together: Enjoy the warm soup with a side of whole-grain bread.

KITCHEN TOOLS NEEDED
- Pot or microwave-safe bowl
- Soup spoon

DINNER: GRILLED LAMB CHOPS WITH STEAMED GREEN BEANS AND QUINOA TABBOULEH

INGREDIENTS

- 2-3 lamb chops
- 1 cup green beans
- 1 cup cooked quinoa
- Fresh herbs, tomatoes, cucumber for tabbouleh
- Olive oil, lemon juice, salt, and pepper for seasoning

INSTRUCTIONS

- Grill Lamb Chops: Season lamb chops and grill until desired doneness.
- Steam Green Beans: Steam green beans until tender-crisp.
- Prepare Quinoa Tabbouleh: Mix cooked quinoa with chopped herbs, tomatoes, cucumber, olive oil, and lemon juice.
- Serve: Plate the lamb chops with steamed green beans and quinoa tabbouleh.

KITCHEN TOOLS NEEDED
- Grill pan or barbecue grill
- Steamer or pot
- Mixing bowl

DRINK: LEMON AND GINGER WATER

INGREDIENTS
- 1 lemon
- 1-inch piece of fresh ginger
- 1 liter of water

INSTRUCTIONS
- Prepare Ingredients: Slice the lemon and ginger.
- Infuse Water: Add lemon and ginger slices to water, let it infuse for an hour or more.
- Serve: Enjoy chilled or at room temperature.

KITCHEN TOOLS NEEDED
- Pitcher or large bottle
- Knife and cutting board

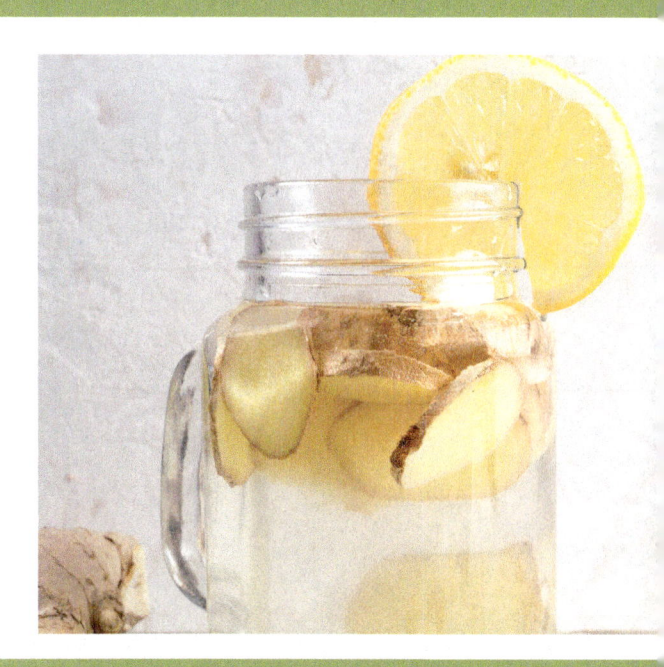

SNACK: ORANGE SLICES

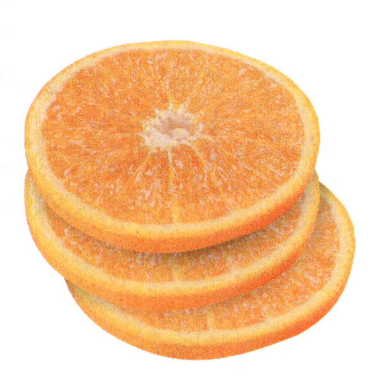

INGREDIENTS
- 1 orange

INSTRUCTIONS
- Slice Orange: Peel and slice the orange into segments.
- Serve: Enjoy the fresh, juicy orange slices.

KITCHEN TOOLS NEEDED
- Knife and cutting board

SNACK: CARROT STICKS WITH ALMOND BUTTER

INGREDIENTS
- 2-3 large carrots
- 2 tablespoons almond butter

INSTRUCTIONS
- Prepare Carrot Sticks: Peel and cut carrots into sticks.
- Serve with Almond Butter: Enjoy the carrot sticks dipped in almond butter.

KITCHEN TOOLS NEEDED
- Knife and cutting board

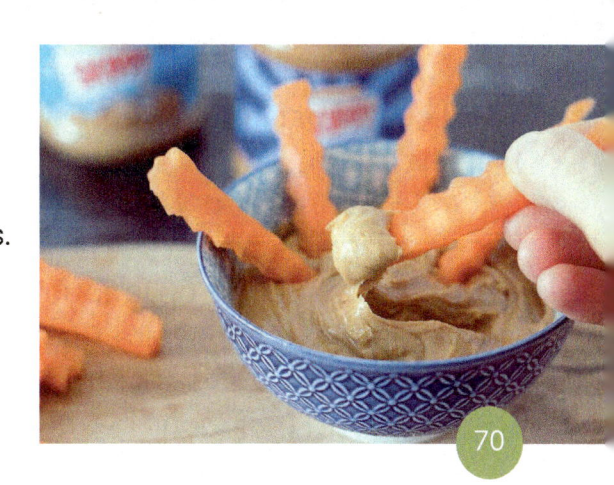

GREEN BEANS – THE VIBRANT VEGGIE ALLY

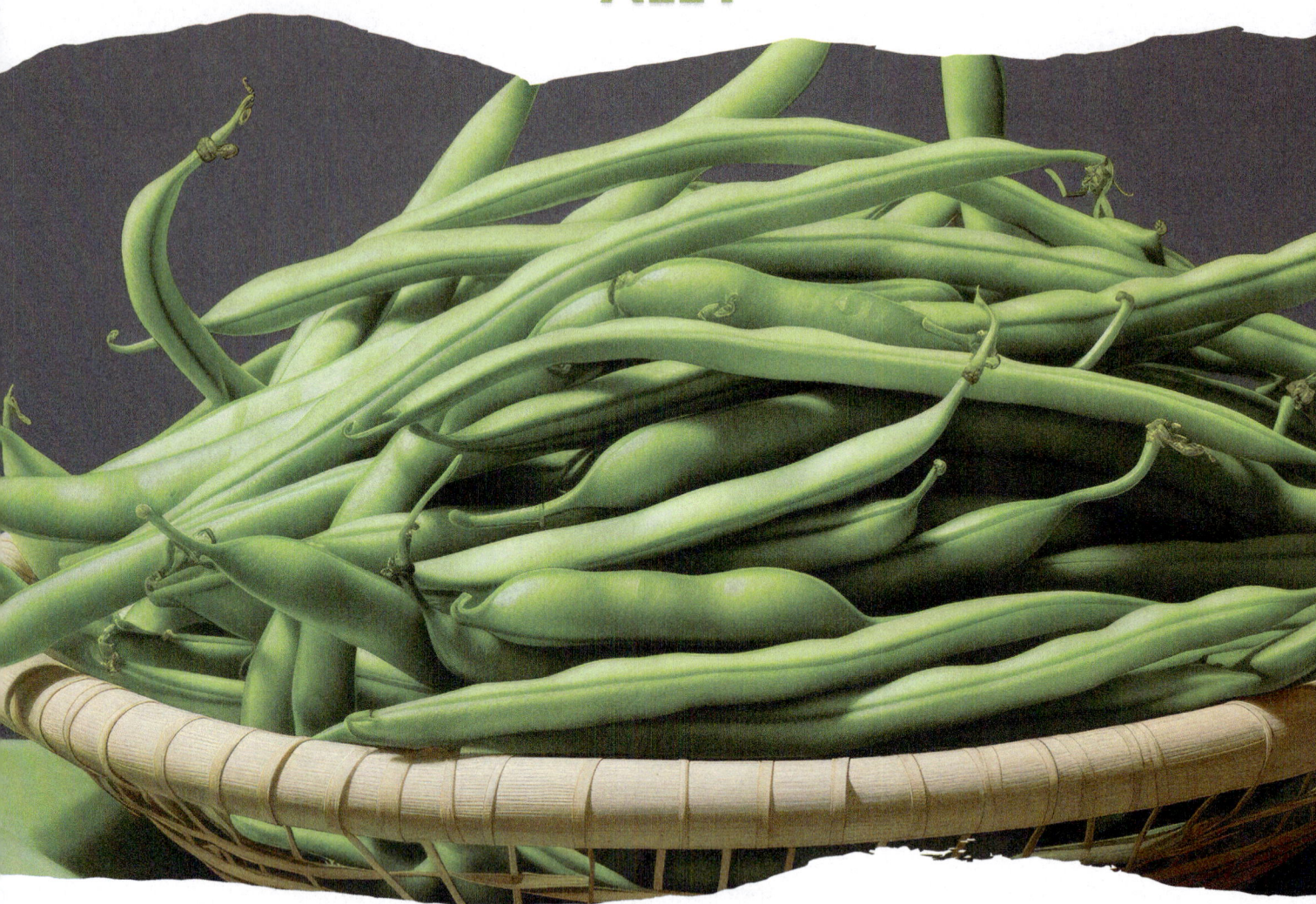

As we progress with our Anti-Inflammatory Meal Plan, it's time to focus on green beans, a vibrant and nutritious vegetable. These slender green pods, often a side dish staple, are much more than just an accompaniment; they are a nutritional powerhouse essential for anyone aiming to reduce inflammation and enhance their overall health.

The Health-Boosting Advantages of Green Beans

- Rich in Nutrients: Green beans are loaded with vital nutrients including vitamin C, dietary fiber, folate, vitamin K, and silicon (necessary for healthy bones, skin, and hair).
- Anti-Inflammatory Benefits: The antioxidants in green beans, such as flavonoids and carotenoids, play a key role in anti-inflammatory processes. This is crucial for reducing the risk of various chronic diseases.
- Promotes Heart Health: Regular consumption of green beans has been associated with a reduced risk of heart diseases due to their ability to lower bad cholesterol levels and their rich fiber content.

Integrating Green Beans into Daily Meals

- Culinary Versatility: Green beans can be steamed, boiled, stir-fried, or even eaten raw in salads, making them a versatile ingredient to include in various meals.
- Enhancing Lunch and Dinner Options: They can complement a wide range of dishes, from grilled meats to vegetarian stews, adding both nutrition and color.

Paving the Way for a Nutritious Future

- A Vegetable for Everyone: Green beans are low in calories yet high in essential nutrients, making them ideal for weight management and overall health maintenance.
- Encouraging a Balanced Diet: Including green beans in our meal plan encourages the consumption of a variety of vegetables, which is key to a balanced and anti-inflammatory diet.

In conclusion, green beans are a fantastic addition to an anti-inflammatory diet. Their nutritional value, coupled with their versatility in cooking, makes them an excellent choice for enhancing meals both in flavor and health benefits. As you continue exploring healthy eating options, let green beans be a regular feature in your meals, contributing to your journey towards a healthier, more balanced lifestyle.

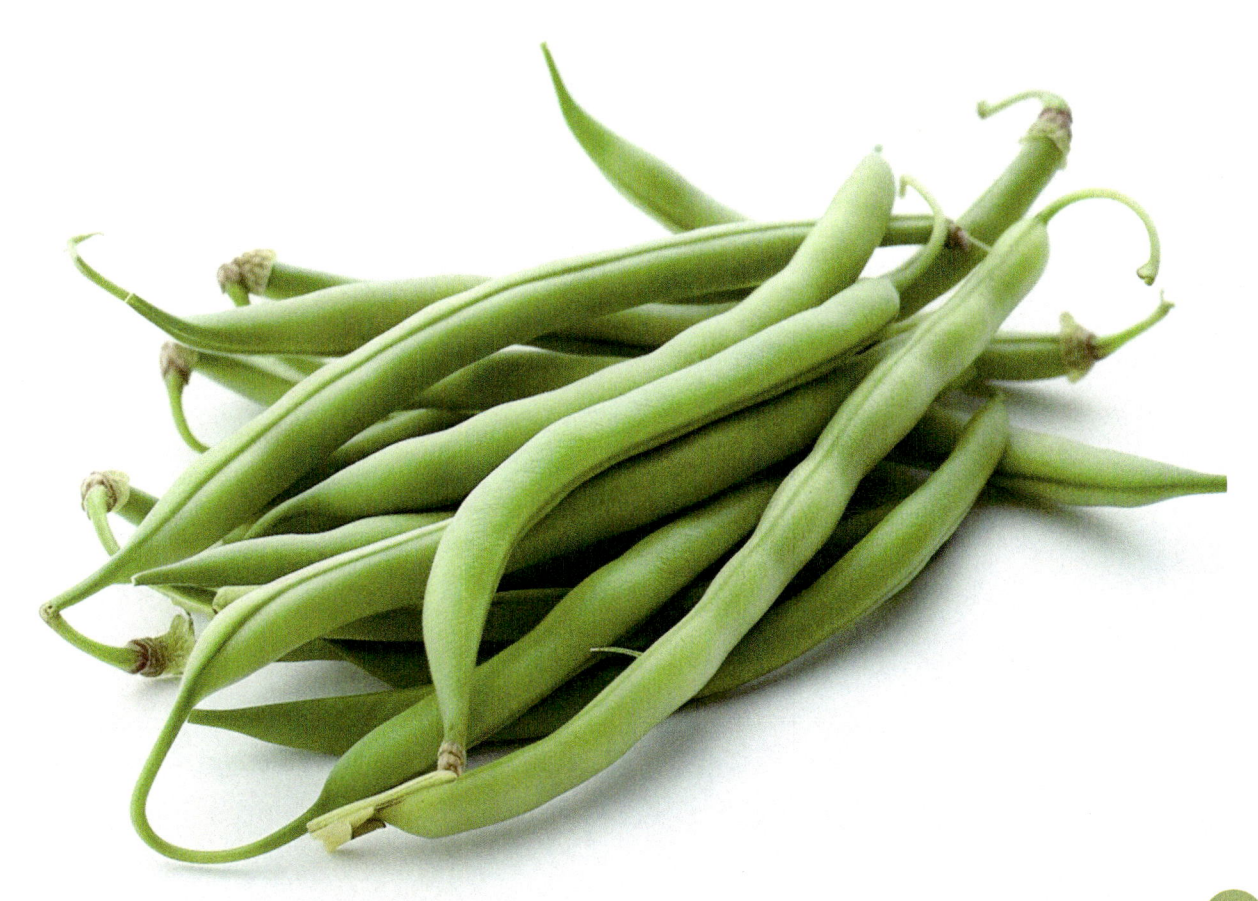

DAY 11 MEAL PLAN

BREAKFAST: AVOCADO TOAST WITH POACHED EGGS
LUNCH: RAINBOW WRAP WITH HUMMUS
DINNER: VEGETABLE STIR-FRY WITH TOFU AND BROWN RICE
SNACK: A HANDFUL OF MIXED NUTS
SNACK: PEACHES
DRINK: PEPPERMINT TEA

BREAKFAST: AVOCADO TOAST WITH POACHED EGGS

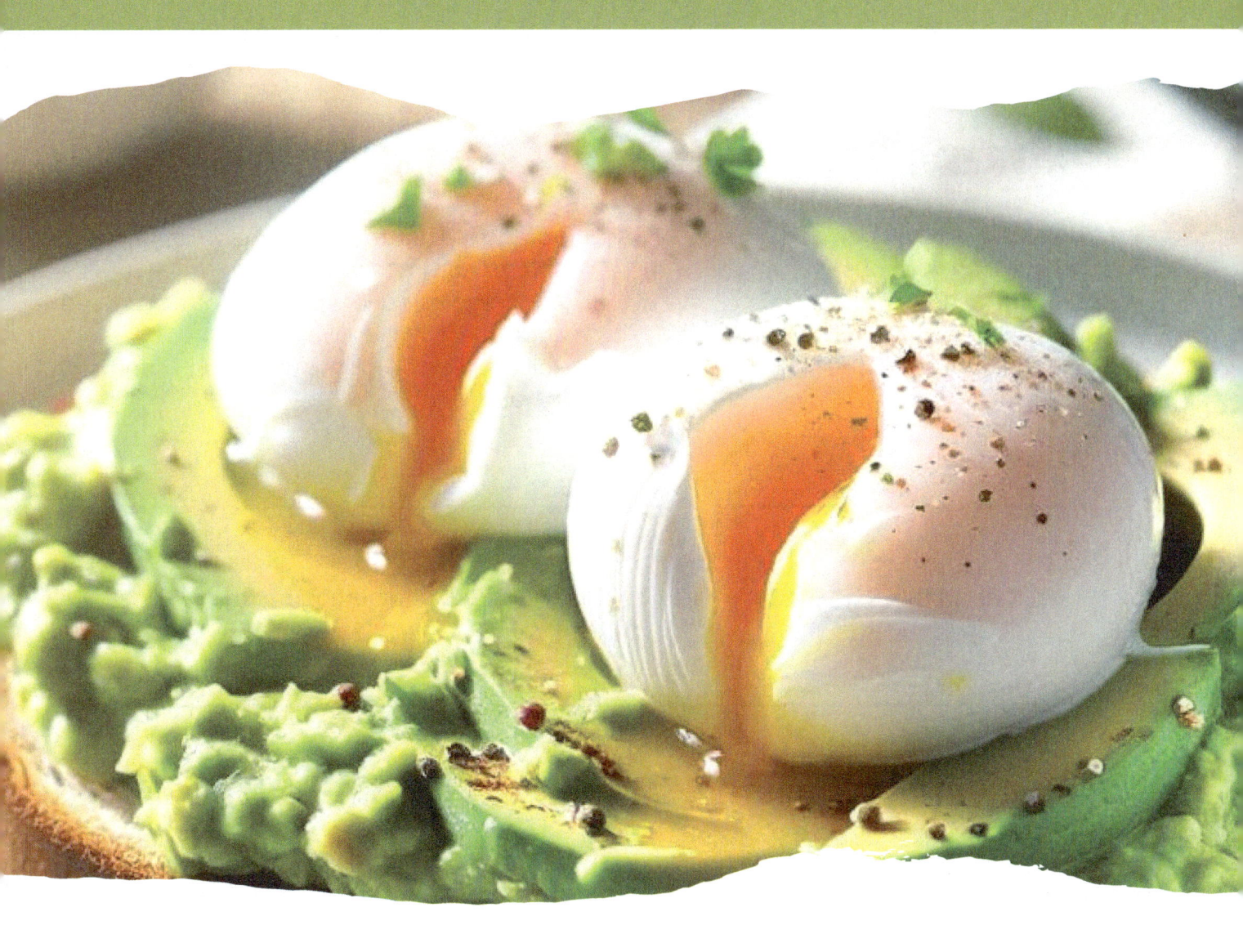

INGREDIENTS

- 1 ripe avocado
- 2 eggs
- 2 slices of whole-grain bread
- Salt, pepper, and other desired seasonings (like chili flakes or lemon juice)

INSTRUCTIONS

- Poach Eggs: Bring water to a simmer in a pot and poach eggs to desired doneness.
- Prepare Avocado Toast: Mash avocado on toasted whole-grain bread, season as desired.
- Assemble and Serve: Top each toast with a poached egg.

KITCHEN TOOLS NEEDED

- Pot for poaching eggs
- Toaster
- Knife and cutting board

LUNCH: RAINBOW WRAP WITH HUMMUS

INGREDIENTS

- 1 whole-grain or spinach wrap
- 2 tablespoons hummus
- Handful of spinach
- Shredded carrot
- Sliced red cabbage

INSTRUCTIONS

- Spread Hummus: Lay out the wrap and spread hummus over it.
- Add Veggies: Layer spinach, carrot, and red cabbage.
- Roll and Serve: Roll the wrap tightly and cut in half.

KITCHEN TOOLS NEEDED

- Knife and cutting board

DINNER: VEGETABLE STIR-FRY WITH TOFU AND BROWN RICE

INGREDIENTS

- 1 block of tofu, cubed
- Assorted vegetables (broccoli, bell peppers, carrots, etc.)
- 1 cup brown rice, cooked
- Tamari-sesame sauce (tamari, sesame oil, garlic, ginger)

INSTRUCTIONS

- Cook Rice: Prepare brown rice as per package instructions.
- Prepare Stir-Fry: Stir-fry tofu and vegetables, add tamari-sesame sauce.
- Serve: Serve the stir-fry over a bed of brown rice.

KITCHEN TOOLS NEEDED

- Frying pan or wok
- Pot for cooking rice
- Knife and cutting board

DRINK: PEPPERMINT TEA

INGREDIENTS

- 1 peppermint tea bag
- 1 cup boiling water

INSTRUCTIONS

- Boil Water: Heat the water.
- Steep Tea: Place the tea bag in a mug and pour hot water over it.

KITCHEN TOOLS NEEDED

- Kettle or pot for boiling water
- Mug

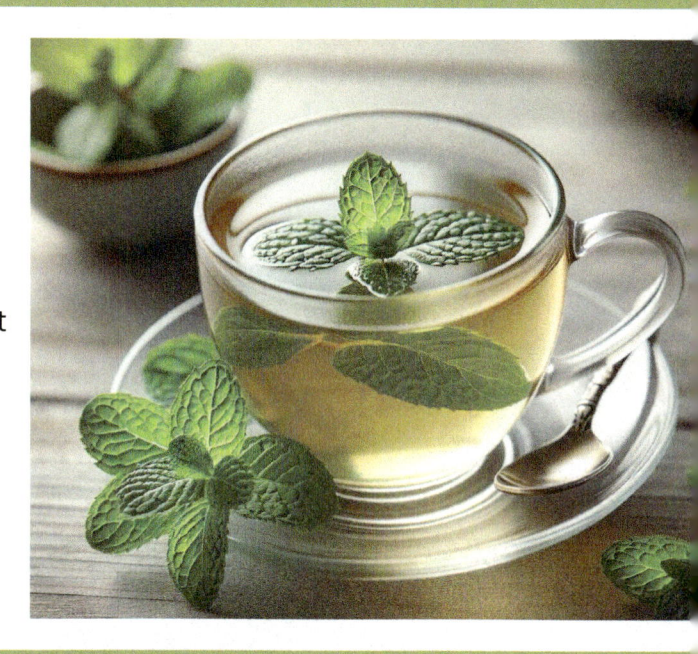

SNACK: PEACHES

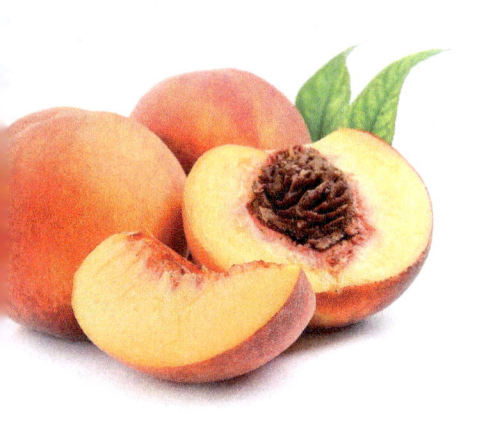

INGREDIENTS

- 1-2 ripe peaches

PREPARATION TIME: NONE, READY TO EAT.

SNACK: A HANDFUL OF MIXED NUTS

INGREDIENTS

- A handful of mixed nuts (almonds, walnuts, cashews, etc.)

PREPARATION TIME: NONE, READY TO EAT.

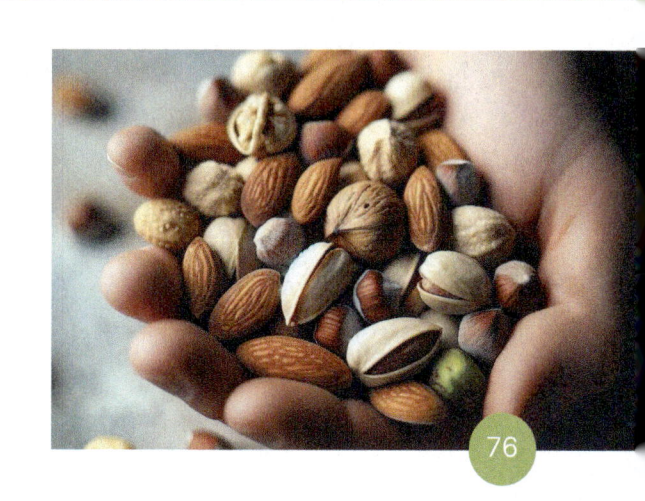

PEACHES: THE SWEET ALLY IN ANTI-INFLAMMATORY EATING

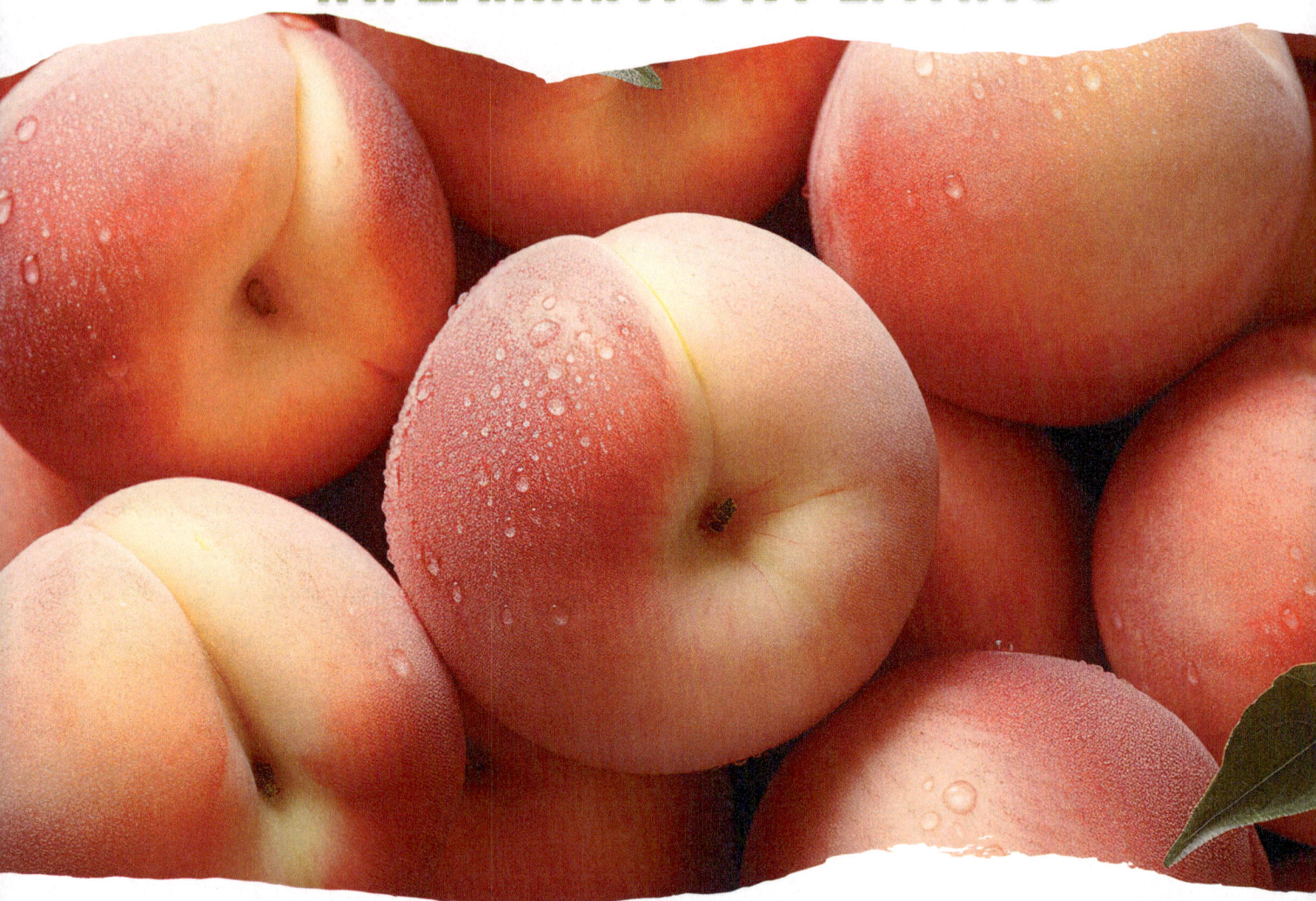

The Role of Peaches in Reducing Inflammation
As we explore diverse foods in our Anti-Inflammatory Meal Plan, peaches stand out for their unique blend of flavors and health benefits. These luscious fruits do more than add a touch of sweetness to your diet; they offer a myriad of nutrients that are key in combating inflammation and enhancing overall well-being.

Unveiling the Health Benefits of Peaches

- Nutrient Powerhouse: Loaded with essential vitamins like A and C, peaches are a natural antioxidant source. They also provide fiber and potassium, which contribute to overall health.
- Combatting Inflammation Naturally: The antioxidant properties in peaches help in neutralizing free radicals, reducing oxidative stress and inflammation in the body.
- Nourishing Skin and Eyes: The rich beta-carotene content in peaches promotes healthy skin and good vision, highlighting their role in maintaining overall health.

Incorporating Peaches into Your Diet

- Versatility in the Kitchen: Whether enjoyed fresh as a juicy snack, blended into a smoothie, or incorporated into salads and desserts, peaches add a delightful sweetness to various dishes.
- Balancing Meals with Natural Sweetness: Their natural sugary flavor can enhance both sweet and savory recipes, providing a healthy alternative to added sugars.

Moving Forward with Healthier Choices

- Enjoying Peaches Year-Round: While fresh peaches are seasonal, canned (in juice) or dried varieties offer a way to enjoy their benefits throughout the year.
- A Step Towards Diverse, Nutritious Eating: Regularly including fruits like peaches in your diet is a delicious strategy for achieving a balanced and anti-inflammatory diet.

Peaches exemplify how nature's sweetness can be seamlessly aligned with health goals. Their delightful flavor and nutritional profile make them an excellent addition to a diet focused on reducing inflammation and enhancing overall health. Enjoy the burst of flavor and health benefits that peaches bring to your culinary creations!

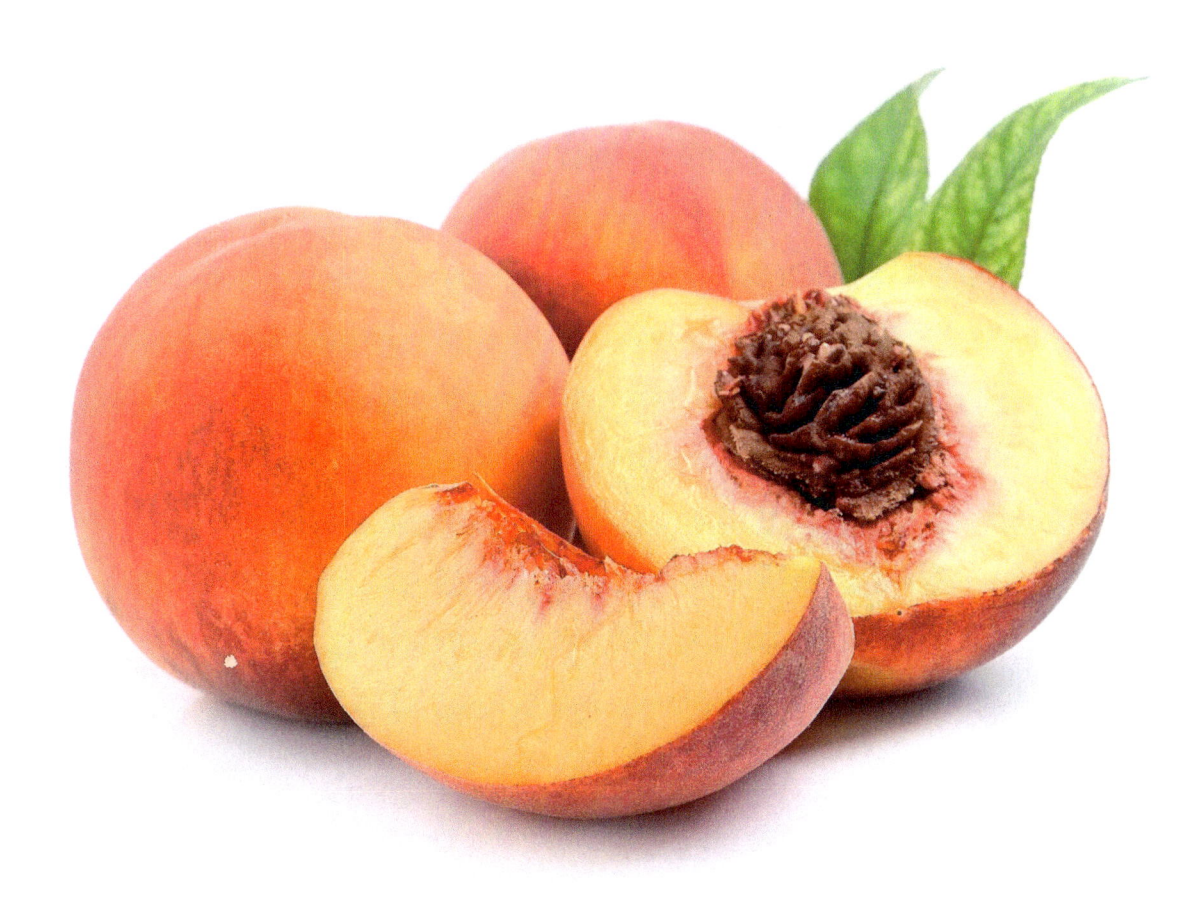

DAY 12 MEAL PLAN

BREAKFAST: GREEK YOGURT PARFAIT WITH GRANOLA, CHIA SEEDS, AND KIWI
LUNCH: ROASTED BEET AND GOAT CHEESE SALAD WITH WALNUTS
DINNER: BEEF AND VEGETABLE KEBABS WITH MIXED SALAD
SNACK: CUCUMBER SLICES WITH TZATZIKI DIP
SNACK: DRIED APRICOTS
DRINK: CHAMOMILE AND HONEY TEA

BREAKFAST: GREEK YOGURT PARFAIT WITH GRANOLA, CHIA SEEDS, AND KIWI

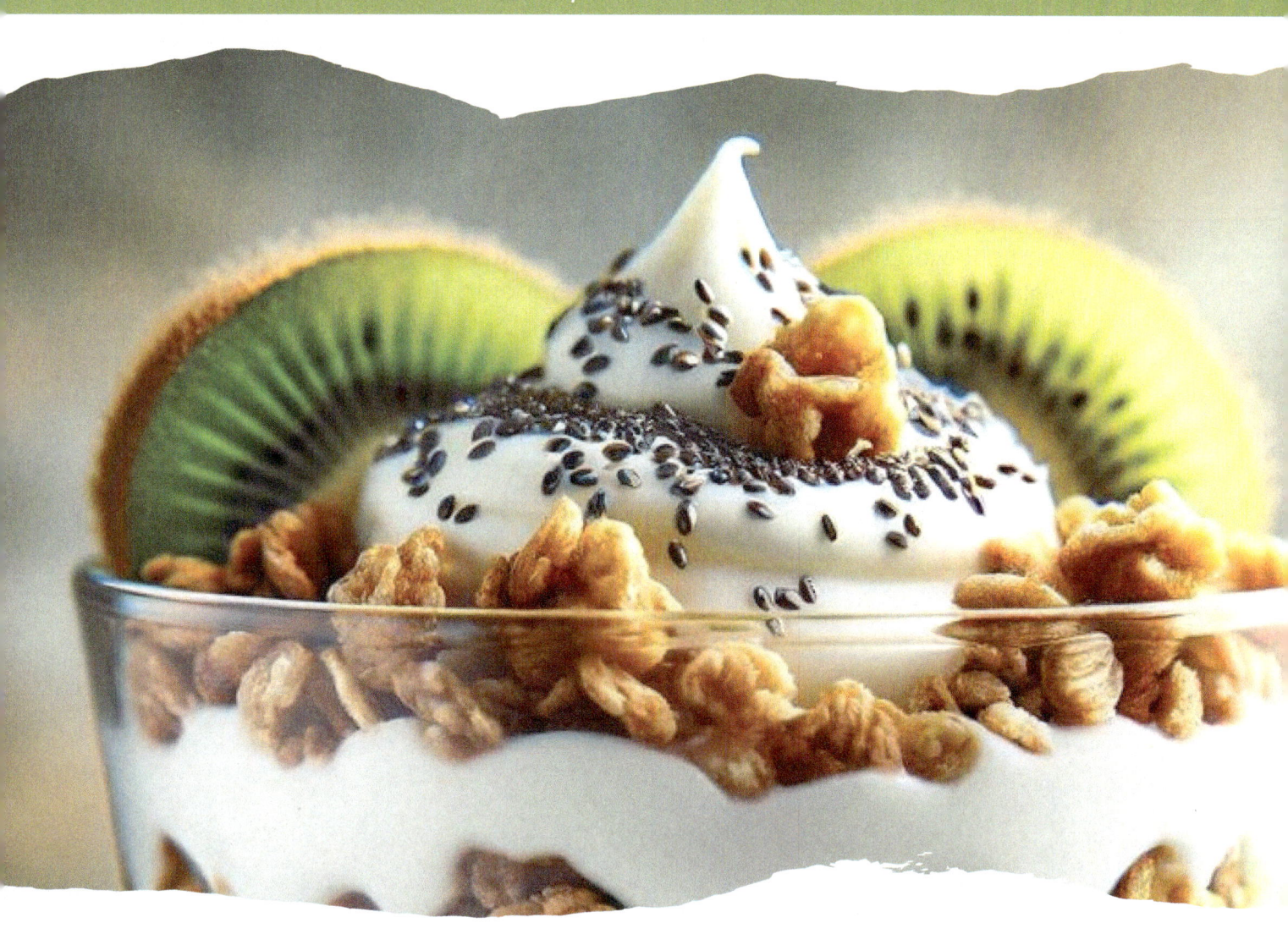

INGREDIENTS

- 1 cup Greek yogurt (plain or unsweetened)
- ½ cup granola
- 1 tablespoon chia seeds
- 1-2 kiwis, peeled and sliced

INSTRUCTIONS

- Layer the Parfait: Start with a layer of Greek yogurt in the glass or bowl.
- Add Granola and Chia Seeds: Sprinkle a layer of granola and chia seeds.
- Add Kiwi Slices: Place a layer of kiwi slices.
- Repeat Layers: Repeat the layers until the glass or bowl is full.
- Serve: Enjoy this nutritious and delicious breakfast.

KITCHEN TOOLS NEEDED
- Knife and cutting board
- Serving glass or bowl

LUNCH: ROASTED BEET AND GOAT CHEESE SALAD WITH WALNUTS

INGREDIENTS

- 2-3 medium beets, roasted and sliced
- ¼ cup goat cheese, crumbled
- ¼ cup walnuts, chopped
- Mixed greens for the salad base
- Olive oil and balsamic vinegar for dressing

INSTRUCTIONS

- Roast Beets: Roast beets in the oven, then slice them.
- Prepare Salad: Arrange mixed greens in a bowl, top with roasted beets, goat cheese, and walnuts.
- Dress Salad: Drizzle with olive oil and balsamic vinegar.

KITCHEN TOOLS NEEDED
- Oven for roasting beets
- Knife and cutting board
- Mixing bowl

DINNER: BEEF AND VEGETABLE KEBABS WITH MIXED SALAD

INGREDIENTS

- Beef cubes (suitable for skewering)
- Vegetables for kebabs (bell peppers, onions, cherry tomatoes)
- Mixed salad ingredients
- Olive oil, herbs, and spices for seasoning

INSTRUCTIONS

- Prepare Kebabs: Thread beef and vegetables onto skewers, season as desired.
- Grill Kebabs: Grill until beef is cooked to your preference.
- Prepare Salad: Toss together mixed salad ingredients.
- Serve: Enjoy the kebabs with the fresh salad on the side.

KITCHEN TOOLS NEEDED
- Skewers (wooden or metal)
- Grill or grill pan
- Mixing bowl

DRINK: CHAMOMILE AND HONEY TEA

INGREDIENTS

- 1 chamomile tea bag
- 1 cup boiling water
- Honey to taste

INSTRUCTIONS

- Boil Water: Heat the water.
- Steep Tea: Place the tea bag in a mug, pour hot water over it.
- Add Honey: Sweeten with honey as desired.

KITCHEN TOOLS NEEDED

- Kettle or pot for boiling water
- Mug

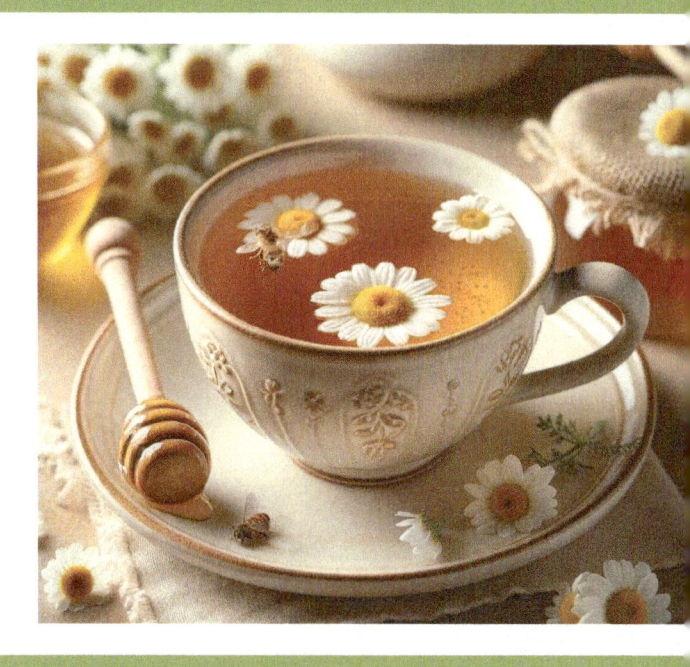

SNACK: CUCUMBER SLICES WITH TZATZIKI DIP

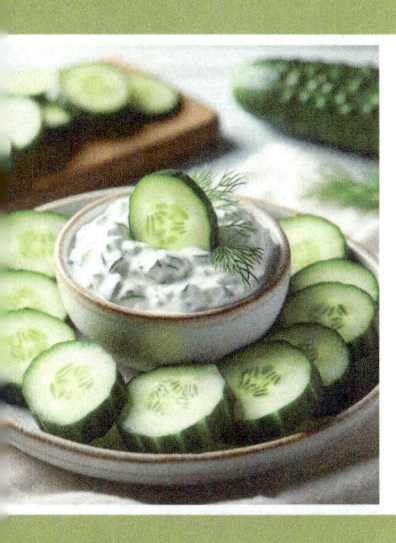

INGREDIENTS

- 1 large cucumber
- ½ cup tzatziki dip

INSTRUCTIONS

- Slice Cucumber: Cut the cucumber into thin slices.
- Serve with Dip: Enjoy the cucumber slices with tzatziki for dipping.

KITCHEN TOOLS NEEDED

- Knife and cutting board

SNACK: DRIED APRICOTS

INGREDIENTS

- A small handful of dried apricots

PREPARATION TIME: NONE, READY TO EAT.

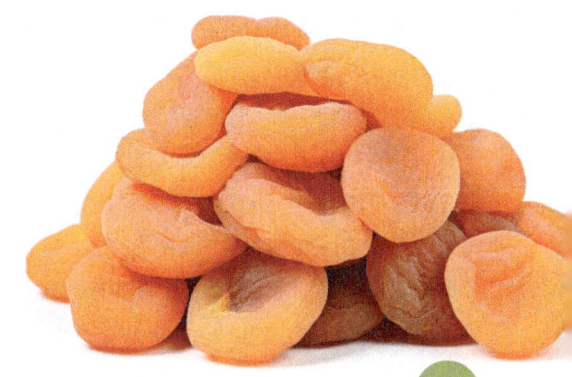

GOAT CHEESE – THE TANGY AND NUTRITIOUS DELIGHT

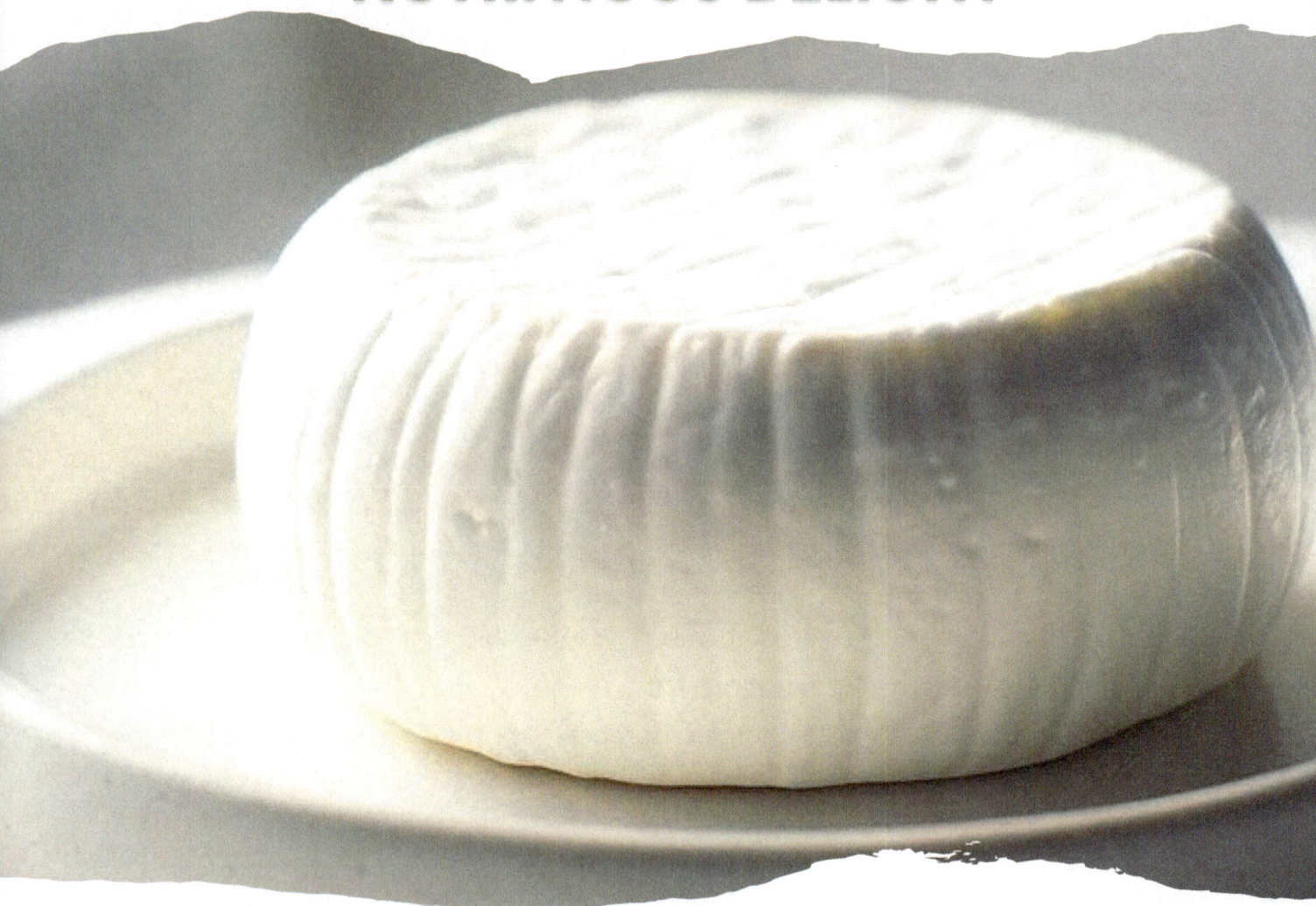

On Day 12 of our Anti-Inflammatory Meal Plan, let's spotlight goat cheese, a tangy and creamy addition to our diet. Known for its distinctive flavor, goat cheese is more than just a culinary indulgence; it offers several health benefits that make it a valuable component in an anti-inflammatory diet.

The Health Perks of Goat Cheese

- Nutrient Profile: Goat cheese is rich in essential nutrients like calcium, protein, and phosphorus. It also contains less lactose than cow's milk cheese, making it a better choice for those with lactose sensitivity.
- Rich in Anti-Inflammatory Fatty Acids: It contains a type of fatty acid that may help reduce inflammation in the body. Additionally, its high levels of probiotics are beneficial for gut health, further supporting anti-inflammatory processes.
- Bone Strengthening Benefits: The calcium in goat cheese is vital for bone health, aiding in the prevention of osteoporosis and bone density loss.

Incorporating Goat Cheese into Meals

- Culinary Versatility: Its creamy texture and distinct flavor make goat cheese a versatile ingredient. It can be crumbled over salads, like the roasted beet and goat cheese salad in our lunch plan, spread on toast, or even incorporated into sauces.
- Enhancing Flavor and Nutrition: Goat cheese adds a rich, tangy flavor to dishes while boosting their nutritional value, making it a great addition to both savory and sweet recipes.

A Step Toward a Balanced Diet

- A Healthier Cheese Option: For those who enjoy cheese but are mindful of their health, goat cheese offers a nutritious alternative with its lower lactose content and beneficial nutrients.
- Encouraging Varied Cheese Consumption: Including different types of cheese like goat cheese in your diet can diversify your nutrient intake and add new flavors to your meals.

Goat cheese is an excellent addition to an anti-inflammatory diet, thanks to its combination of taste and health benefits. Whether it's enhancing the flavors of a salad or being enjoyed as a simple spread, goat cheese can elevate your meals while contributing positively to your health. As you continue exploring diverse and nutritious foods in your meal plan, consider goat cheese as a flavorful and healthful choice.

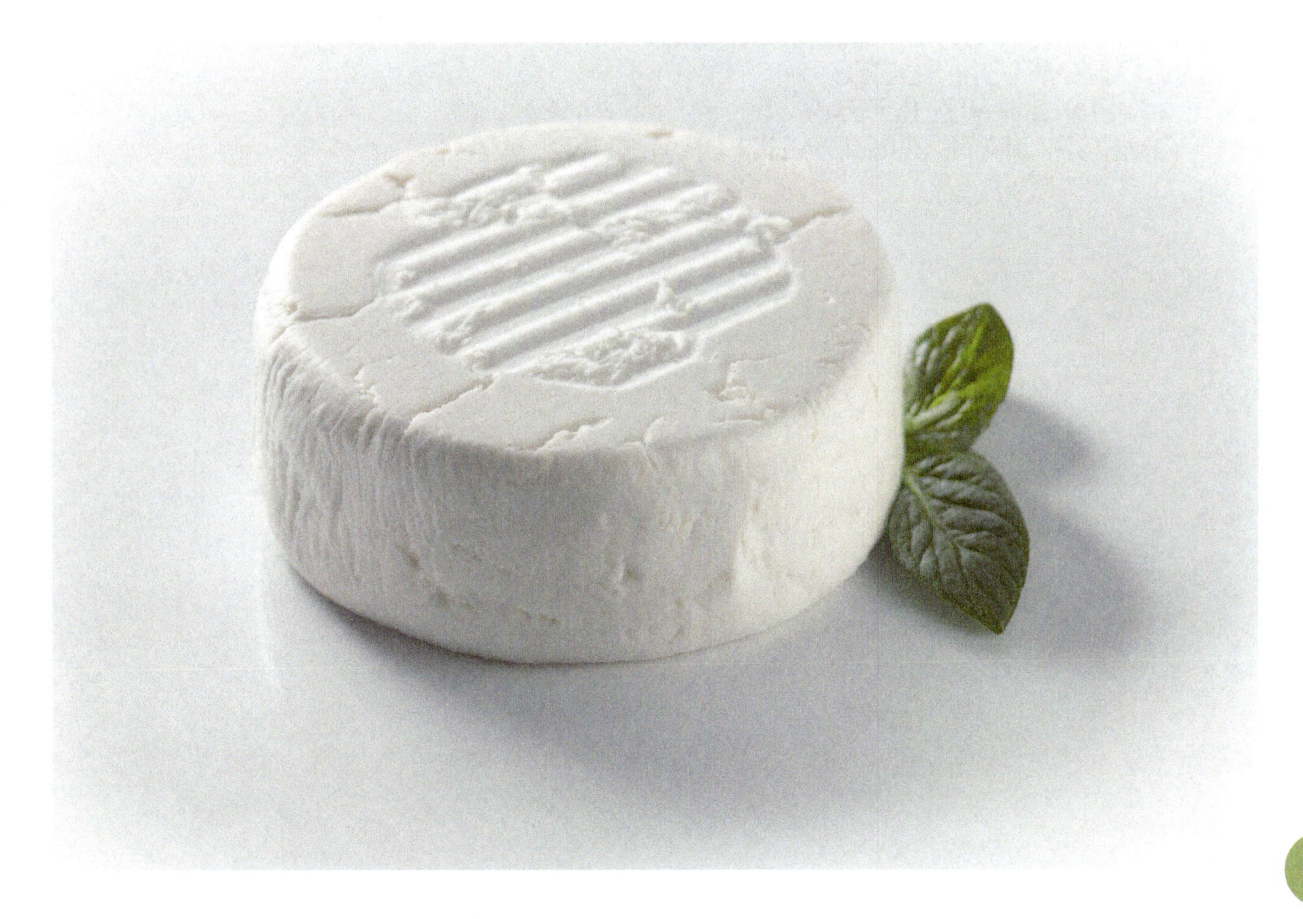

DAY 13 MEAL PLAN

BREAKFAST: SCRAMBLED TOFU WITH SPINACH, TOMATOES, AND TURMERIC
LUNCH: SARDINE SALAD
DINNER: QUINOA-STUFFED BELL PEPPERS
SNACK: WATERMELON SLICES
SNACK: A MEDIUM-SIZED PEAR
DRINK: POMEGRANATE JUICE WITH SPARKLING WATER

BREAKFAST: SCRAMBLED TOFU WITH SPINACH, TOMATOES, AND TURMERIC

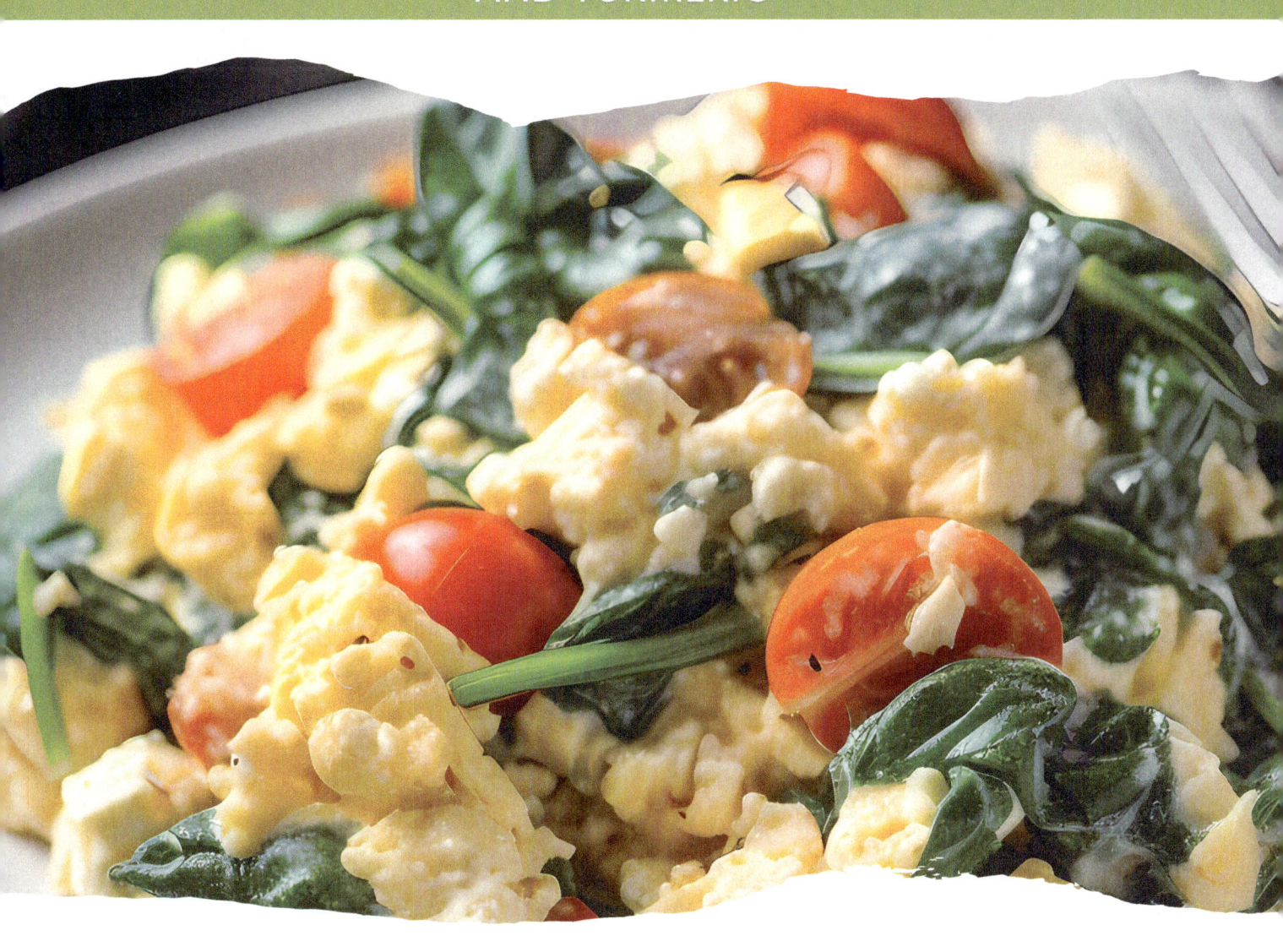

INGREDIENTS

- 1 block of firm tofu, crumbled
- 1 cup fresh spinach, chopped
- 1 tomato, diced
- ½ teaspoon turmeric
- Salt and pepper to taste
- Olive oil for cooking

INSTRUCTIONS

- Cook Tofu: In a pan, heat olive oil and add crumbled tofu. Cook until slightly browned.
- Add Veggies and Spices: Mix in spinach, tomatoes, turmeric, salt, and pepper. Cook until vegetables are tender.
- Serve: Enjoy the flavorful and nutritious scrambled tofu.

KITCHEN TOOLS NEEDED

- Frying pan
- Spatula
- Knife and cutting board

LUNCH: SARDINE SALAD

INGREDIENTS

- 1 can of sardines, drained
- Mixed greens (lettuce, arugula, spinach)
- ½ avocado, sliced
- Lemon juice and olive oil for dressing
- Salt and pepper to taste

INSTRUCTIONS

- Prepare Salad Base: Toss mixed greens in a bowl.
- Add Sardines and Avocado: Place sardines and avocado slices on top of the greens.
- Dress Salad: Drizzle with lemon juice and olive oil, season with salt and pepper.

KITCHEN TOOLS NEEDED

- Mixing bowl
- Knife and cutting board

DINNER: BEEF QUINOA-STUFFED BELL PEPPERS

INGREDIENTS

- 2-3 bell peppers, halved and seeded
- 1 cup cooked quinoa
- Optional fillings: sautéed onion, garlic, tomatoes, corn, beans
- Seasonings: salt, pepper, herbs
- Olive oil

INSTRUCTIONS

- Prepare Filling: Mix cooked quinoa with chosen fillings and seasonings.
- Stuff Peppers: Fill the bell pepper halves with the quinoa mixture.
- Bake: Drizzle with olive oil and bake until peppers are tender.

KITCHEN TOOLS NEEDED

- Oven and baking tray
- Mixing bowl
- Knife and cutting board

DRINK: POMEGRANATE JUICE WITH SPARKLING WATER

INGREDIENTS
- ½ cup pomegranate juice
- ½ cup sparkling water

INSTRUCTIONS
- Mix Drinks: Pour pomegranate juice and sparkling water into a glass.
- Serve: Stir gently and enjoy this refreshing beverage.

KITCHEN TOOLS NEEDED
- Glass

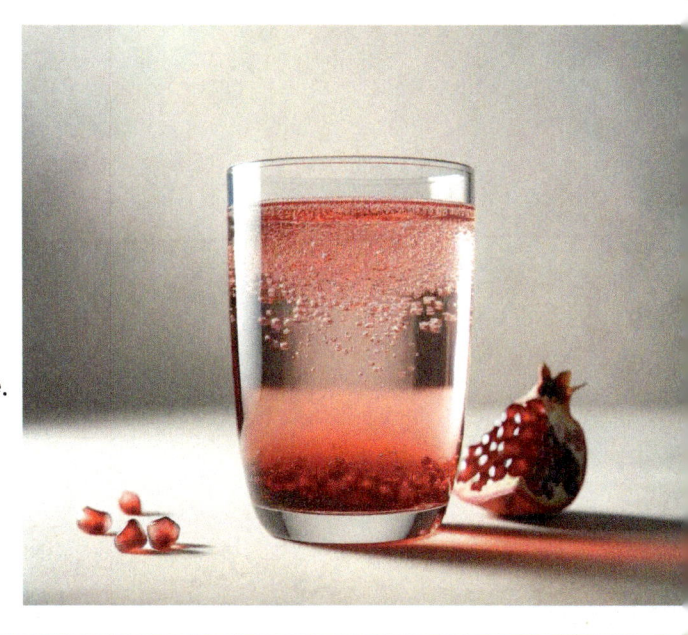

SNACK: WATERMELON SLICES

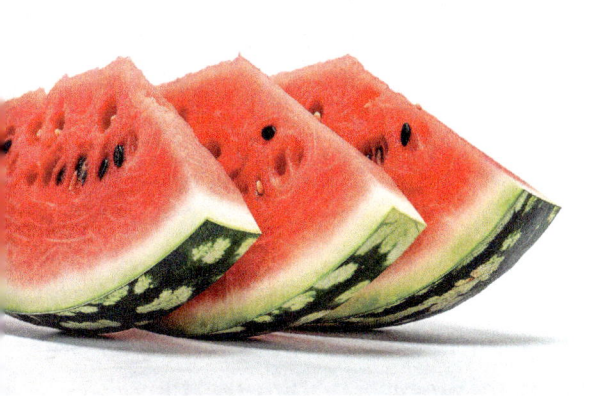

INGREDIENTS
- A few slices of watermelon

INSTRUCTIONS
- Slice Watermelon: Cut the watermelon into easy-to-eat slices.
- Serve: Enjoy the refreshing and hydrating snack.

KITCHEN TOOLS NEEDED
- Knife and cutting board

SNACK: A MEDIUM-SIZED PEAR

INGREDIENTS
- 1 medium-sized pear

PREPARATION TIME: NONE, READY TO EAT.

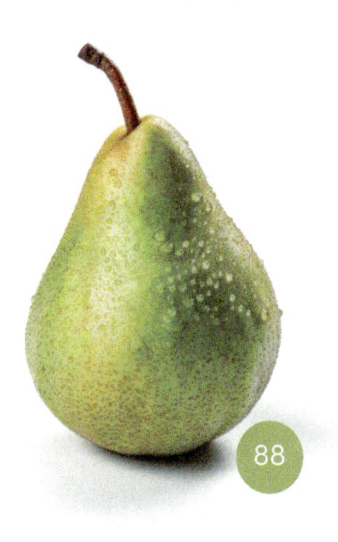

SPARKLING WATER – THE EFFERVESCENT HYDRATOR

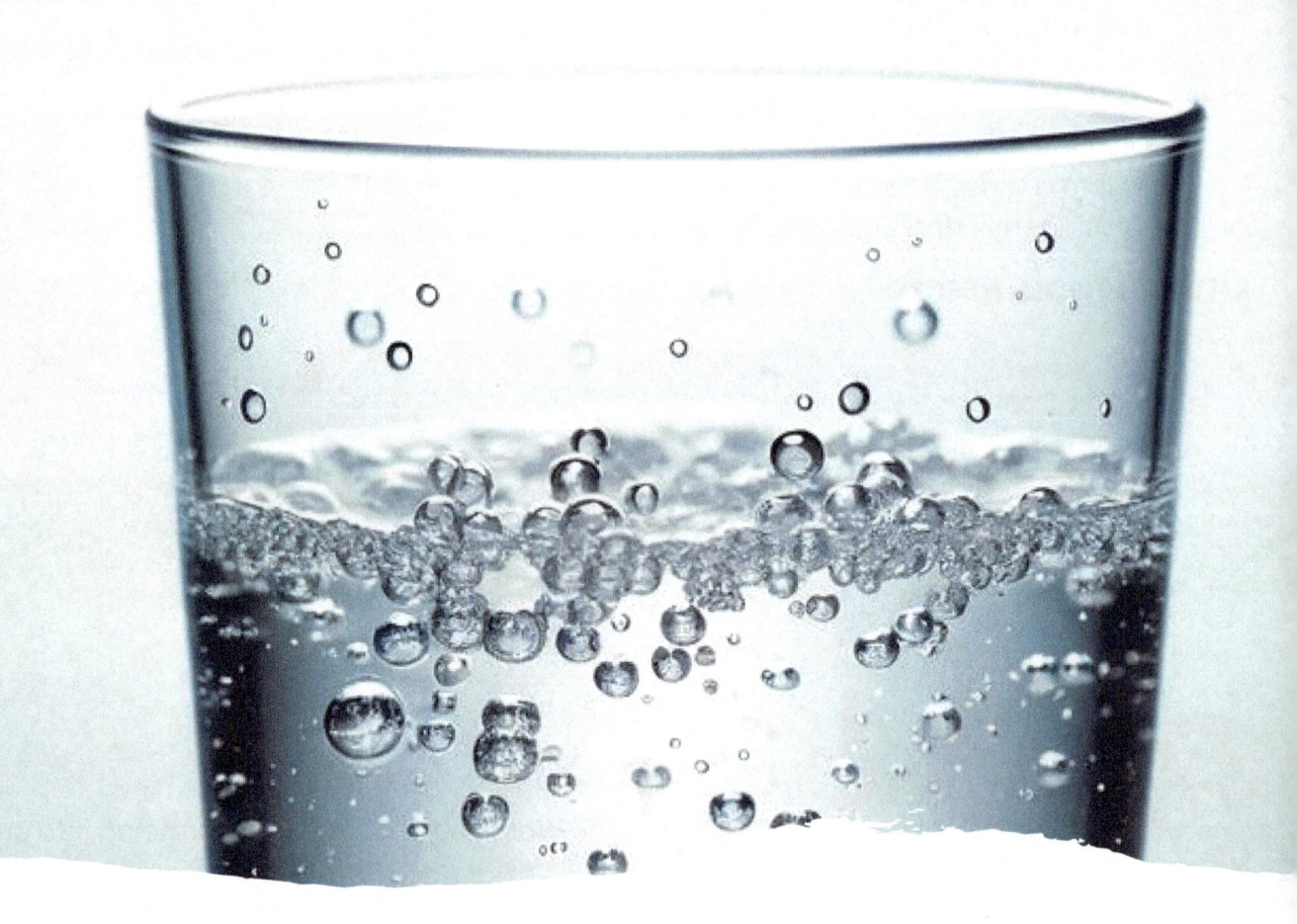

As we continue with Day 13 of our Anti-Inflammatory Meal Plan, let's turn our focus to sparkling water, a refreshing and hydrating choice. This bubbly alternative to still water is not just about quenching thirst; it also plays a role in a healthy, inflammation-conscious diet.

The Refreshing Benefits of Sparkling Water

- Hydration Made Enjoyable: Sparkling water provides all the hydration benefits of regular water but with a fizzy twist that can make staying hydrated more enjoyable, especially for those who find regular water too plain.
- Digestive Aid: The carbonation in sparkling water can aid in digestion. It's often used as a remedy for indigestion and can help in feeling full, which might aid in weight management.
- Zero Calories, Pure Hydration: Unlike many carbonated drinks, plain sparkling water is calorie-free and doesn't contain sugars or artificial sweeteners, making it a healthier choice for maintaining optimal hydration.

Integrating Sparkling Water into Your Routine

- A Versatile Beverage: Sparkling water can be enjoyed on its own, used as a base for healthy beverages like the pomegranate juice drink in our meal plan, or infused with fruits and herbs for added flavor without extra calories.
- Elevating Hydration Moments: Its effervescence makes it a great choice for dining occasions, offering a more exciting alternative to still water without resorting to sugary sodas.

Sparkling Water as Part of a Balanced Diet

- Encouraging Regular Water Intake: Including sparkling water in your diet can help meet your daily hydration needs in a more appealing way, ensuring you stay well-hydrated, which is crucial for overall health and well-being.
- A Healthy Substitute for Sugary Drinks: For those looking to reduce their intake of sugary beverages, sparkling water is a fantastic alternative, offering the satisfaction of a fizzy drink without the health drawbacks of added sugars.

In conclusion, sparkling water is a delightful addition to an anti-inflammatory diet, providing essential hydration in a more enticing form. Whether sipped on its own or used as a mixer for healthy drinks, it's a great way to ensure adequate fluid intake throughout the day. As you explore various ways to stay hydrated, consider sparkling water as a tasty and health-conscious choice.

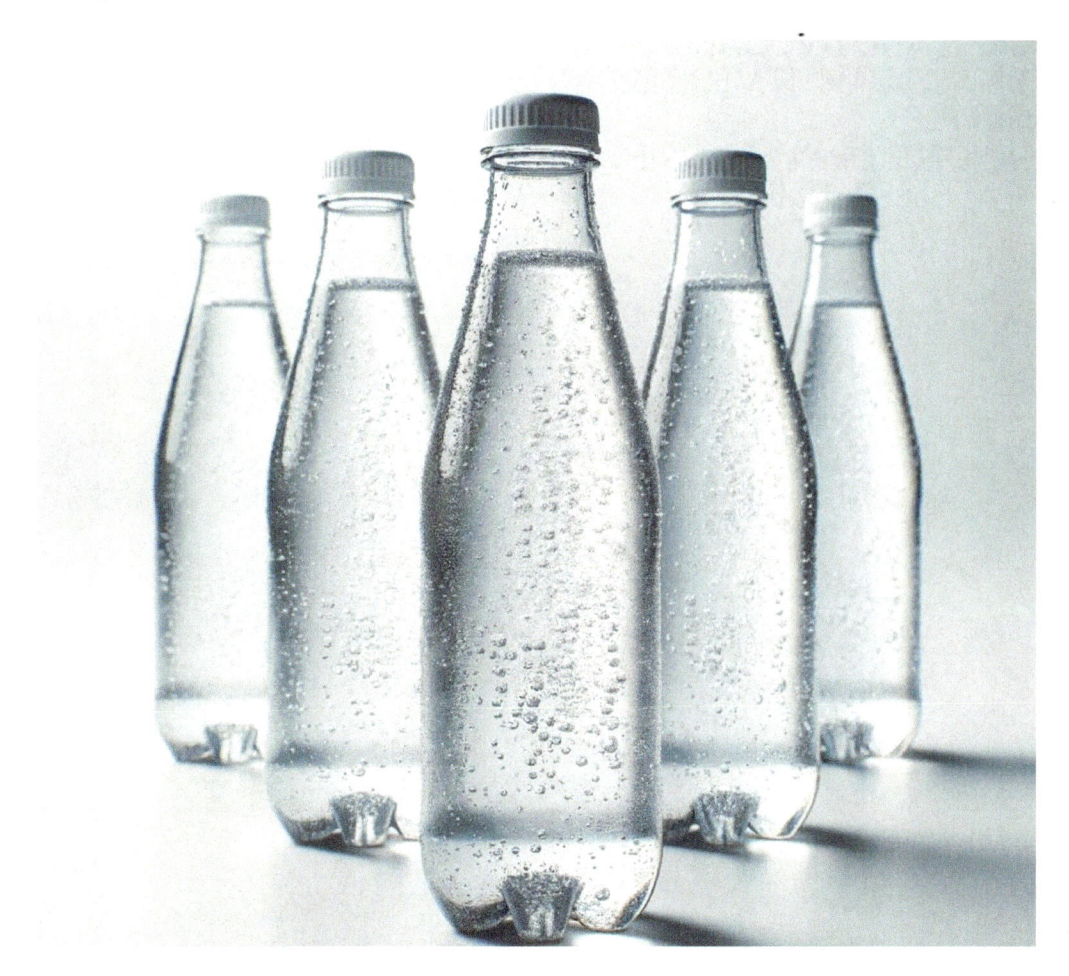

DAY 14 MEAL PLAN

BREAKFAST: ALMOND MILK AND OAT PORRIDGE WITH BANANA AND CINNAMON
LUNCH: CHICKEN AND AVOCADO SANDWICH
DINNER: BAKED COD WITH MEDITERRANEAN TOPPING AND ROASTED ASPARAGUS
SNACK: PINEAPPLE
SNACK: A HANDFUL OF BLUEBERRIES
DRINK: HERBAL SLEEP-TIME TEA

BREAKFAST: ALMOND MILK AND OAT PORRIDGE WITH BANANA AND CINNAMON

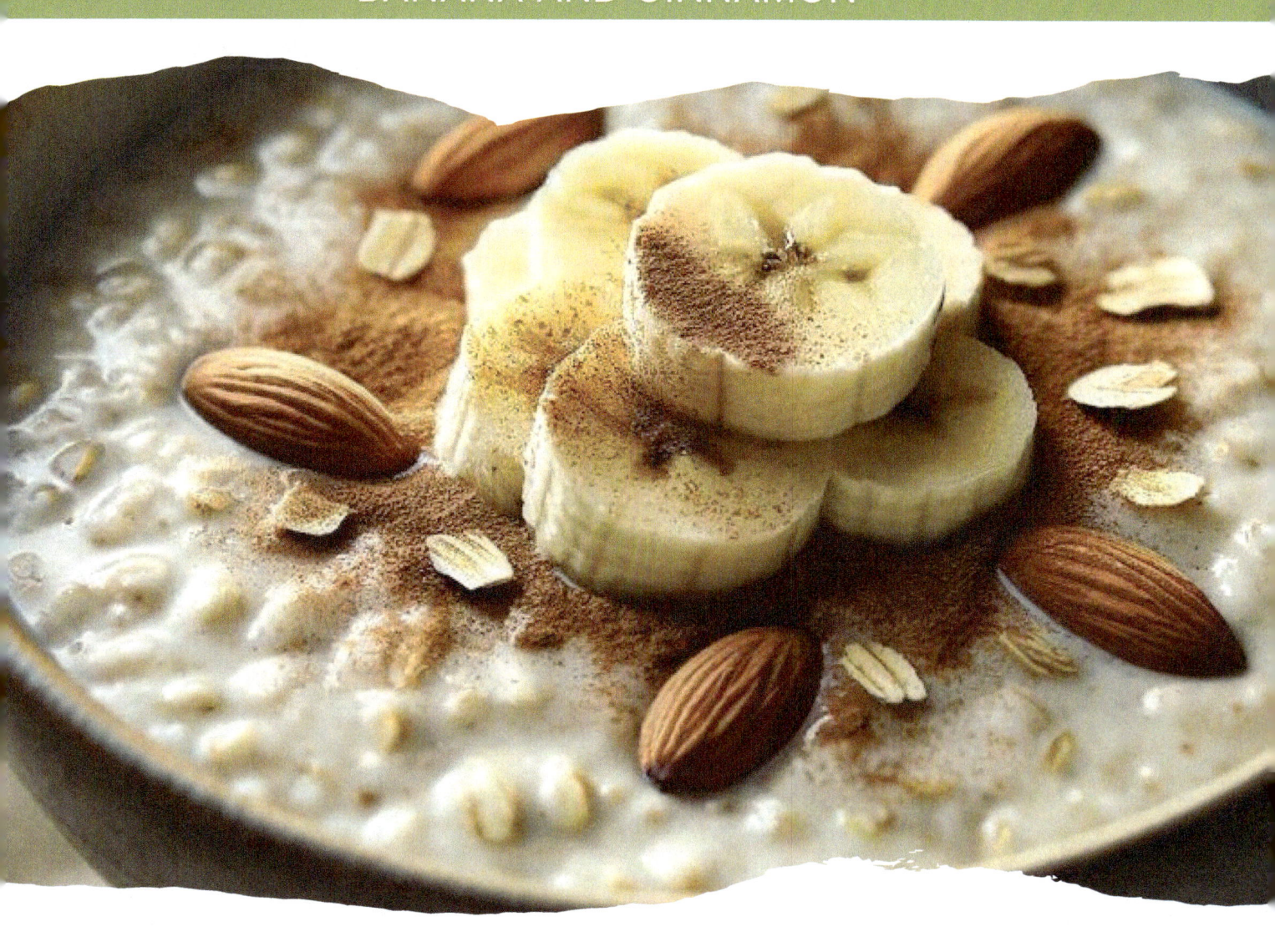

INGREDIENTS

- ½ cup rolled oats
- 1 cup almond milk
- 1 banana, sliced
- A sprinkle of cinnamon

INSTRUCTIONS

- Cook Porridge: Combine oats and almond milk in a pot. Cook over medium heat until the oats are soft and creamy.
- Add Toppings: Top the porridge with sliced banana and a sprinkle of cinnamon.
- Serve: Enjoy this warm and nourishing breakfast.

KITCHEN TOOLS NEEDED

- Pot
- Stirring spoon
- Knife and cutting board

LUNCH: CHICKEN AND AVOCADO SANDWICH

INGREDIENTS

- 2 slices of whole-grain bread
- 1 small chicken breast, cooked and sliced
- ½ avocado, sliced
- Lettuce, tomato, and mustard or mayonnaise (optional)

INSTRUCTIONS

- Assemble Sandwich: Layer chicken and avocado slices on one slice of bread, add lettuce and tomato if desired.
- Add Condiments: Spread mustard or mayonnaise on the other slice of bread.
- Complete Sandwich: Place the second slice of bread on top and cut in half.

KITCHEN TOOLS NEEDED

- Knife and cutting board

DINNER: BAKED COD WITH MEDITERRANEAN TOPPING AND ROASTED ASPARAGUS

INGREDIENTS

- 1 cod fillet
- Cherry tomatoes, olives, garlic, and herbs for the topping
- 1 bunch of asparagus
- Olive oil, salt, and pepper for seasoning

INSTRUCTIONS

- Prepare Cod: Place cod on a baking tray, top with sliced tomatoes, olives, minced garlic, and herbs.
- Roast Asparagus: Toss asparagus with olive oil, salt, and pepper. Roast in the oven.
- Bake Cod: Bake the cod and asparagus together until the fish is cooked through.

KITCHEN TOOLS NEEDED

- Oven and baking tray
- Knife and cutting board

DRINK: HERBAL SLEEP-TIME TEA

INGREDIENTS
- 1 bag of herbal sleep-time tea (like chamomile or lavender)
- 1 cup boiling water

INSTRUCTIONS
- Boil Water: Heat the water.
- Steep Tea: Place the tea bag in a mug, pour hot water over it.

KITCHEN TOOLS NEEDED
- Kettle or pot for boiling water
- Mug

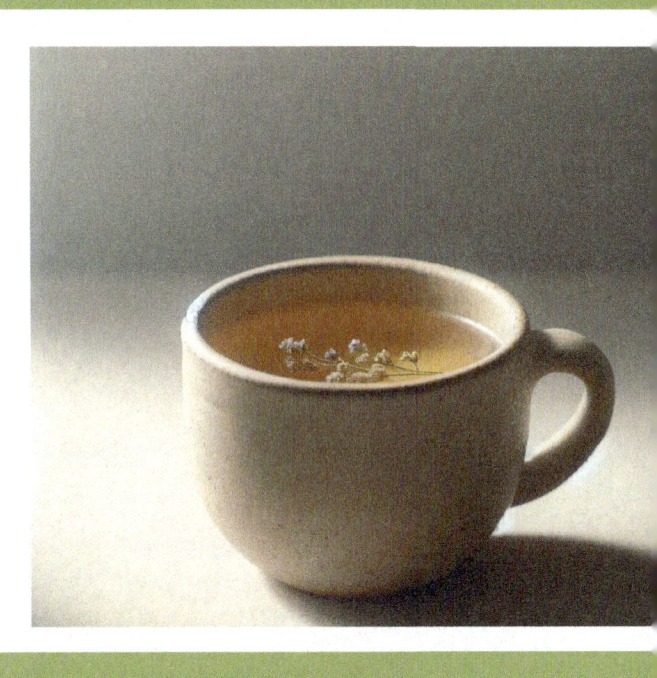

SNACK: PINEAPPLE

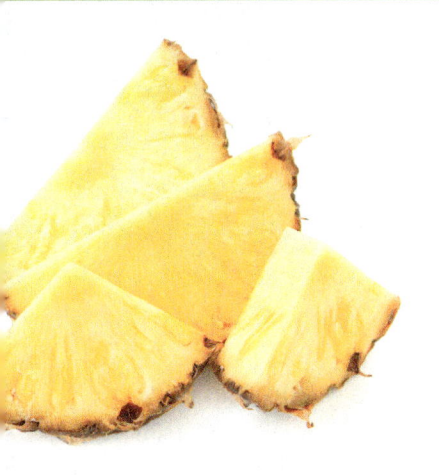

INGREDIENTS
- A small serving of pineapple (fresh or canned in juice)

INSTRUCTIONS
- Prepare Pineapple: If fresh, peel and cut the pineapple into chunks. If canned, drain the juice.

KITCHEN TOOLS NEEDED
- Knife and cutting board (if using fresh pineapple)

SNACK: A HANDFUL OF BLUEBERRIES

INGREDIENTS
- A handful of blueberries

PREPARATION TIME: NONE, READY TO EAT.

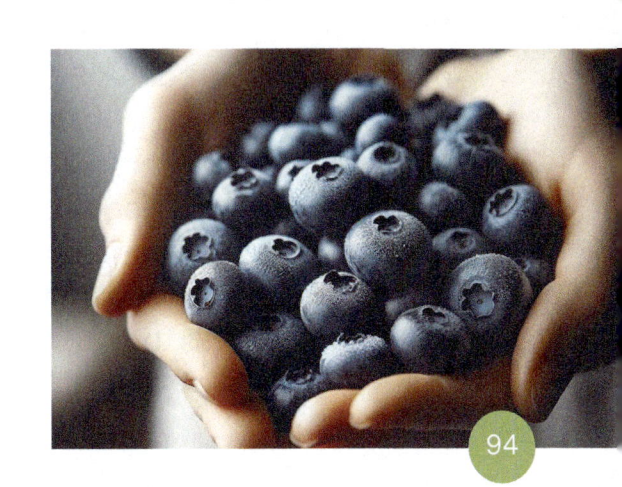

BLUEBERRIES - THE BRAIN-BOOSTING, ANTI-INFLAMMATORY SUPERFRUIT

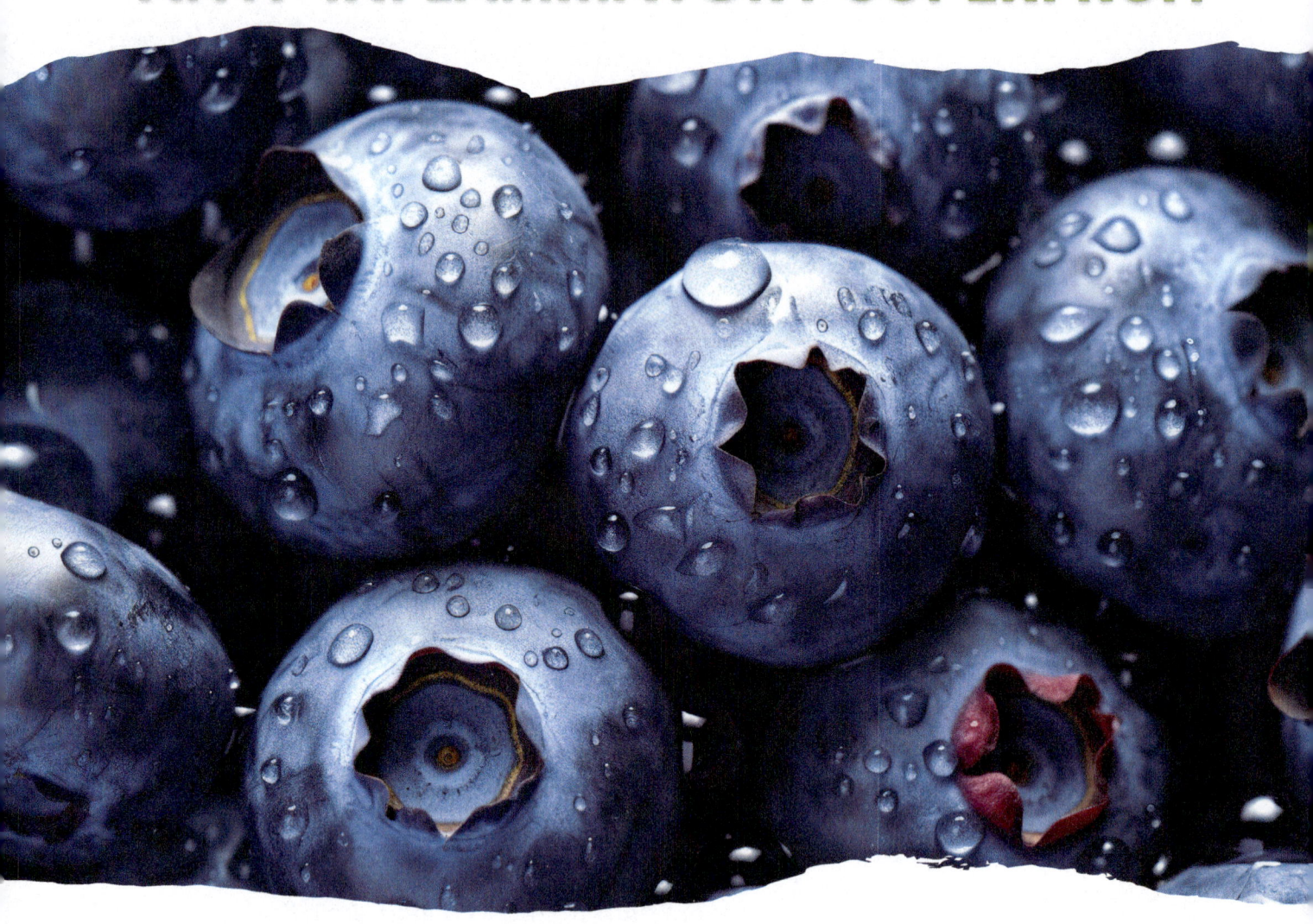

On Day 14 of our Anti-Inflammatory Meal Plan, we highlight blueberries, a small but mighty fruit. These little blue jewels are renowned not just for their deliciousness but also for their impressive array of health benefits, particularly in combating inflammation and supporting brain health.

The Dual Power of Blueberries

- Antioxidant Powerhouse: Blueberries are incredibly rich in antioxidants, particularly anthocyanins, which give them their vibrant color. These antioxidants are known for their anti-inflammatory properties, helping to reduce oxidative stress and inflammation in the body.
- Brain Food: Regular consumption of blueberries has been linked to improved brain function. They are believed to enhance memory, cognitive performance, and neural functioning, thanks to their high antioxidant content.

Incorporating Blueberries into Daily Meals

- Versatile and Delicious: Blueberries can be enjoyed in various ways – as a fresh snack, blended into smoothies, mixed into yogurt or oatmeal, or used as a natural sweetener in baked goods.
- Enhancing Meals with a Nutritional Punch: Adding a handful of blueberries to your breakfast, like the almond milk and oat porridge in our plan, not only elevates the taste but also boosts the meal's nutritional value.

Blueberries as a Staple in Healthy Eating

- A Fruit for Cognitive and Physical Health: Including blueberries in your diet is a simple yet effective way to support both brain health and reduce inflammation, contributing to overall well-being.
- Promoting a Diverse, Antioxidant-Rich Diet: Their inclusion in our meal plan emphasizes the importance of consuming a variety of fruits, particularly those high in antioxidants, for their unique health benefits and flavors.

In summary, blueberries are a standout ingredient in an anti-inflammatory diet. Their combination of brain-boosting and anti-inflammatory properties makes them an invaluable addition to your dietary routine. As you continue your journey toward a health-conscious lifestyle, let blueberries be a regular feature in your meals, offering both delightful flavors and a host of health benefits.

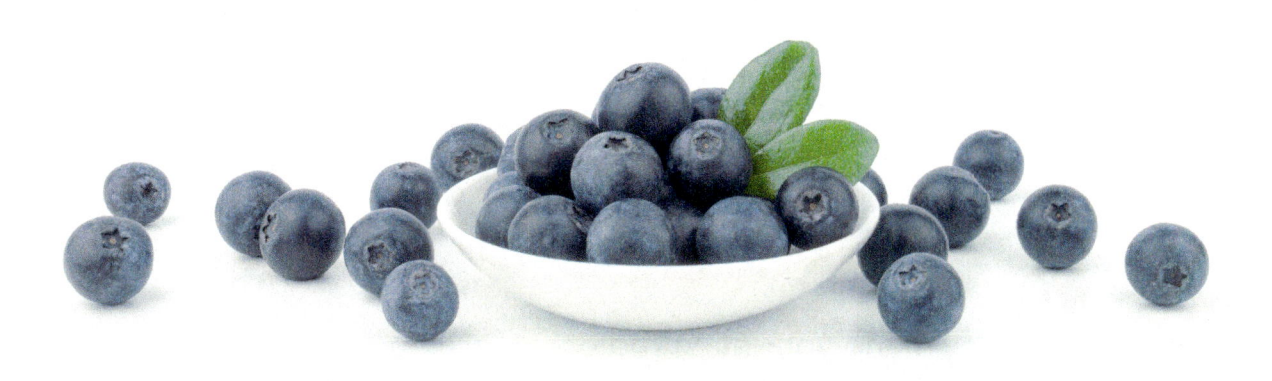

COMPLETION OF WEEK 2: A GRATITUDE MESSAGE

Congratulations on Finishing Week 2!

You've just crossed the halfway mark of the Anti-Inflammatory Meal Plan, and it's time to celebrate your dedication. Thank you for continuing this journey with us through Week 2's Flavorful Foods Fiesta!

Acknowledging Your Efforts and Adaptability

- Gratitude for Your Participation: Your commitment to trying new, diverse foods and integrating them into your diet is truly admirable. We are grateful for your enthusiasm and openness to this culinary adventure.
- Recognizing Your Adaptability: We understand that introducing a variety of new foods can be both exciting and challenging. Your adaptability and willingness to explore different flavors and ingredients are key to making this journey a success.

Looking Forward to the Next Phase

- Encouragement for Week 3: As you step into Week 3, where we 'Mix It Up' even more, remember that each new food and recipe is an opportunity to further reduce inflammation and enhance your overall well-being.
- Celebrating Every Step: Each day brings you closer to a healthier lifestyle. Continue to embrace these changes, and don't forget to acknowledge the progress you're making.

Please take a moment to reflect on how your body has felt during Week 2 using the Body Awareness Scale. Your observations and experiences are crucial in understanding the impact of these dietary changes and in preparing for the exciting week ahead. Keep up the great work, and thank you for being an integral part of this journey!

WEEK 2 REFLECTION

After completing Week 2 of the Anti-Inflammatory Meal Plan, it's important to reflect on how your body has responded to the dietary changes. Use the following scale to rate your experiences in various aspects of your health and well-being. Rate each category from 1 to 10 (where 1 is 'no improvement' and 10 is 'significant improvement').

1. Digestive Comfort

- Question: How would you rate the overall comfort of your digestive system this week?
- Rating (1-10): _____

2. Energy Levels

- Question: How do you feel about your energy levels after following the meal plan for a week?
- Rating (1-10): _____

3. Sleep Quality

- Question: Have you noticed any changes in the quality of your sleep?
- Rating (1-10): _____

4. Mood and Mental Clarity

- Question: How has your mood and mental clarity been affected by the dietary changes?
- Rating (1-10): _____

5. Physical Comfort and Pain Levels

- Question: If you previously experienced any physical discomfort or pain, have you noticed any changes in its intensity or frequency?
- Rating (1-10): _____

6. Skin Health

- Question: Have there been any noticeable changes in your skin health/appearance?
- Rating (1-10): _____

7. Cravings and Appetite Control

- Question: How would you rate your control over cravings and appetite this week?
- Rating (1-10): _____

8. Overall Well-being

- Question: Considering all factors, how would you rate your overall well-being after Week 1?
- Rating (1-10): _____

Notes

Notes

- Daily Observations: Note any specific reactions or feelings on a day-to-day basis. This can include changes in mood, energy levels, digestive reactions, or any other physical or mental responses you notice.

- Dietary Adaptations: If you made any modifications to the meal plan, such as substituting ingredients or altering meal times, document these changes. This can help you understand how different foods or eating patterns affect you.

- Challenges and Successes: Reflect on any challenges you faced, such as cravings or difficulty in meal preparation, and how you addressed them. Also, celebrate successes, like resisting a particular craving or noticing positive changes in your health.

- Physical and Emotional Well-being: Expand on the ratings you provided by describing in more detail how you feel physically and emotionally. This could include noting any reduction in pain, improvements in skin health, or changes in mental clarity and mood.

- Future Adjustments: Based on your week's experience, jot down any thoughts on what you might want to try differently in the upcoming week. This could be trying new recipes, adjusting portion sizes, or incorporating more of a particular type of food.

- Questions and Research: If you have questions or areas of curiosity that arose during the week, such as the effects of certain foods or why you experienced specific reactions, note these down. You can then research these topics or discuss them with a healthcare professional.

- Overall Reflection: Conclude with a general reflection on how the week went, what you learned about your body's response to the diet, and how you feel about continuing with the meal plan.

DAY 15 MEAL PLAN

BREAKFAST: CHIA SEED AND BERRY COMPOTE PARFAIT
LUNCH: COLD RICE NOODLE SALAD WITH CHICKEN
DINNER: MOROCCAN-SPICED LAMB STEW WITH COUSCOUS
SNACK: A MEDIUM-SIZED BANANA
SNACK: POMEGRANATE SEEDS
DRINK: ICED GREEN TEA WITH LEMON

BREAKFAST: CHIA SEED AND BERRY COMPOTE PARFAIT

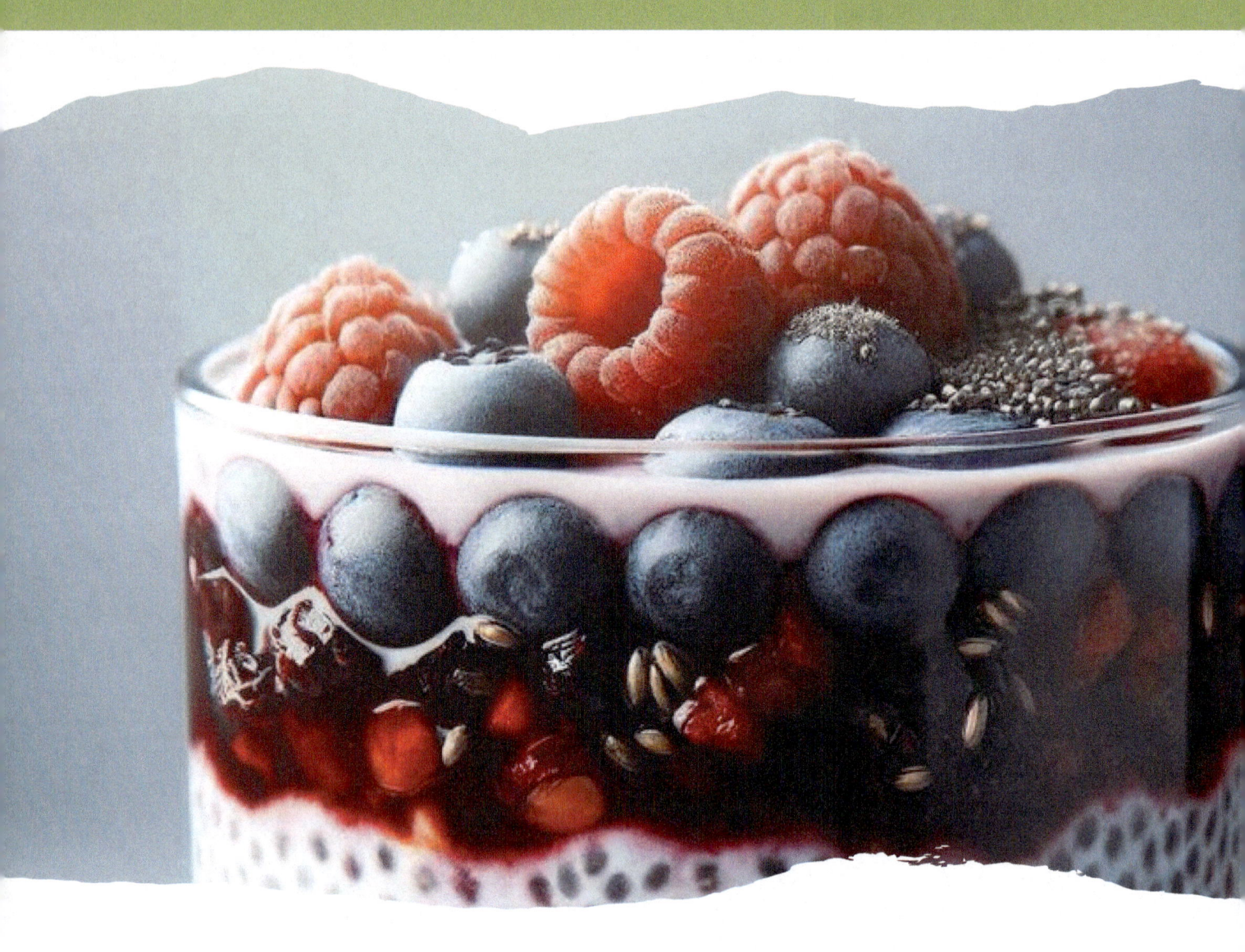

INGREDIENTS

- ¼ cup chia seeds
- 1 cup almond or coconut milk
- ½ cup berry compote or mixed berries
- Optional: honey or maple syrup for sweetness

INSTRUCTIONS

- Prepare Chia Pudding: Mix chia seeds with milk and let it sit until it achieves a pudding-like consistency.
- Layer the Parfait: In a glass or jar, layer the chia pudding and berry compote.
- Serve: Optionally, sweeten with honey or maple syrup.

KITCHEN TOOLS NEEDED
- Bowl for mixing
- Glass or jar for serving

LUNCH: COLD RICE NOODLE SALAD WITH CHICKEN

INGREDIENTS

- 1 cup cooked rice noodles
- ½ cup shredded chicken
- ½ cup shredded carrots
- ½ cucumber, sliced
- Ginger-lime dressing (lime juice, grated ginger, olive oil, salt)

INSTRUCTIONS

- Prepare Salad: Combine rice noodles, chicken, carrots, and cucumber in a bowl.
- Add Dressing: Toss with ginger-lime dressing.

KITCHEN TOOLS NEEDED
- Mixing bowl
- Knife and cutting board

DINNER: MOROCCAN-SPICED LAMB STEW WITH COUSCOUS

INGREDIENTS

- Lamb stew meat
- Moroccan spices (cumin, coriander, cinnamon)
- Vegetables for stew (carrots, onions, tomatoes)
- 1 cup couscous
- Broth or water for cooking couscous

INSTRUCTIONS

- Cook Lamb Stew: Cook lamb with spices and vegetables until tender.
- Prepare Couscous: Cook couscous in broth or water as per package instructions.
- Serve: Enjoy the flavorful stew with a side of fluffy couscous.

KITCHEN TOOLS NEEDED
- Pot for stew
- Pot for couscous
- Knife and cutting board

DRINK: ICED GREEN TEA WITH LEMON

INGREDIENTS
- 1 bag of green tea
- 1 cup cold water
- Ice cubes
- 1 slice of lemon

INSTRUCTIONS
- Steep Tea: Brew green tea in hot water, then cool it down.
- Serve Iced: Fill a glass with ice, pour in the cooled tea, and add a slice of lemon.

KITCHEN TOOLS NEEDED
- Kettle or pot for boiling water
- Glass

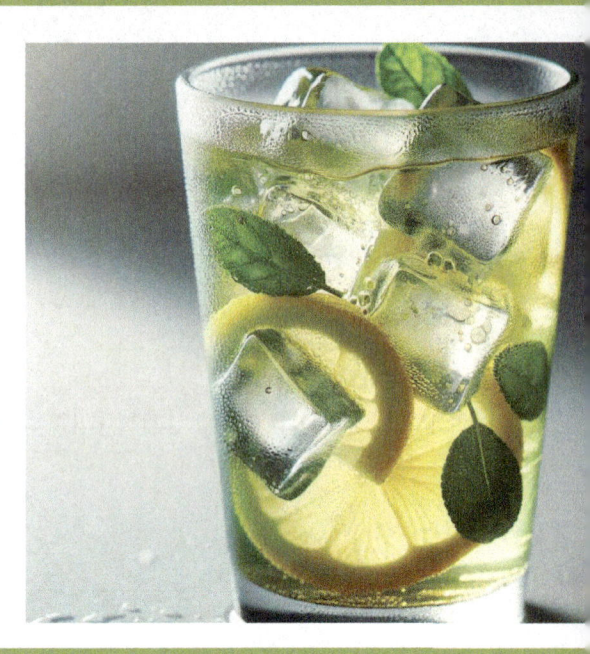

SNACK: A MEDIUM-SIZED BANANA

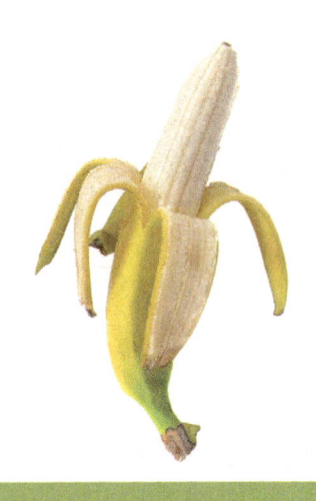

INGREDIENTS
- 1 medium-sized banana

PREPARATION TIME: NONE, READY TO EAT.

SNACK: POMEGRANATE SEEDS

INGREDIENTS

PREPARATION TIME: NONE, READY TO EAT.

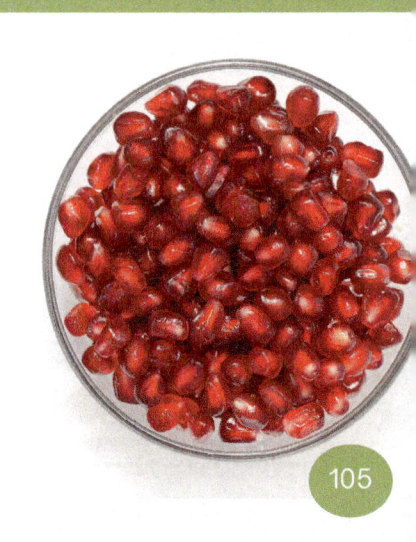

CHIA SEEDS – THE TINY TITANS OF NUTRITION

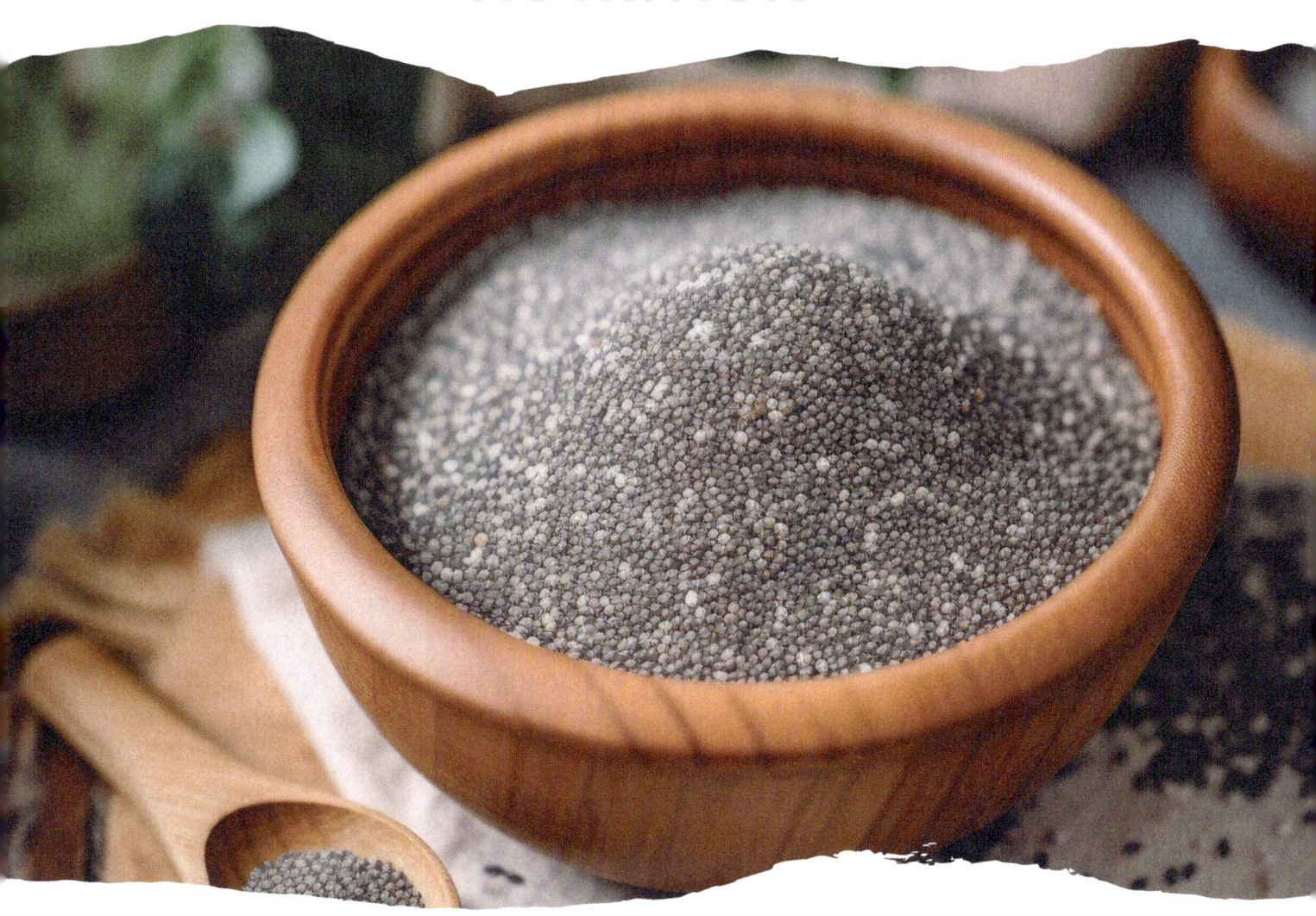

On Day 15, we spotlight chia seeds, a central ingredient in our chia seed and berry compote parfait. These tiny seeds are a nutritional powerhouse, offering a multitude of health benefits. They are especially valuable in an anti-inflammatory diet, thanks to their unique combination of nutrients.

The Mighty Benefits of Chia Seeds

- Omega-3 Fatty Acids: Chia seeds are an excellent plant-based source of omega-3 fatty acids, known for their anti-inflammatory properties. Omega-3s are crucial for heart and brain health and play a key role in reducing inflammation throughout the body.
- Rich in Fiber: High in dietary fiber, chia seeds are beneficial for digestive health, aiding in regular bowel movements and maintaining a healthy gut – a critical aspect of controlling inflammation.
- Loaded with Antioxidants: These seeds are rich in antioxidants, which help combat oxidative stress and reduce the risk of chronic diseases.

Incorporating Chia Seeds into Daily Meals

- Versatile in Use: Chia seeds can be added to almost anything – from smoothies and yogurts to baked goods and salads. They have a mild, nutty flavor and absorb liquid, creating a gel-like texture, which is great for thickening recipes.
- Boosting Breakfast and Beyond: In our breakfast parfait, chia seeds not only add texture and nutrition but also enhance the dish's ability to keep you full and satisfied throughout the morning.

Chia Seeds as a Cornerstone in Healthy Eating

- A Nutrient-Dense Addition: Incorporating chia seeds into your diet is an easy way to boost your intake of several key nutrients, particularly if you're following a plant-based diet.
- Promoting Balanced, Inflammation-Fighting Meals: Their inclusion in our meal plan underscores the importance of adding diverse, nutrient-rich foods that support an anti-inflammatory lifestyle.

In conclusion, chia seeds are an incredibly versatile and nutritious addition to an anti-inflammatory diet. Their ability to support digestive health, coupled with their rich omega-3 and antioxidant content, makes them an ideal choice for anyone looking to improve their overall health and well-being. As you explore various ways to incorporate these tiny seeds into your diet, enjoy the plethora of benefits they bring to your meals.

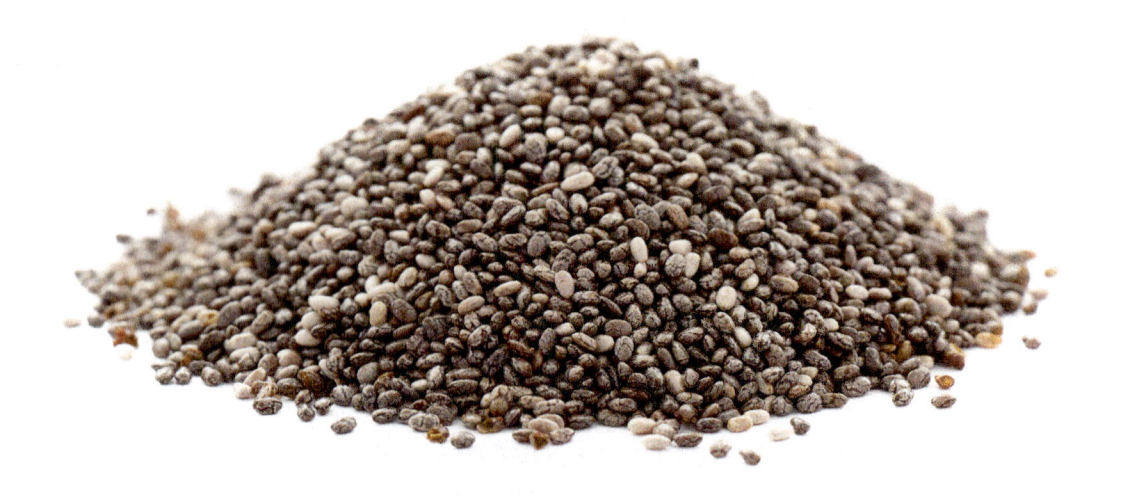

DAY 16 MEAL PLAN

BREAKFAST: BUCKWHEAT PANCAKES WITH STEWED APPLES AND CINNAMON
LUNCH: GRILLED VEGETABLE AND HALLOUMI CHEESE SKEWERS
DINNER: LEMON-GARLIC SHRIMP OVER ZUCCHINI NOODLES
SNACK: SLICED MANGO
SNACK: A HANDFUL OF WALNUTS
DRINK: KOMBUCHA

BREAKFAST: BUCKWHEAT PANCAKES WITH STEWED APPLES AND CINNAMON

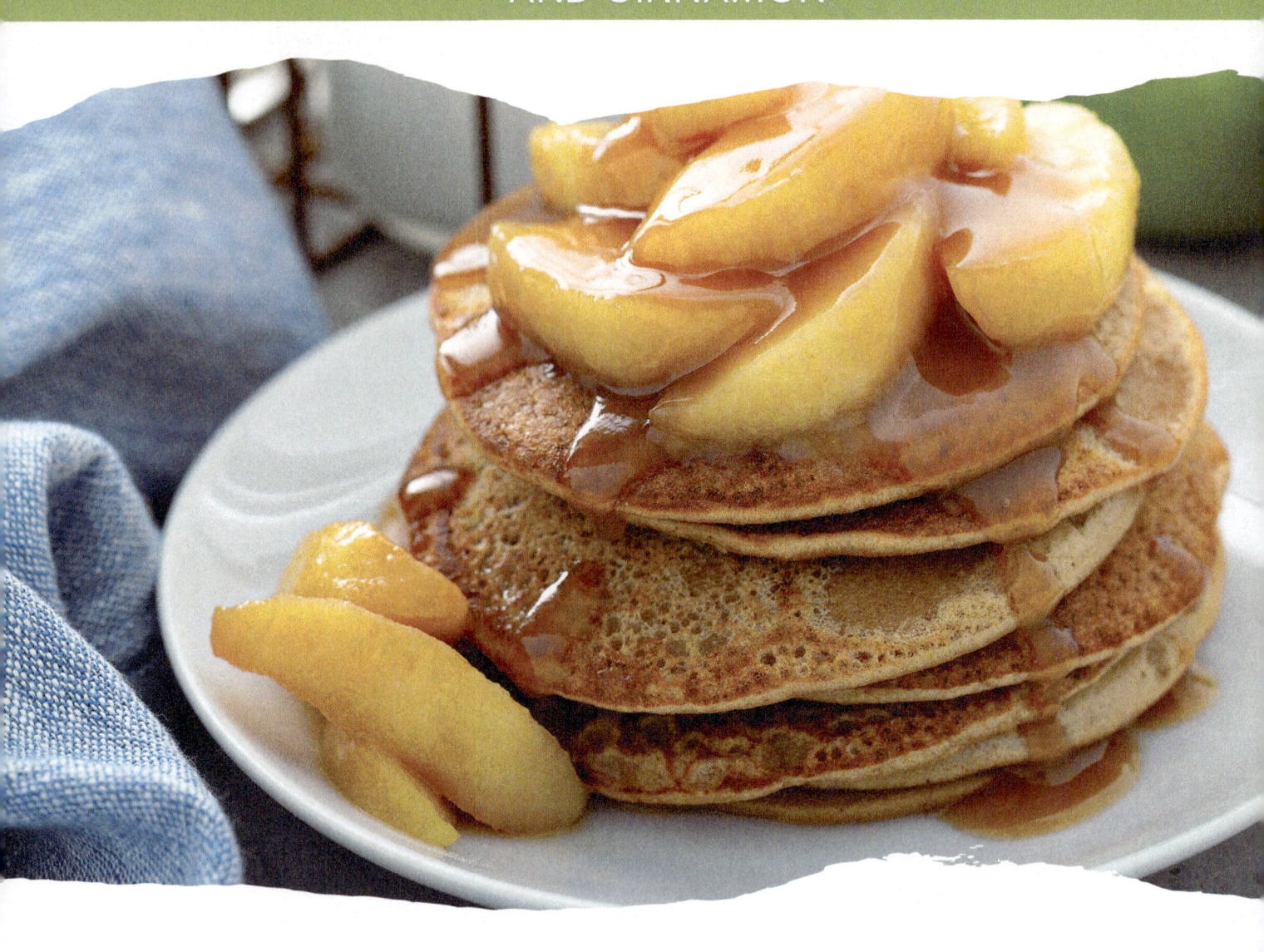

INGREDIENTS

- Buckwheat pancake mix (prepare as per package instructions)
- 2 apples, peeled and sliced
- Cinnamon to taste
- Optional: honey or maple syrup for sweetness

INSTRUCTIONS

- Cook Pancakes: Make buckwheat pancakes according to the package instructions.
- Stew Apples: In a saucepan, cook apple slices with a bit of water and cinnamon until soft.
- Serve: Top pancakes with stewed apples. Sweeten with honey or syrup if desired.

KITCHEN TOOLS NEEDED
- Frying pan or griddle
- Saucepan
- Mixing bowl

LUNCH: GRILLED VEGETABLE AND HALLOUMI CHEESE SKEWERS

INGREDIENTS

- Assorted vegetables (bell peppers, zucchini, cherry tomatoes)
- Halloumi cheese, cut into cubes
- Olive oil, salt, and pepper for seasoning

INSTRUCTIONS

- Prepare Skewers: Thread vegetables and halloumi cubes onto skewers.
- Grill: Brush with olive oil and season. Grill until vegetables are tender and cheese is golden.

KITCHEN TOOLS NEEDED
- Skewers (wooden or metal)
- Grill or grill pan

DINNER: LEMON-GARLIC SHRIMP OVER ZUCCHINI NOODLES

INGREDIENTS

- Shrimp, peeled and deveined
- 2-3 zucchinis, spiralized into noodles
- Garlic, minced
- Lemon juice and zest
- Olive oil for cooking
- Salt and pepper to taste

INSTRUCTIONS

- Cook Shrimp: Sauté shrimp with garlic, lemon juice, and zest until cooked.
- Prepare Zucchini Noodles: Sauté spiralized zucchini in olive oil until tender.
- Serve: Place zucchini noodles on a plate, top with lemon-garlic shrimp.

KITCHEN TOOLS NEEDED
- Frying pan
- Spiralizer or vegetable peeler

DRINK: KOMBUCHA

INGREDIENTS

- 1 bottle of kombucha (flavor of your choice)

PREPARATION TIME: NONE, READY TO EAT.

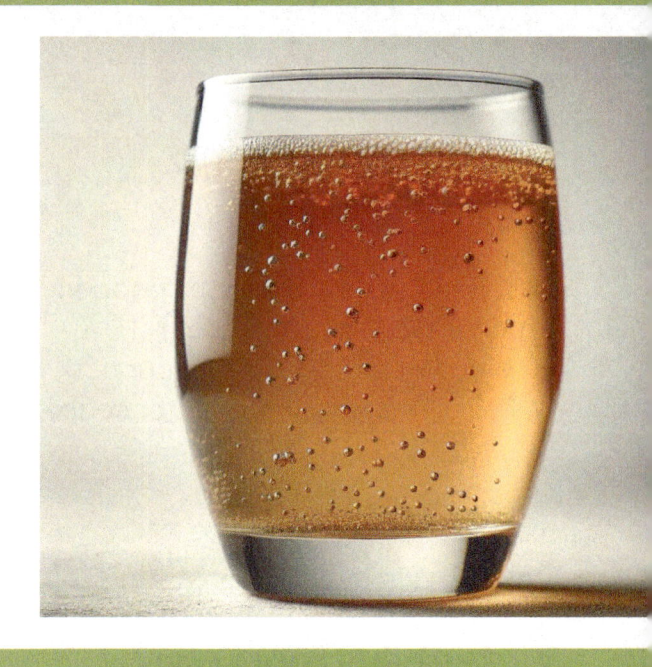

SNACK: SLICED MANGO

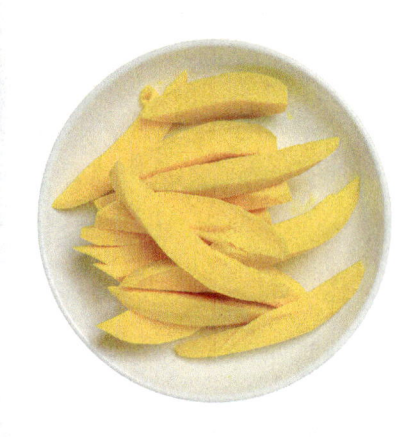

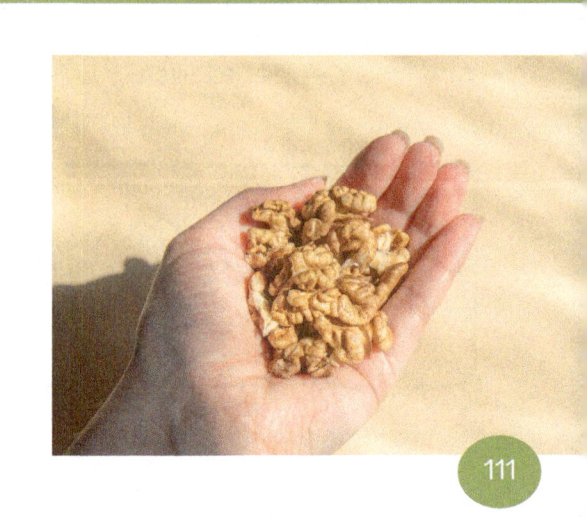

INGREDIENTS

- 1 ripe mango

INSTRUCTIONS

- Slice Mango: Peel and slice the mango into wedges.
- Serve: Enjoy the sweet and juicy mango slices.

KITCHEN TOOLS NEEDED

- Knife and cutting board

SNACK: A HANDFUL OF WALNUTS

INGREDIENTS

- A handful of walnuts

PREPARATION TIME: NONE, READY TO EAT.

ZUCCHINI – THE VERSATILE VEGETABLE FOR HEALTH

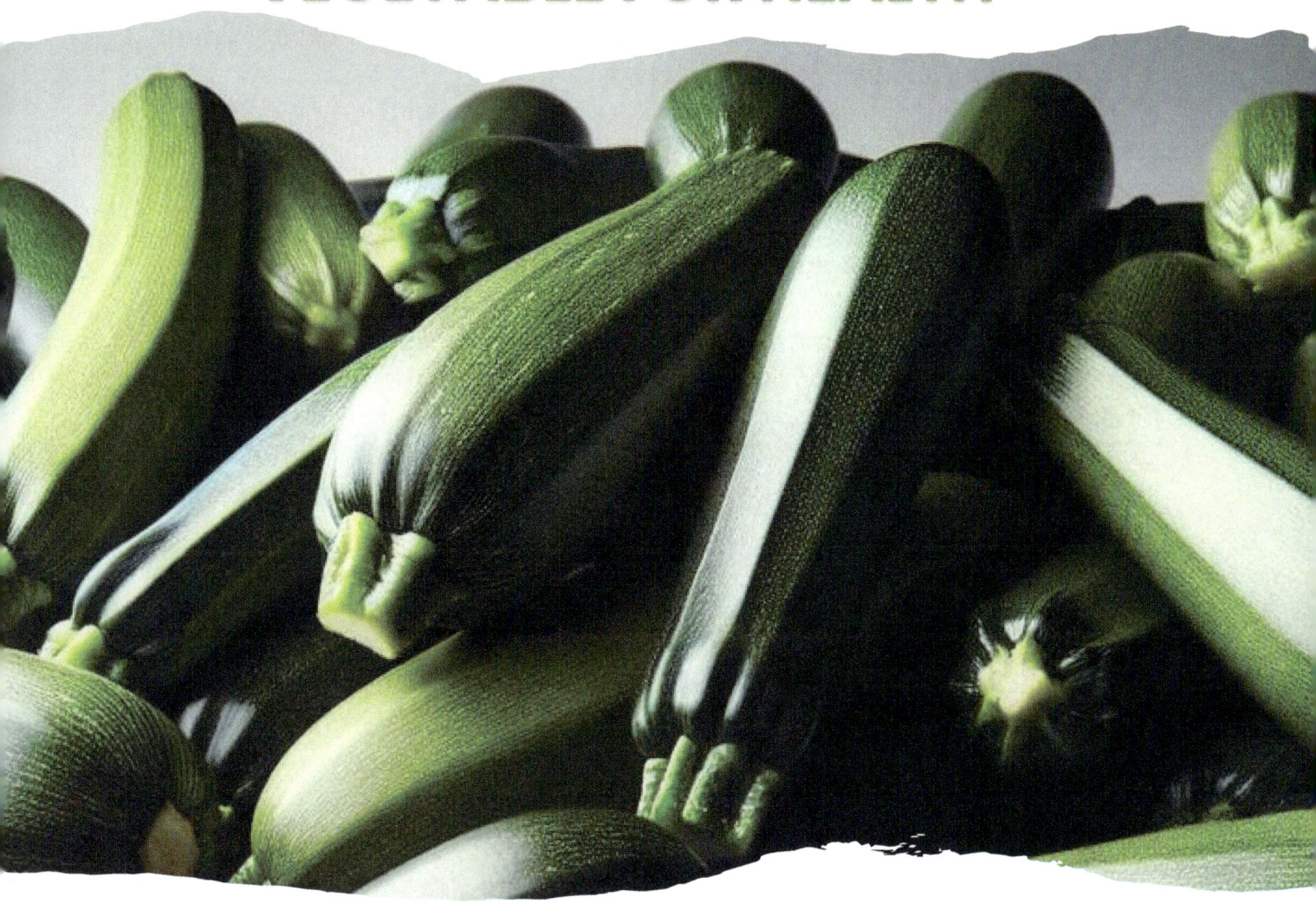

As we explore Day 16 of our Anti-Inflammatory Meal Plan, let's focus on zucchini, a key ingredient in our dinner recipe. This versatile and mild-flavored vegetable is a valuable addition to any diet, especially for its anti-inflammatory properties and nutrient richness.

The Nutritional Power of Zucchini

- Low in Calories, High in Nutrients: Zucchini is low in calories but high in essential vitamins and minerals, such as vitamin C, potassium, manganese, and antioxidants. These nutrients contribute to reducing inflammation and support overall health.
- Hydration and Digestive Health: Being high in water content and fiber, zucchini aids in hydration and promotes healthy digestion, which is vital for reducing inflammation.
- Heart Health Benefits: The fiber, potassium, and antioxidants in zucchini are beneficial for heart health, helping to lower cholesterol and blood pressure levels.

Incorporating Zucchini into Your Diet

- **Adaptable to Many Dishes:** Zucchini can be grilled, roasted, sautéed, or even turned into zucchini noodles, as in our dinner recipe. Its mild flavor makes it a perfect addition to both savory and sweet dishes.
- **A Perfect Pair for Many Flavors:** Whether it's combined with lemon and garlic in shrimp dishes or mixed into salads, zucchini complements a wide range of flavors, enhancing the overall taste and nutrition of meals.

Embracing Zucchini for a Balanced Diet

- **Ideal for Weight Management:** Zucchini's low calorie and high water content make it excellent for those focusing on weight management without sacrificing nutrient intake.
- **Encouraging a Diverse Vegetable Intake:** Regularly including vegetables like zucchini in your diet contributes to a varied and balanced nutritional intake, essential for combating inflammation and maintaining overall health.

In conclusion, zucchini is a fantastic vegetable for those seeking to reduce inflammation and enhance their overall well-being. Its versatility in the kitchen and wide range of health benefits make it an indispensable ingredient in your anti-inflammatory meal plan. Enjoy it in a variety of dishes to reap its full health benefits while adding delicious variety to your meals.

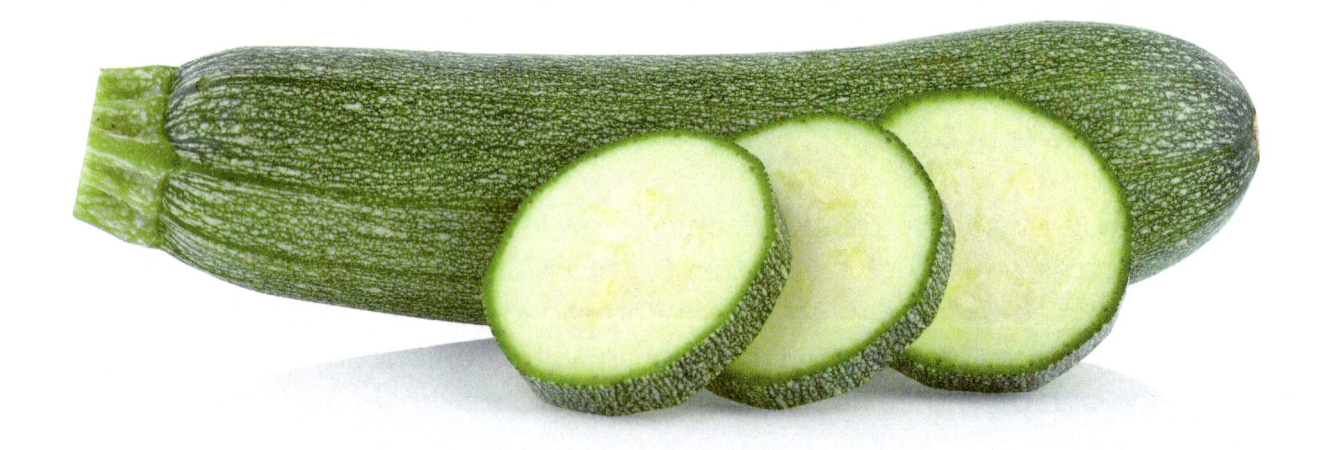

DAY 17 MEAL PLAN

BREAKFAST: SAVORY OATMEAL WITH SAUTÉED MUSHROOMS, SPINACH, AND A POACHED EGG
LUNCH: MEDITERRANEAN CHICKPEA AND QUINOA BOWL
DINNER: SLOW-COOKED BEEF RAGU OVER WHOLE-GRAIN PASTA
SNACK: DARK CHOCOLATE CHIPS
SNACK: SLICES OF KIWI
DRINK: SPARKLING WATER WITH CRANBERRY JUICE

BREAKFAST: SAVORY OATMEAL WITH SAUTÉED MUSHROOMS, SPINACH, AND A POACHED EGG

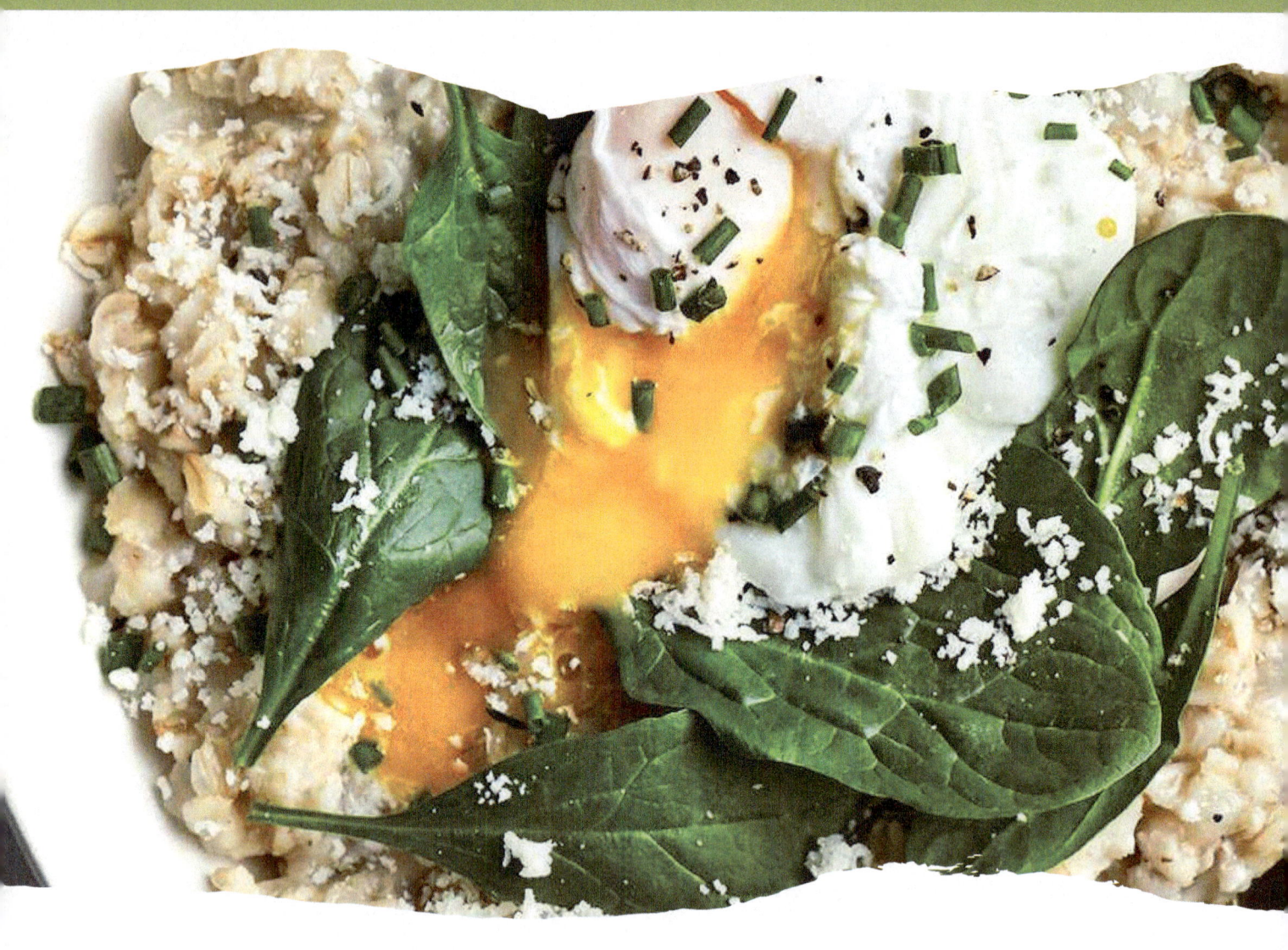

INGREDIENTS

- ½ cup rolled oats
- 1 cup water or broth
- 1 cup mushrooms, sliced
- 1 cup spinach
- 1 egg
- Salt and pepper to taste
- Olive oil for sautéing

INSTRUCTIONS

- Cook Oatmeal: Prepare oatmeal with water or broth as per package instructions.
- Sauté Vegetables: In a pan, sauté mushrooms and spinach in olive oil.
- Poach Egg: Poach the egg in simmering water.
- Assemble and Serve: Combine oatmeal with veggies, top with a poached egg.

KITCHEN TOOLS NEEDED
- Pot for oatmeal
- Frying pan
- Pot for poaching egg

LUNCH: MEDITERRANEAN CHICKPEA AND QUINOA BOWL

INGREDIENTS

- 1 cup cooked quinoa
- 1 cup chickpeas, cooked or canned
- Mixed vegetables (cucumbers, tomatoes, bell peppers)
- Hummus for topping
- Olive oil, lemon juice, herbs for dressing

INSTRUCTIONS

- Combine Bowl Ingredients: In a bowl, mix quinoa, chickpeas, and chopped vegetables.
- Add Dressing and Hummus: Drizzle with olive oil, lemon juice, and herbs. Top with a dollop of hummus.

KITCHEN TOOLS NEEDED
- Mixing bowl
- Knife and cutting board

DINNER: SLOW-COOKED BEEF RAGU OVER WHOLE-GRAIN PASTA

INGREDIENTS

- Beef for ragu (such as chuck or stew meat)
- Tomato sauce and herbs for ragu
- Whole-grain pasta
- Parmesan cheese for topping (optional)

INSTRUCTIONS

- Prepare Ragu: Cook beef with tomato sauce and herbs in a slow cooker until tender.
- Cook Pasta: Boil whole-grain pasta as per package instructions.
- Serve: Plate pasta, top with beef ragu, and sprinkle Parmesan cheese if desired.

KITCHEN TOOLS NEEDED
- Slow cooker or large pot
- Pot for pasta

DRINK: SPARKLING WATER WITH CRANBERRY JUICE

INGREDIENTS
- Sparkling water
- Cranberry juice

INSTRUCTIONS
- Mix Drink: Fill a glass with sparkling water and add a splash of cranberry juice for flavor.

KITCHEN TOOLS NEEDED
- Glass

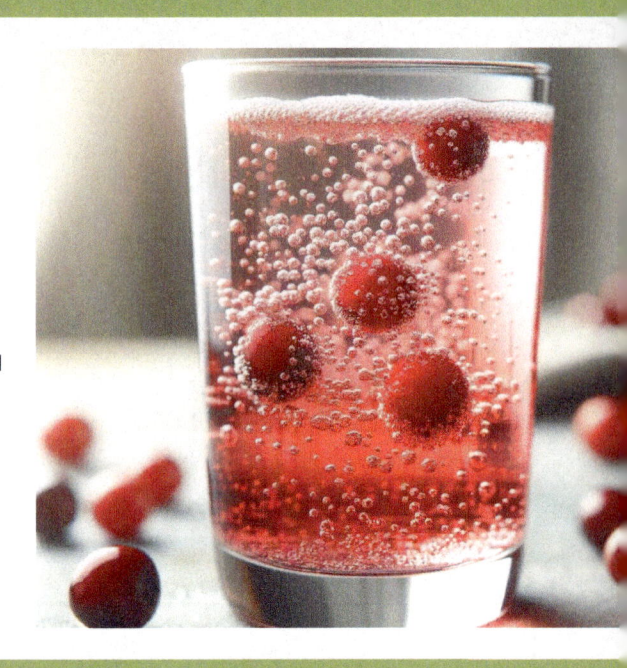

SNACK: SLICES OF KIWI

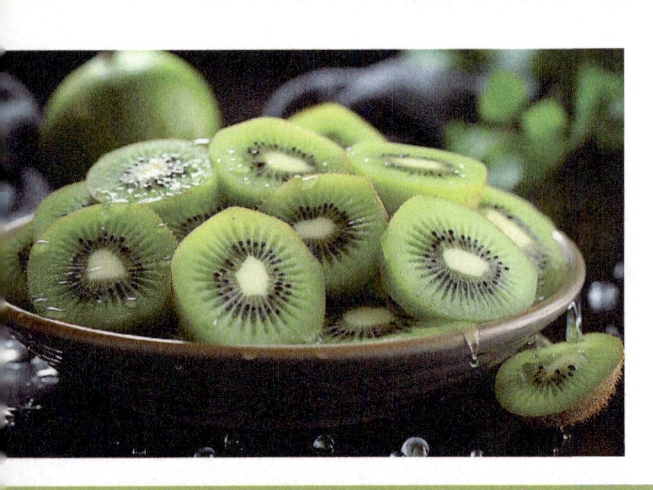

INGREDIENTS
- 1-2 kiwis, peeled and sliced

INSTRUCTIONS
- Prepare Kiwi: Slice the kiwi into rounds or wedges.
- Serve: Enjoy the tangy and refreshing kiwi slices.

KITCHEN TOOLS NEEDED
- Knife and cutting board

SNACK: DARK CHOCOLATE CHIPS

INGREDIENTS
- A small handful of dark chocolate chips

PREPARATION TIME: NONE, READY TO EAT.

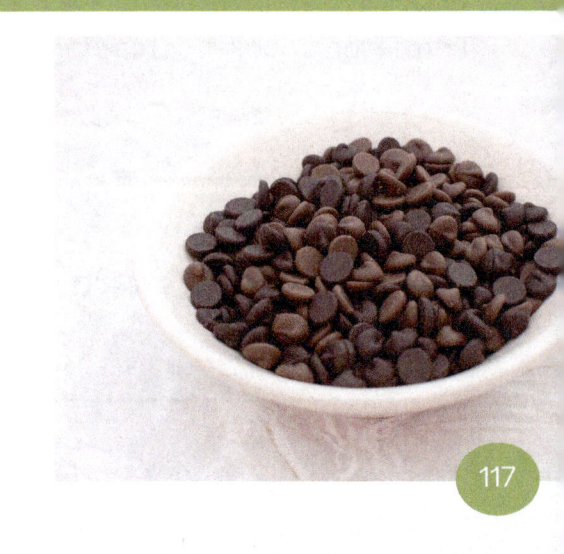

KIWI - THE TANGY VITAMIN POWERHOUSE

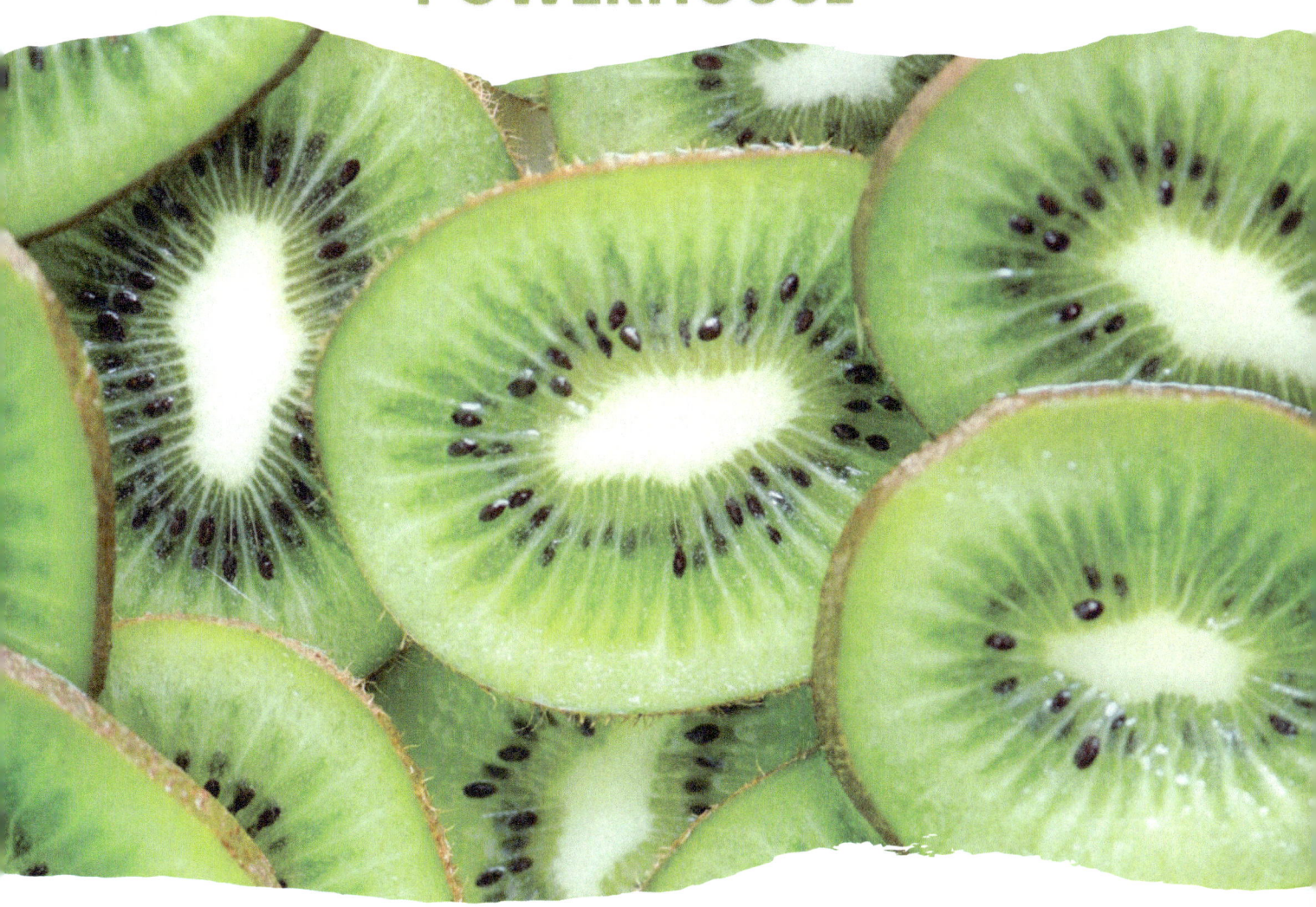

On Day 17, let's spotlight the kiwi, a vibrant and tangy fruit that features in our snack. Beyond its bright green hue and unique taste, kiwi is a nutritional treasure, packed with vitamins and antioxidants that are essential in an anti-inflammatory diet.

The Nutrient-Rich Profile of Kiwi

- Vitamin C Galore: Kiwi is an excellent source of vitamin C, even outdoing oranges. This powerful antioxidant is vital for boosting the immune system, enhancing skin health, and reducing inflammation.
- Digestive Health Ally: The fruit contains a good amount of dietary fiber, aiding in digestion and promoting gut health, which is key in managing inflammation.
- Rich in Other Nutrients: Kiwi also provides vitamin K, vitamin E, potassium, and folate, contributing to overall health and wellness.

Incorporating Kiwi into Your Diet

- A Refreshing Snack or Addition: Kiwi can be enjoyed on its own, added to fruit salads, blended into smoothies, or used as a natural sweetener in desserts and breakfast bowls.
- Enhancing Meals with Kiwi: Its sweet and tangy flavor makes it a delightful addition to a variety of dishes, adding a burst of flavor and nutrition.

Kiwi's Role in a Balanced Diet

- Supporting Heart Health: The antioxidants and fiber in kiwi are beneficial for heart health, helping to manage blood pressure and cholesterol levels.
- Promoting Diverse Fruit Intake: Regularly including a variety of fruits like kiwi in your diet ensures a wide range of nutrients and antioxidants, essential for reducing inflammation and boosting overall health.

In summary, kiwi is a standout fruit in an anti-inflammatory diet. Its combination of essential nutrients, particularly vitamin C, and digestive benefits make it an excellent choice for anyone seeking to improve their health and reduce inflammation. Enjoy the lively taste and health benefits of kiwi as a regular part of your meal plan.

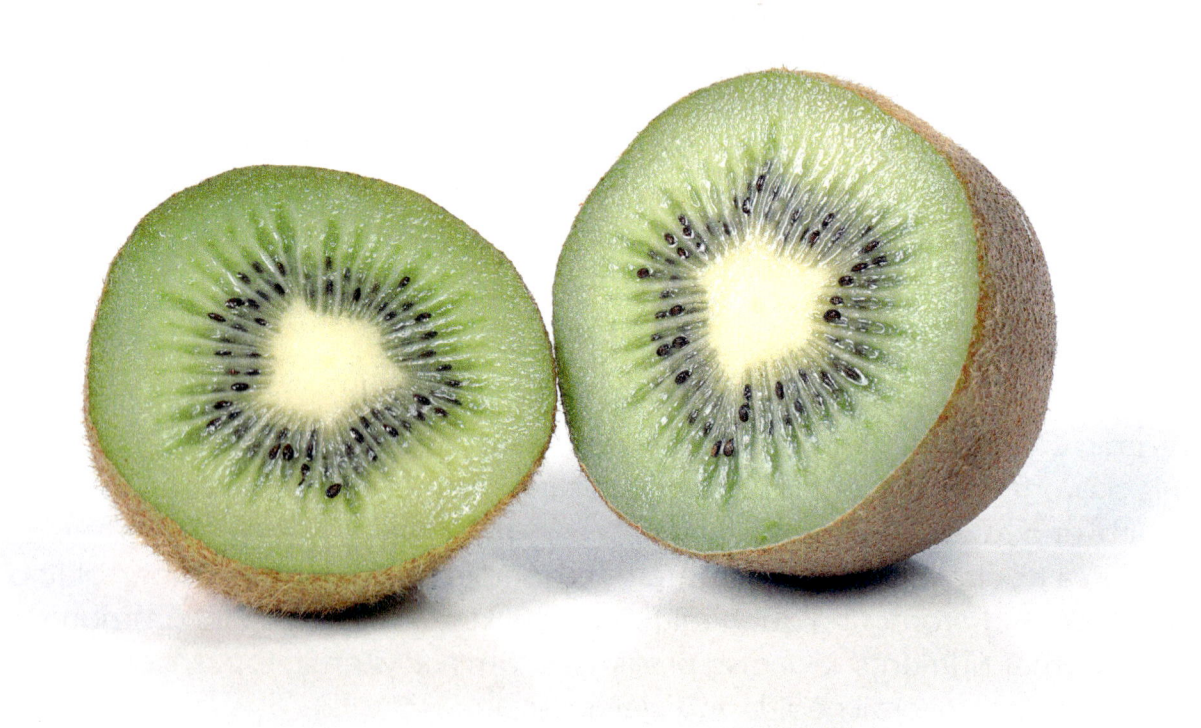

DAY 18 MEAL PLAN

BREAKFAST: GREEN SMOOTHIE WITH KALE, AVOCADO, AND PINEAPPLE
LUNCH: ROASTED BUTTERNUT SQUASH SOUP WITH WHOLE-GRAIN TOAST
DINNER: GRILLED TROUT WITH WILD RICE AND STEAMED GREEN BEANS
SNACK: A FEW DATES
SNACK: A MEDIUM-SIZED ORANGE
DRINK: HERBAL CHAMOMILE TEA

BREAKFAST: GREEN SMOOTHIE WITH KALE, AVOCADO, AND PINEAPPLE

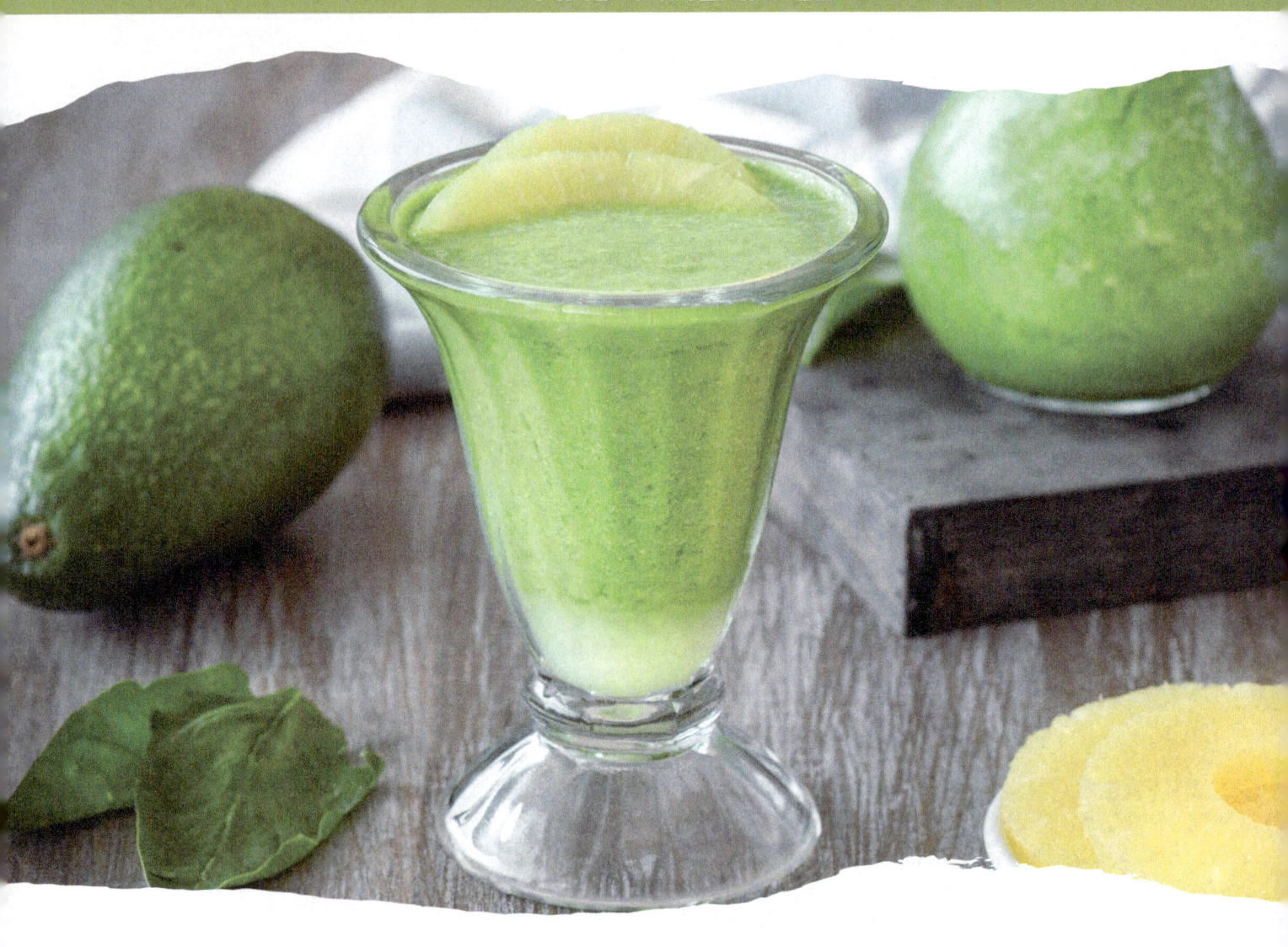

INGREDIENTS

- 1 cup kale, stems removed
- ½ avocado
- ½ cup pineapple chunks
- 1 cup water or coconut water

INSTRUCTIONS

- Blend Ingredients: Add kale, avocado, pineapple, and water/coconut water to the blender.
- Blend until Smooth: Blend until you achieve a smooth consistency.
- Serve: Pour into a glass and enjoy this nutritious smoothie.

KITCHEN TOOLS NEEDED
- Blender
- Measuring cup

LUNCH: ROASTED BUTTERNUT SQUASH SOUP WITH WHOLE-GRAIN TOAST

INGREDIENTS

- 1 butternut squash, peeled and cubed
- Vegetable broth
- Onion, garlic, herbs (for flavor)
- Whole-grain bread for side toast

INSTRUCTIONS

- Roast Squash: Roast butternut squash until tender.
- Cook Soup: Sauté onion and garlic, add roasted squash and broth, then blend until smooth.
- Toast Bread: Toast whole-grain bread as a side.
- Serve: Enjoy the creamy soup with a slice of toasted bread.

KITCHEN TOOLS NEEDED
- Oven for roasting squash
- Pot for soup
- Blender or immersion blender
- Toaster

DINNER: GRILLED TROUT WITH WILD RICE AND STEAMED GREEN BEANS

INGREDIENTS

- 1 trout fillet
- 1 cup wild rice
- 1 cup green beans
- Olive oil, lemon, herbs for seasoning

INSTRUCTIONS

- Grill Trout: Season trout and grill until cooked through.
- Cook Wild Rice: Prepare wild rice as per package instructions.
- Steam Green Beans: Steam green beans until tender-crisp.
- Serve: Plate the grilled trout with wild rice and steamed green beans.

KITCHEN TOOLS NEEDED
- Grill or grill pan
- Pot for rice
- Steamer or pot for green beans

DRINK: HERBAL CHAMOMILE TEA

INGREDIENTS

- 1 chamomile tea bag
- 1 cup boiling water

INSTRUCTIONS

- Boil Water: Heat the water.
- Steep Tea: Place the tea bag in a mug, pour hot water over it.

KITCHEN TOOLS NEEDED

- Kettle or pot for boiling water
- Mug

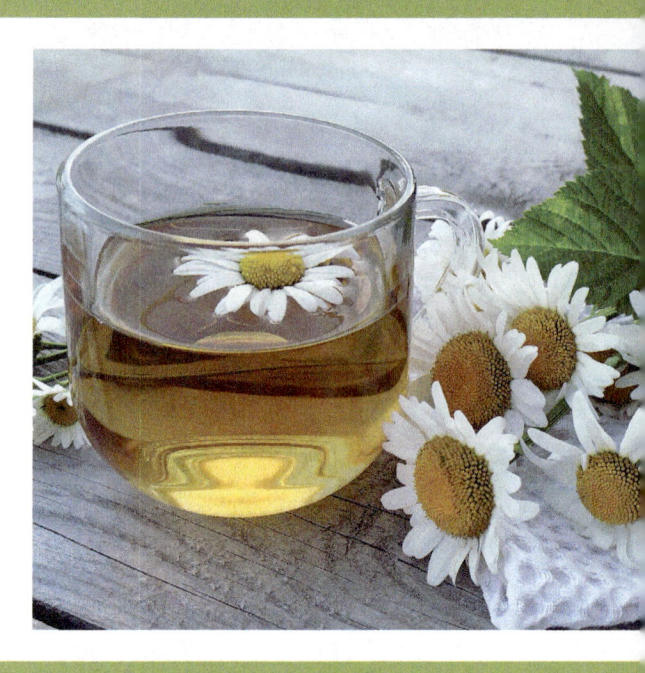

SNACK: A MEDIUM-SIZED ORANGE

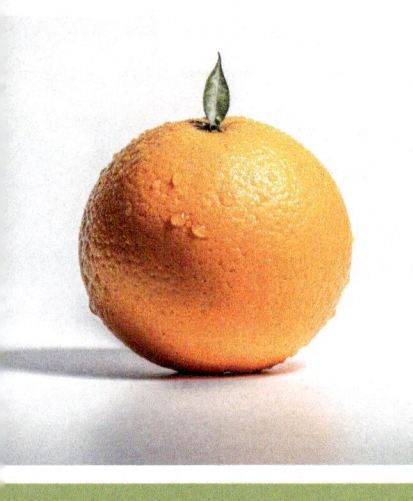

INGREDIENTS

- 1 medium-sized orange

PREPARATION TIME: NONE, READY TO EAT.

SNACK: A FEW DATES

INGREDIENTS

- A few dates

PREPARATION TIME: NONE, READY TO EAT.

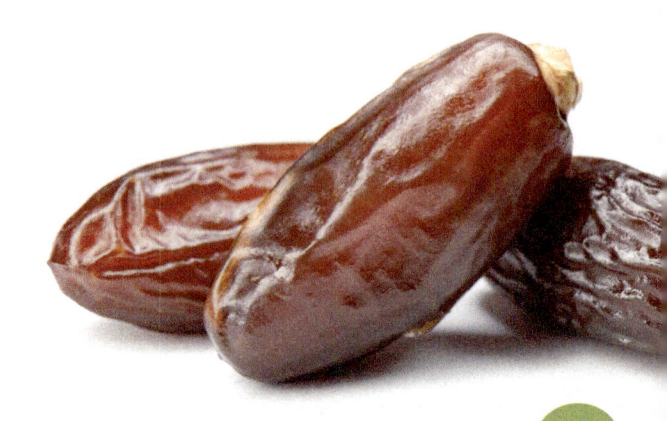

TROUT - THE NUTRIENT-RICH, LEAN PROTEIN

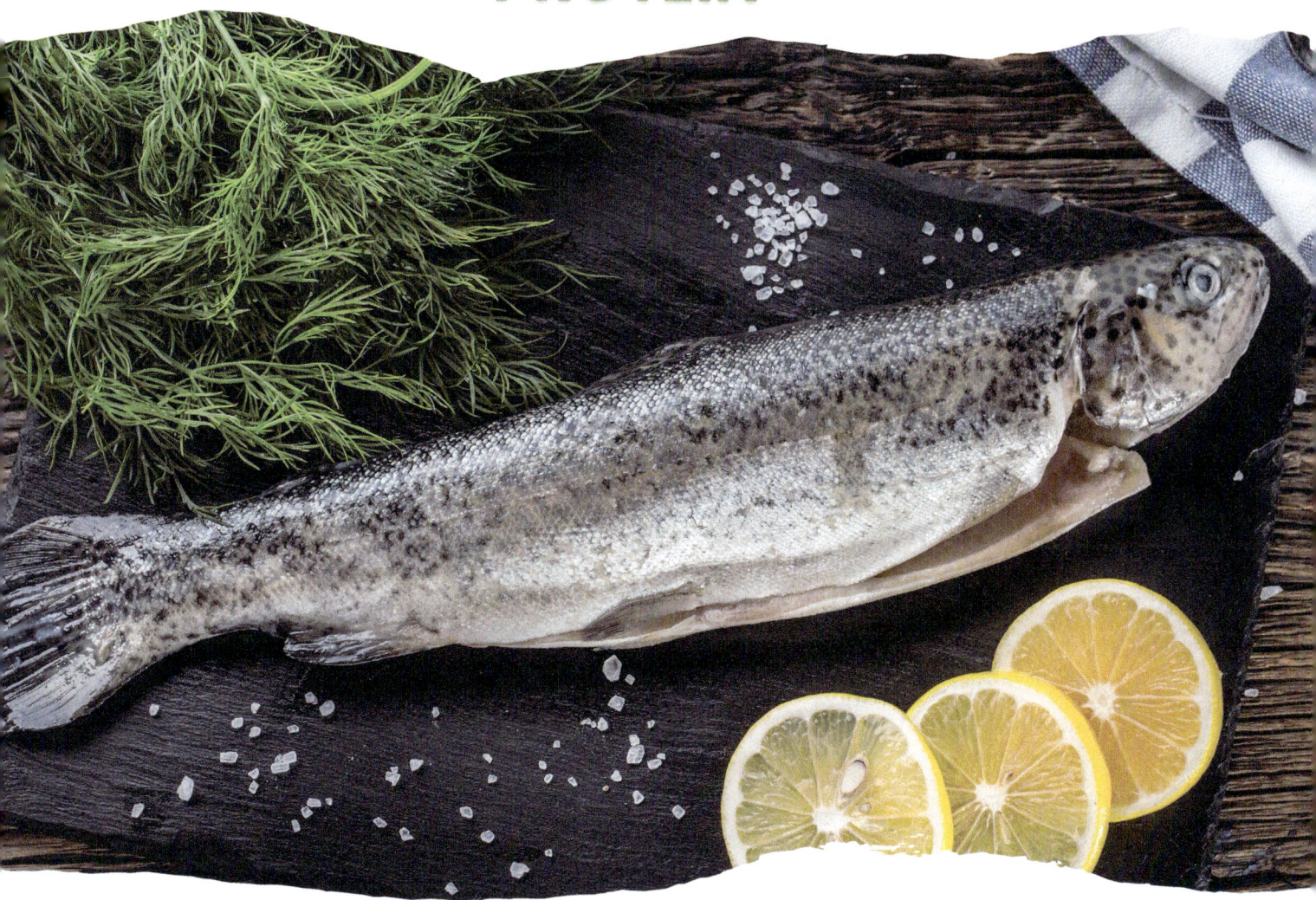

As we continue on Day 18 of our Anti-Inflammatory Meal Plan, let's focus on trout, our choice for dinner. Trout, a freshwater fish, is not only delicious but also packed with essential nutrients that make it a valuable component of any health-conscious diet, particularly for its anti-inflammatory properties.

The Health Benefits of Trout

- Omega-3 Fatty Acids: Trout is an excellent source of omega-3 fatty acids, which are crucial for reducing inflammation in the body. These healthy fats are known for their benefits to heart and brain health.
- High-Quality Protein: It provides lean protein, essential for muscle repair and growth, and overall body function. This makes trout an excellent choice for a satisfying and nutritious meal.
- Rich in Vitamins and Minerals: Trout is also a good source of B vitamins, vitamin D, potassium, and selenium, contributing to its overall nutritional profile.

Incorporating Trout into Your Diet

- Versatile Cooking Options: Trout can be prepared in various ways – grilled, as in our dinner recipe, baked, broiled, or pan-seared. It pairs well with a range of seasonings and sides, making it a versatile protein choice for any meal.
- A Delicious and Healthy Dinner Choice: Paired with wild rice and steamed green beans, grilled trout creates a balanced and nourishing meal, rich in both flavor and nutrients.

Trout's Role in a Wholesome Diet

- Ideal for Heart-Healthy Diets: Given its high omega-3 content, trout is particularly beneficial for those looking to maintain or improve heart health and reduce inflammation.
- Supporting Diverse Protein Sources: Including a variety of protein sources like trout in your diet ensures a broader intake of essential nutrients. It's especially beneficial for those looking to diversify their protein choices beyond red meat and poultry.

In conclusion, trout is an excellent addition to an anti-inflammatory diet. Its rich array of nutrients, particularly omega-3 fatty acids, along with its versatility in cooking, makes it a great choice for anyone seeking to improve their health through diet. Enjoy trout in your meals to benefit from its flavorful and nutritious properties.

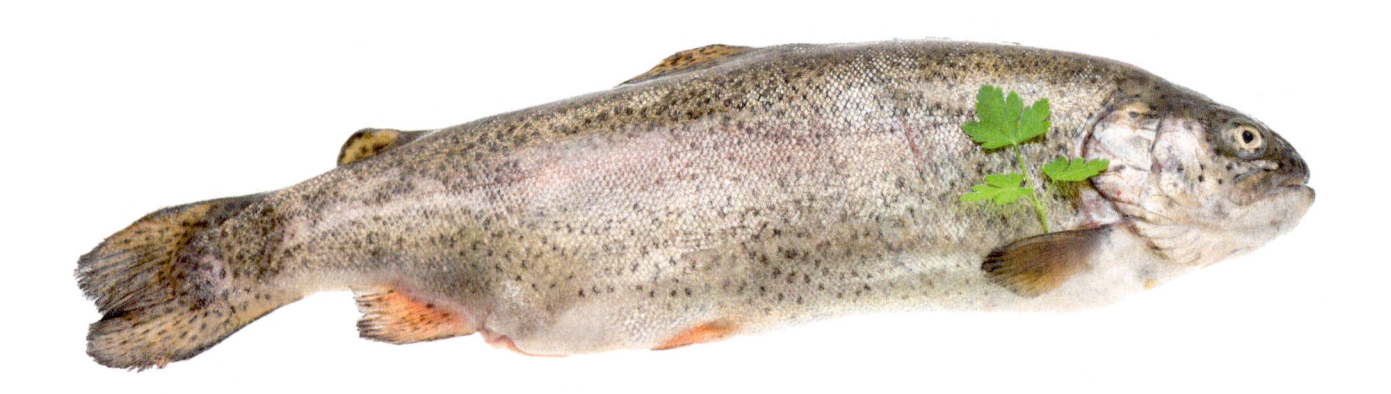

DAY 19 MEAL PLAN

BREAKFAST: YOGURT WITH MIXED NUTS AND HONEY
LUNCH: ROAST CHICKEN WRAP
DINNER: VEGETABLE CURRY WITH BROWN RICE
SNACK: DRIED APRICOTS
SNACK: MIXED BERRIES
DRINK: FRESH GINGER TEA

BREAKFAST: YOGURT WITH MIXED NUTS AND HONEY

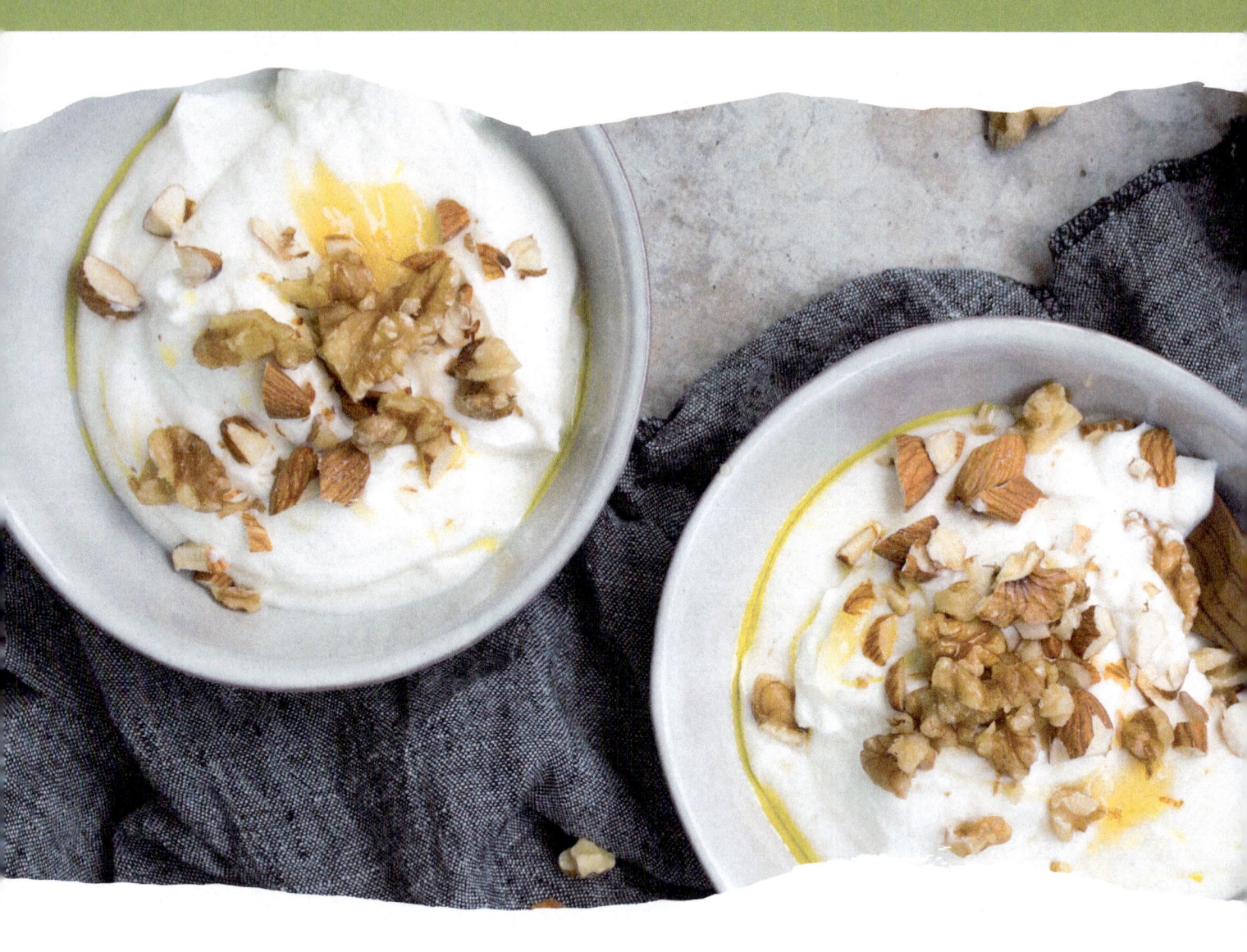

INGREDIENTS

- 1 cup plain or Greek yogurt
- A handful of mixed nuts (almonds, walnuts, cashews)
- Honey for drizzling

INSTRUCTIONS

- Serve Yogurt: Put yogurt in a bowl.
- Add Nuts: Sprinkle mixed nuts on top.
- Drizzle Honey: Finish with a drizzle of honey.

KITCHEN TOOLS NEEDED

- Bowl
- Spoon

LUNCH: ROAST CHICKEN WRAP

INGREDIENTS

- 1 whole-grain or flour tortilla
- Roast chicken, sliced or shredded
- Spinach leaves
- Sliced red onion
- Tzatziki spread

INSTRUCTIONS

- Assemble Wrap: Lay out the tortilla, spread tzatziki, add chicken, spinach, and onion.
- Roll and Serve: Roll up the wrap tightly, cut in half if desired.

KITCHEN TOOLS NEEDED
- Knife and cutting board

DINNER: VEGETABLE CURRY WITH BROWN RICE

INGREDIENTS

- Assorted vegetables (carrots, peas, bell peppers, cauliflower)
- Curry spices (turmeric, cumin, coriander)
- Coconut milk or tomato sauce for curry base
- 1 cup brown rice

INSTRUCTIONS

- Cook Curry: Sauté vegetables, add spices and coconut milk/tomato sauce, simmer until veggies are tender.
- Cook Rice: Prepare brown rice according to package instructions.
- Serve: Enjoy the vegetable curry over a bed of brown rice.

KITCHEN TOOLS NEEDED
- Pot for curry
- Pot for rice
- Knife and cutting board

DRINK: FRESH GINGER TEA

INGREDIENTS

- 1-inch piece of fresh ginger, sliced
- 1 cup water

INSTRUCTIONS

- Prepare Tea: Boil water with ginger slices for a few minutes.
- Serve: Strain the ginger tea into a mug.

KITCHEN TOOLS NEEDED

- Pot for boiling water
- Mug

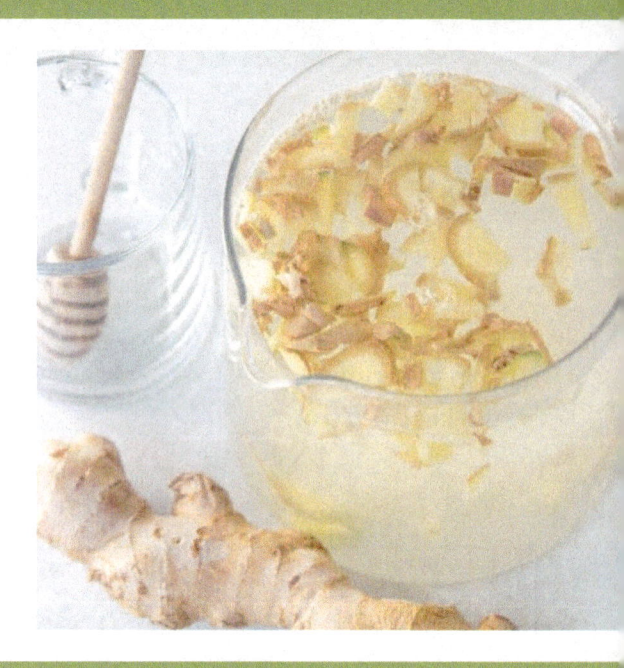

SNACK: MIXED BERRIES

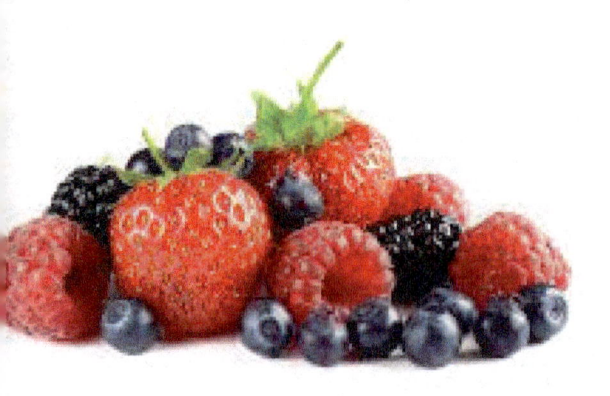

INGREDIENTS

- A small bowl of mixed berries (strawberries, blueberries, raspberries)

PREPARATION TIME: NONE, READY TO EAT.

SNACK: DRIED APRICOTS

INGREDIENTS

- A few dried apricots

PREPARATION TIME: NONE, READY TO EAT.

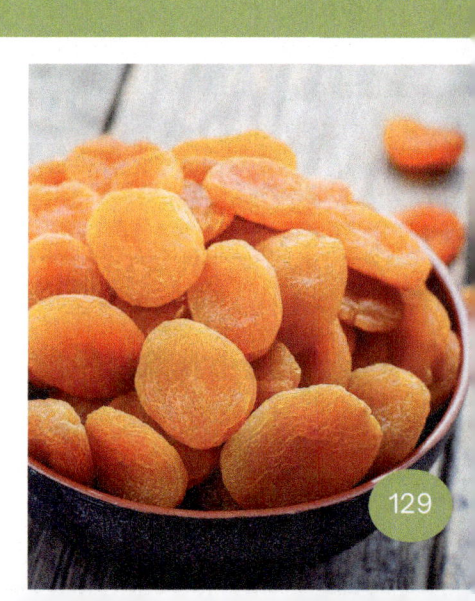

MIXED NUTS – THE HEART-HEALTHY, NUTRIENT-DENSE SNACK

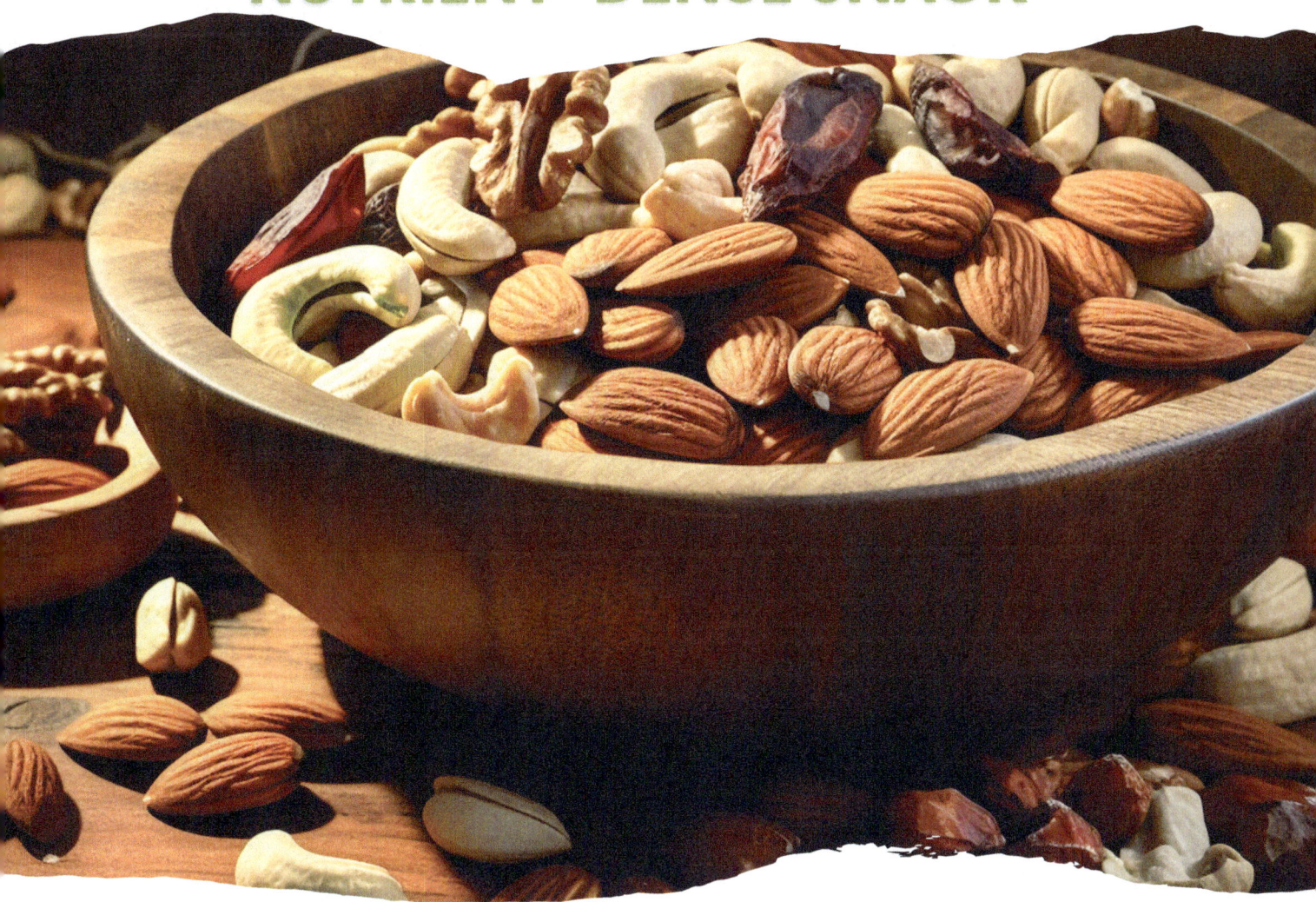

On Day 19 of our Anti-Inflammatory Meal Plan, we highlight mixed nuts, featured in our breakfast. This blend of various nuts is not only a crunchy, satisfying snack but also a nutritional powerhouse. Each type of nut brings its unique set of nutrients, making mixed nuts a multifaceted contributor to an anti-inflammatory diet.

The Diverse Benefits of Mixed Nuts

- Variety of Nutrients: Mixed nuts typically include almonds, walnuts, cashews, pistachios, and more, each offering vitamins, minerals, and healthy fats. They collectively provide a wide spectrum of nutrients like magnesium, zinc, omega-3 fatty acids, and vitamin E.
- Anti-Inflammatory Properties: The omega-3 fatty acids in nuts like walnuts are known for their anti-inflammatory effects. Additionally, nuts contain antioxidants and other compounds that help reduce inflammation in the body.
- Heart Health and More: Regular consumption of mixed nuts has been associated with improved heart health, thanks to their ability to lower bad cholesterol levels and maintain healthy blood vessels.

Integrating Mixed Nuts into Your Diet

- Versatile and Convenient: Mixed nuts are an easy addition to any meal or snack. They can be enjoyed on their own, added to yogurt or salads, or used as a topping for oatmeal and other dishes.
- Boosting Meals with Nutrition and Flavor: Incorporating mixed nuts into your breakfast, like the yogurt with nuts and honey, adds both texture and a nutritional boost to start your day.

Embracing Mixed Nuts for Balanced Eating

- Ideal for Satiety and Weight Management: The protein and fiber content in nuts help in feeling full, which can aid in weight management efforts.
- Promoting Varied Nutrient Intake: Including a mix of different nuts ensures a broader intake of various nutrients, supporting overall health and reducing dietary monotony.

In summary, mixed nuts are a fantastic addition to an anti-inflammatory diet. Their blend of essential nutrients, combined with their versatility and delicious taste, makes them an ideal choice for enhancing meals or enjoying as a standalone snack. As you continue your journey of healthful eating, consider mixed nuts as a go-to source for nutrition and flavor.

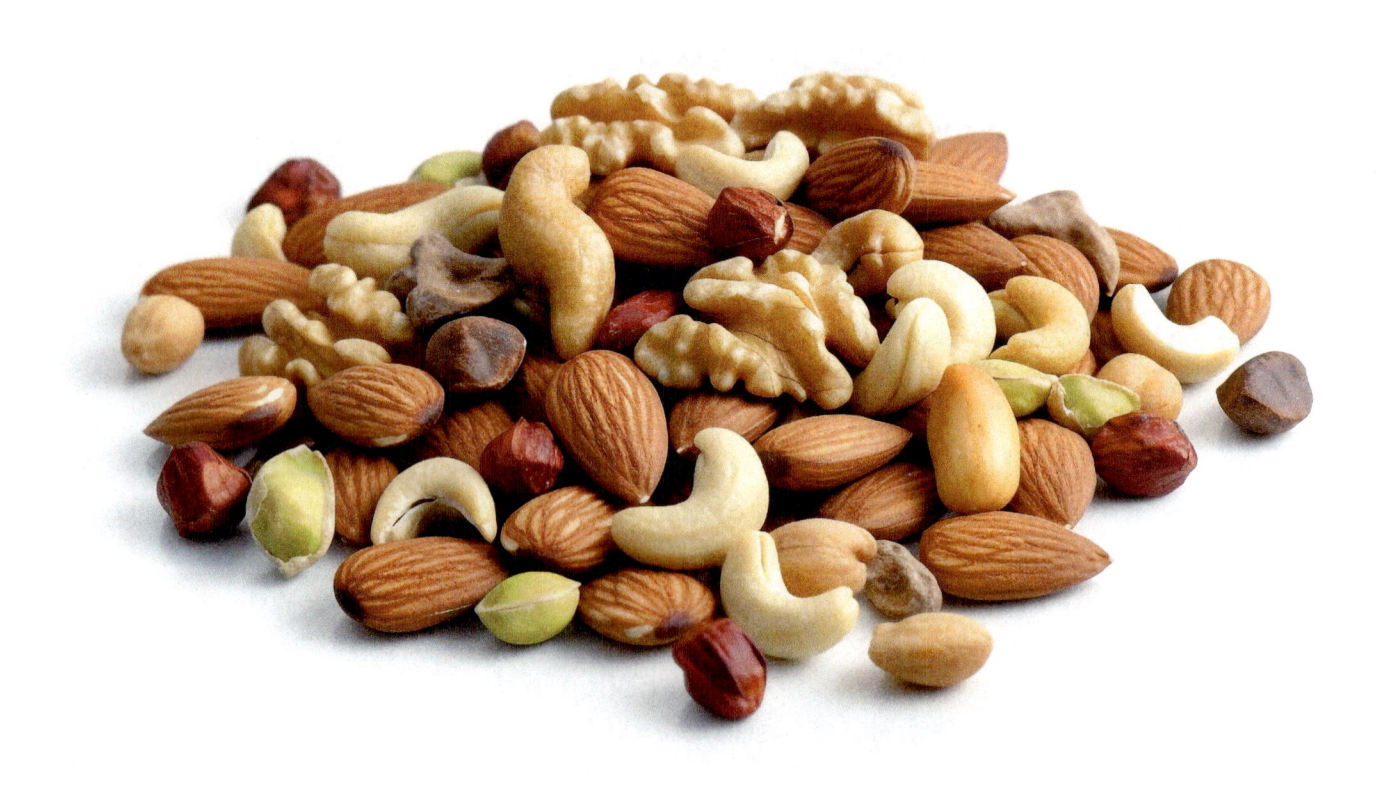

DAY 20 MEAL PLAN

BREAKFAST: QUINOA PORRIDGE WITH ALMOND MILK, PEACHES, AND NUTMEG
LUNCH: TUNA SALAD WITH MIXED GREENS
DINNER: PORK TENDERLOIN WITH ROASTED BRUSSELS SPROUTS AND SWEET POTATOES
SNACK: CELERY STICKS WITH PEANUT BUTTER
SNACK: A SMALL APPLE
DRINK: DANDELION ROOT TEA

BREAKFAST: QUINOA PORRIDGE WITH ALMOND MILK, PEACHES, AND NUTMEG

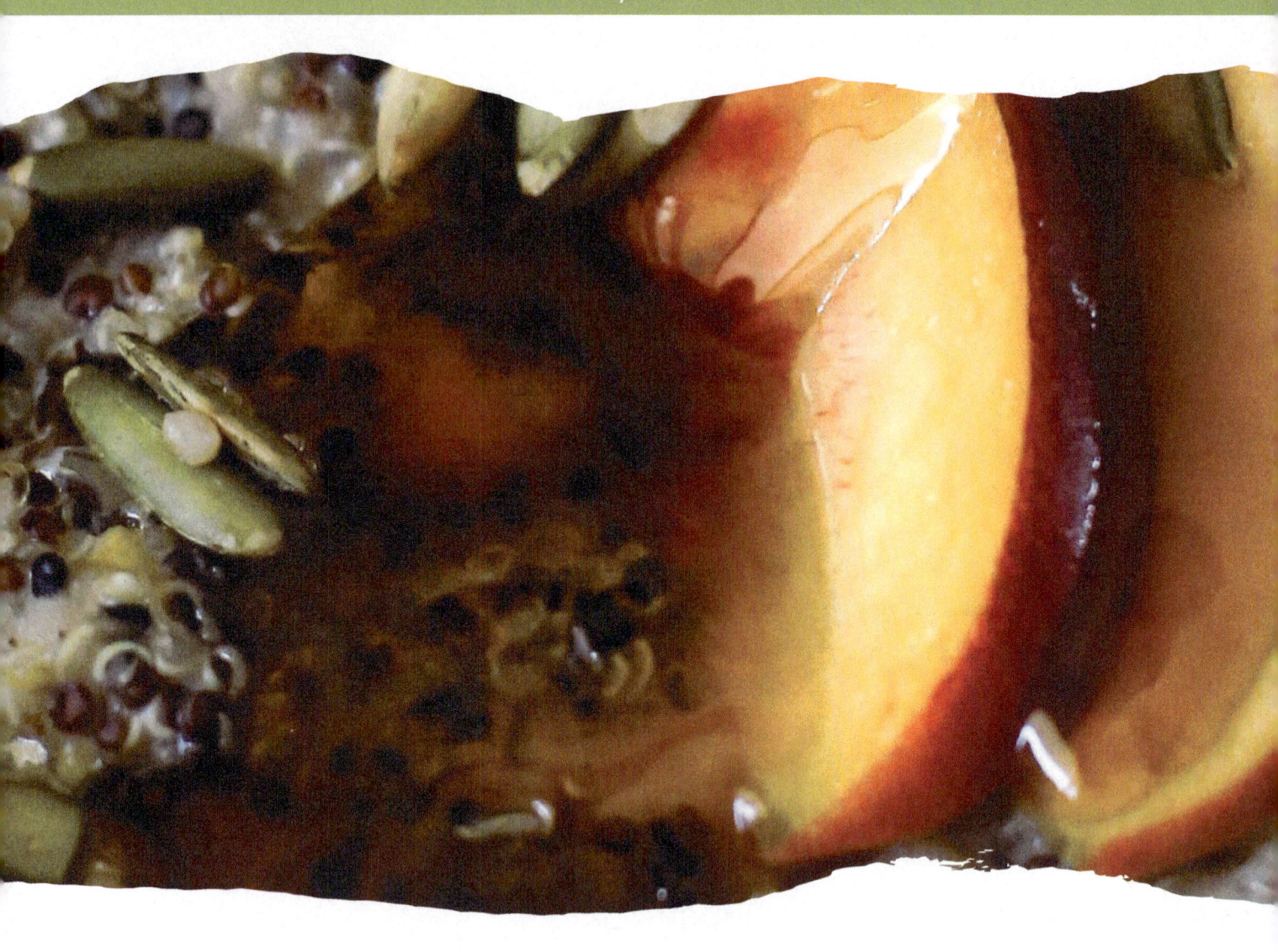

INGREDIENTS

- ½ cup quinoa
- 1 cup almond milk
- 1 peach, sliced
- A sprinkle of nutmeg

INSTRUCTIONS

- Cook Quinoa: Rinse quinoa and cook it in almond milk until soft and porridge-like.
- Add Toppings: Top with sliced peaches and a sprinkle of nutmeg.
- Serve: Enjoy this warm and nutritious breakfast.

KITCHEN TOOLS NEEDED

- Pot
- Knife and cutting board

LUNCH: TUNA SALAD WITH MIXED GREENS

INGREDIENTS

- 1 can of tuna, drained
- Mixed greens (lettuce, spinach, arugula)
- Cherry tomatoes, halved
- Olives
- Olive oil and lemon juice for dressing

INSTRUCTIONS

- Prepare Salad: Combine tuna, greens, tomatoes, and olives in a bowl.
- Dress Salad: Toss with olive oil and lemon juice.

KITCHEN TOOLS NEEDED
- Mixing bowl

DINNER: PORK TENDERLOIN WITH ROASTED BRUSSELS SPROUTS AND SWEET POTATOES

INGREDIENTS

- Pork tenderloin
- Brussels sprouts
- Sweet potatoes, cubed
- Olive oil, herbs, salt, and pepper for seasoning

INSTRUCTIONS

- Prepare Pork: Season the pork tenderloin and roast in the oven.
- Roast Vegetables: Toss Brussels sprouts and sweet potatoes with olive oil and seasonings. Roast until tender.
- Serve: Slice the pork and serve with the roasted vegetables.

KITCHEN TOOLS NEEDED
- Oven and baking tray
- Knife and cutting board

DRINK: DANDELION ROOT TEA

INGREDIENTS

- 1 dandelion root tea bag
- 1 cup boiling water

INSTRUCTIONS

- Boil Water: Heat the water.
- Steep Tea: Place the tea bag in a mug, pour hot water over it.

KITCHEN TOOLS NEEDED

- Kettle or pot for boiling water
- Mug

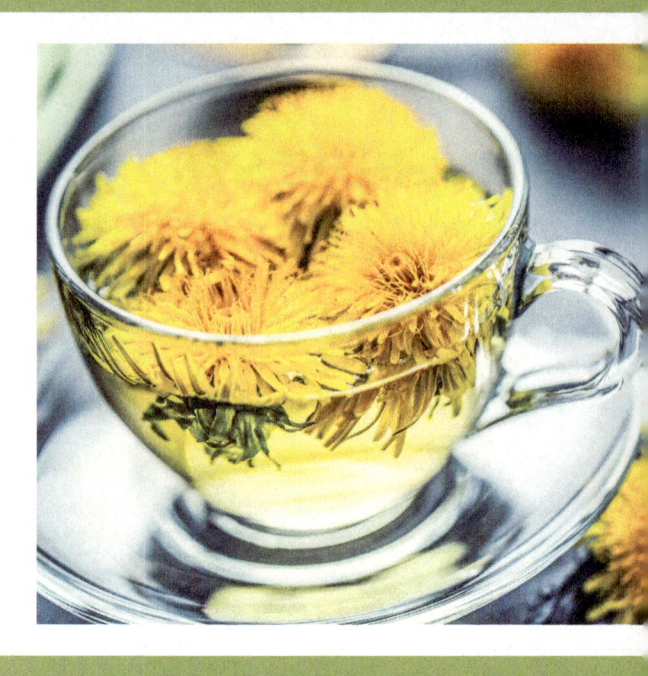

SNACK: CELERY STICKS WITH PEANUT BUTTER

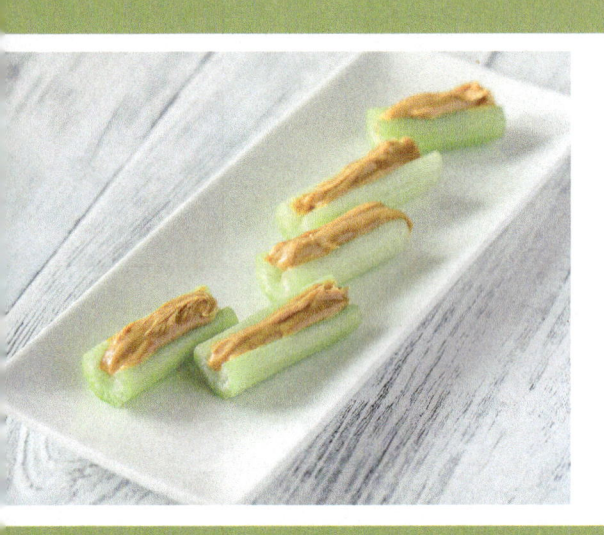

INGREDIENTS

- Celery sticks
- Peanut butter

INSTRUCTIONS

- Prepare Snack: Spread peanut butter on celery sticks.
- Serve: Enjoy this crunchy and protein-rich snack.

KITCHEN TOOLS NEEDED

- Knife

SNACK: A SMALL APPLE

INGREDIENTS

- 1 small apple

PREPARATION TIME: NONE, READY TO EAT.

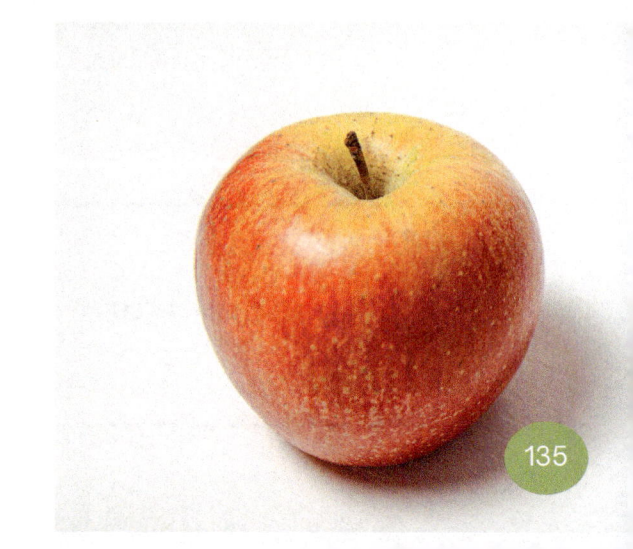

TUNA – THE LEAN PROTEIN WITH OMEGA-3 BENEFITS

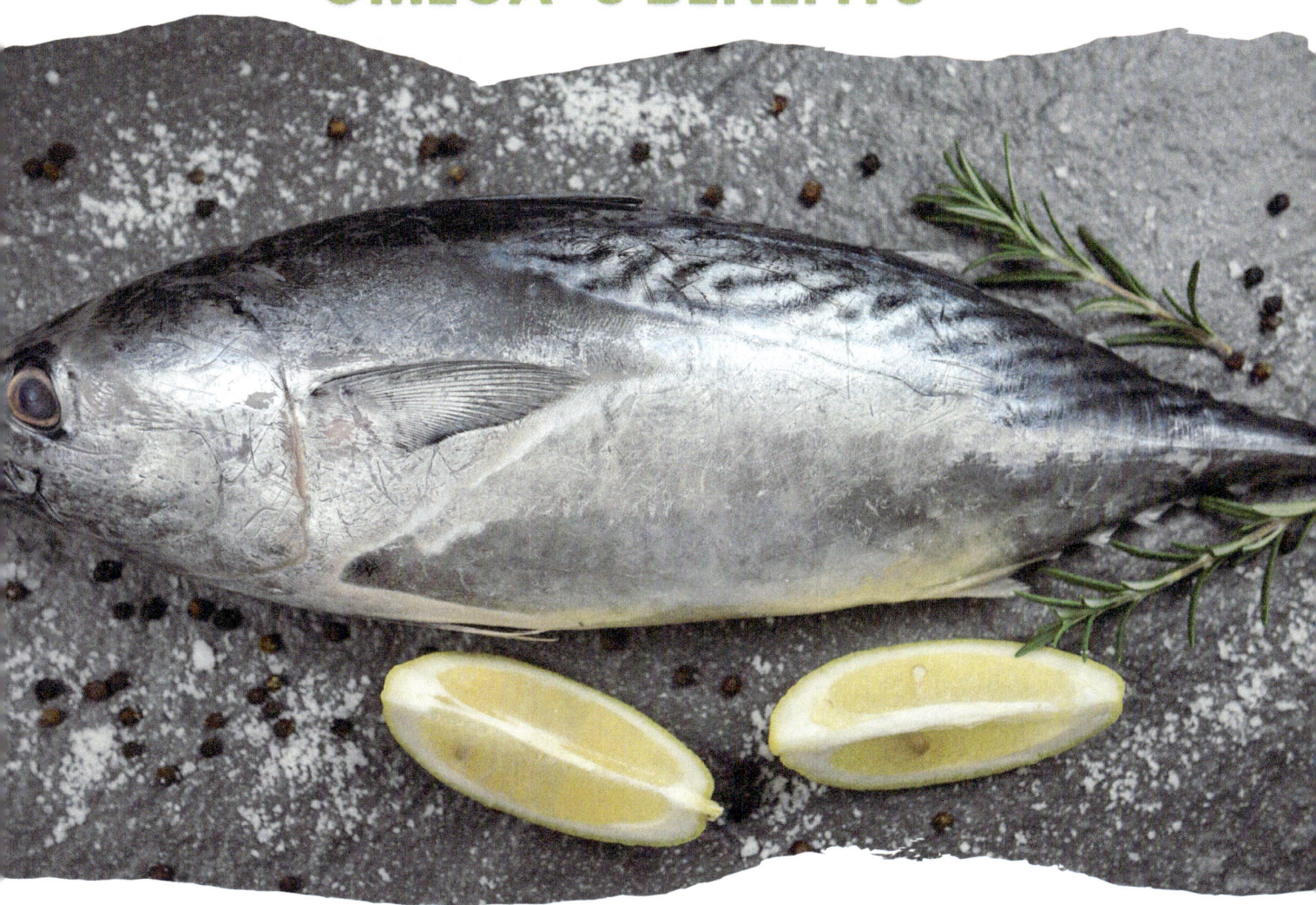

On Day 20 of our Anti-Inflammatory Meal Plan, we focus on tuna, a key ingredient in our lunch. Tuna, a versatile and widely-consumed fish, is not just a culinary favorite but also a nutritionally rich choice, particularly valuable for its anti-inflammatory properties and heart health benefits.

The Nutritional Edge of Tuna

- High in Omega-3 Fatty Acids: Tuna is an excellent source of omega-3 fatty acids, known for their anti-inflammatory effects. These healthy fats are essential for cardiovascular health and cognitive function.
- Quality Protein Source: It provides high-quality protein, necessary for muscle repair, growth, and overall bodily functions.
- Rich in Vitamins and Minerals: Tuna contains a variety of vitamins and minerals, including B vitamins, selenium, and potassium, contributing to its overall health benefits.

Incorporating Tuna into Your Diet

- Flexible and Delicious: Tuna can be enjoyed in many forms – fresh, canned, grilled, or baked. It's perfect for salads, sandwiches, or as a main protein in meals.
- A Nutritious Lunch Option: In our tuna salad with mixed greens, the fish adds a protein punch and omega-3s, making the meal both satisfying and heart-healthy.

Tuna's Role in a Healthy Diet

- Ideal for a Heart-Healthy Diet: Tuna's omega-3 content makes it an excellent food choice for those looking to support heart health and manage inflammation.
- Diversifying Protein Sources: Including various types of fish like tuna in your diet ensures a broad intake of essential nutrients and adds variety to your protein choices.

In conclusion, tuna is an outstanding choice for an anti-inflammatory diet. Its combination of omega-3 fatty acids, high-quality protein, and a spectrum of vitamins and minerals make it a valuable food for maintaining good health. Enjoy tuna in your meals for a delicious way to boost your nutritional intake and support your overall wellness.

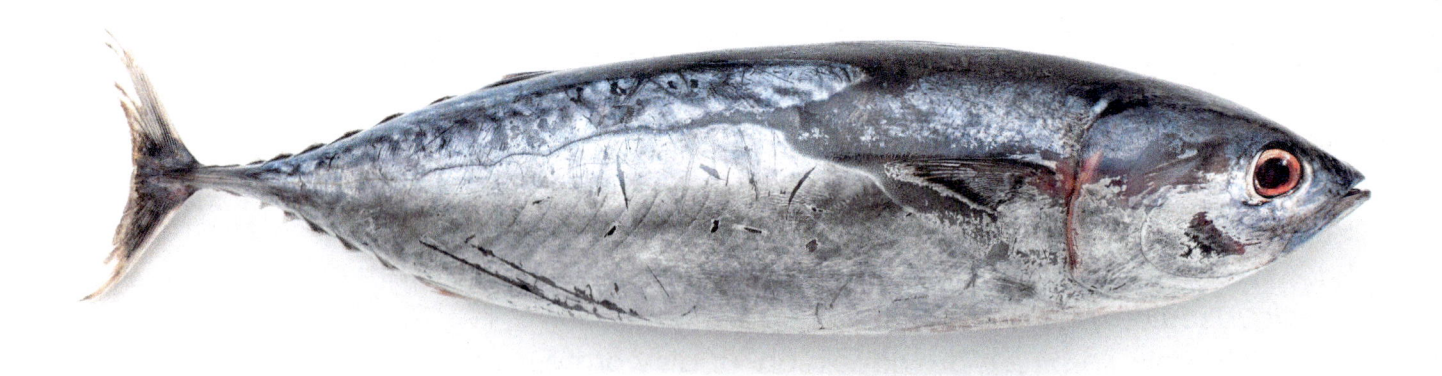

DAY 21 MEAL PLAN

BREAKFAST: EGG MUFFINS WITH SPINACH, BELL PEPPER, AND FETA CHEESE
LUNCH: BALSAMIC GLAZED BEET SALAD WITH GOAT CHEESE AND WALNUTS
DINNER: BAKED CHICKEN WITH QUINOA TABBOULEH AND GRILLED ASPARAGUS
SNACK: WATERMELON SLICES
SNACK: ROASTED PUMPKIN SEEDS
DRINK: LEMON BALM TEA

BREAKFAST: EGG MUFFINS WITH SPINACH, BELL PEPPER, AND FETA CHEESE

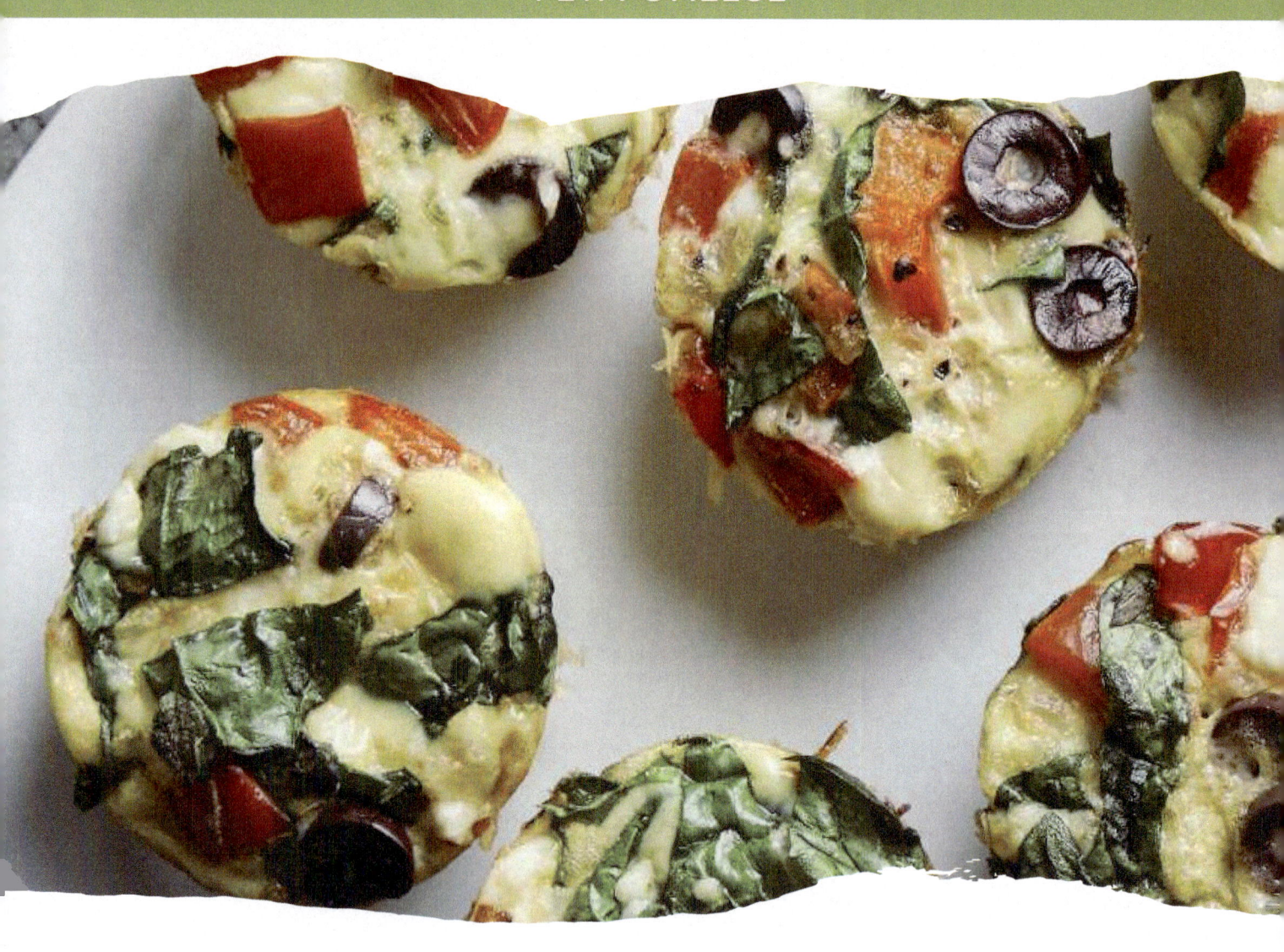

INGREDIENTS

- 6 eggs
- 1 cup spinach, chopped
- 1 bell pepper, diced
- ½ cup feta cheese, crumbled
- Salt and pepper to taste

INSTRUCTIONS

- Preheat Oven: Set your oven to 350ºF (175ºC).
- Prepare Mixture: Whisk eggs in a bowl, mix in spinach, bell pepper, and feta. Season with salt and pepper.
- Bake Egg Muffins: Pour the mixture into muffin tins and bake for 20-25 minutes or until set.

KITCHEN TOOLS NEEDED

- Muffin tin
- Mixing bowl
- Whisk

LUNCH: BALSAMIC GLAZED BEET SALAD WITH GOAT CHEESE AND WALNUTS

INGREDIENTS

- Beets, roasted and sliced
- Goat cheese, crumbled
- Walnuts, chopped
- Mixed greens for salad base
- Balsamic vinegar and olive oil for dressing

INSTRUCTIONS

- Prepare Salad: Arrange mixed greens, top with roasted beets, goat cheese, and walnuts.
- Dress Salad: Drizzle with balsamic vinegar and olive oil.

KITCHEN TOOLS NEEDED
- Oven for roasting beets
- Mixing bowl

DINNER: BAKED CHICKEN WITH QUINOA TABBOULEH AND GRILLED ASPARAGUS

INGREDIENTS

- Chicken breasts
- Quinoa for tabbouleh
- Fresh parsley, mint, tomatoes, cucumber for tabbouleh
- Asparagus
- Olive oil, lemon juice, and spices for seasoning

INSTRUCTIONS

- Bake Chicken: Season chicken breasts and bake until cooked through.
- Prepare Quinoa Tabbouleh: Mix cooked quinoa with chopped parsley, mint, tomatoes, cucumber, olive oil, and lemon juice.
- Grill Asparagus: Grill asparagus with a bit of olive oil and seasoning until tender.
- Serve: Plate the chicken with a side of quinoa tabbouleh and grilled asparagus.

KITCHEN TOOLS NEEDED
- Oven for baking chicken
- Grill or grill pan for asparagus
- Mixing bowl

DRINK: LEMON BALM TEA

INGREDIENTS
- 1 lemon balm tea bag
- 1 cup boiling water

INSTRUCTIONS
- Boil Water: Heat the water.
- Steep Tea: Place the tea bag in a mug, pour hot water over it.

KITCHEN TOOLS NEEDED
- Kettle or pot for boiling water
- Mug

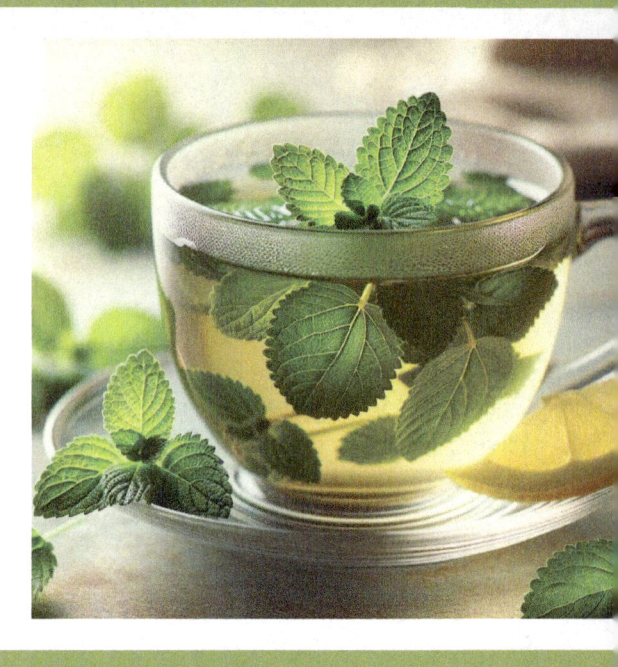

SNACK: WATERMELON SLICES

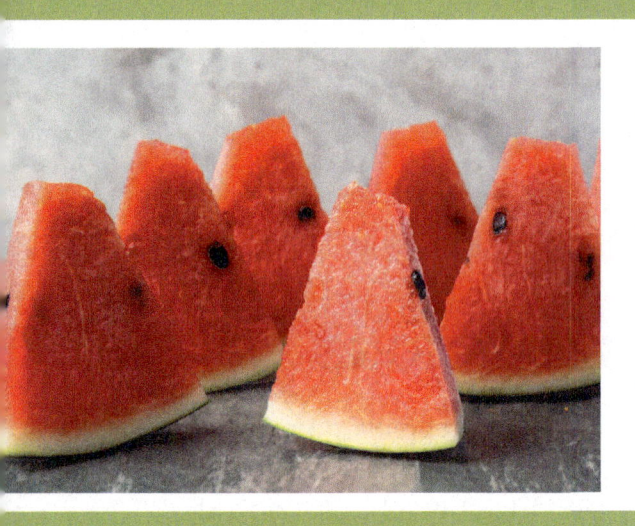

INGREDIENTS
- A few slices of watermelon

INSTRUCTIONS
- Slice Watermelon: Cut the watermelon into easy-to-eat slices.

KITCHEN TOOLS NEEDED
- Knife and cutting board

SNACK: ROASTED PUMPKIN SEEDS

INGREDIENTS
- A handful of roasted pumpkin seeds

PREPARATION TIME: NONE, READY TO EAT.

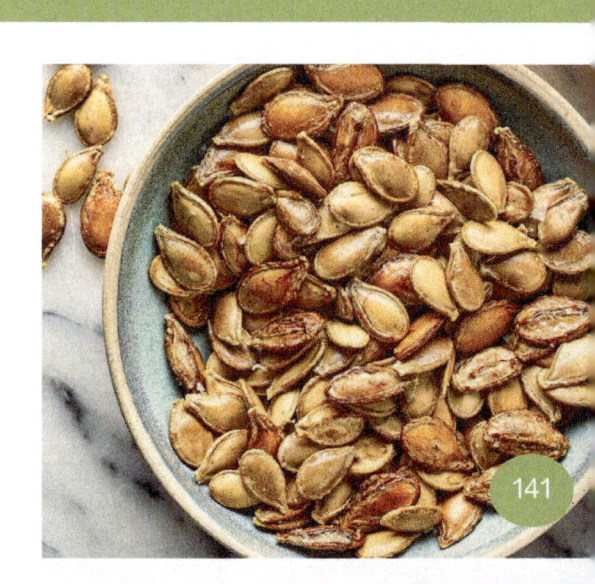

ASPARAGUS – THE ELEGANT AND NUTRITIOUS VEGETABLE

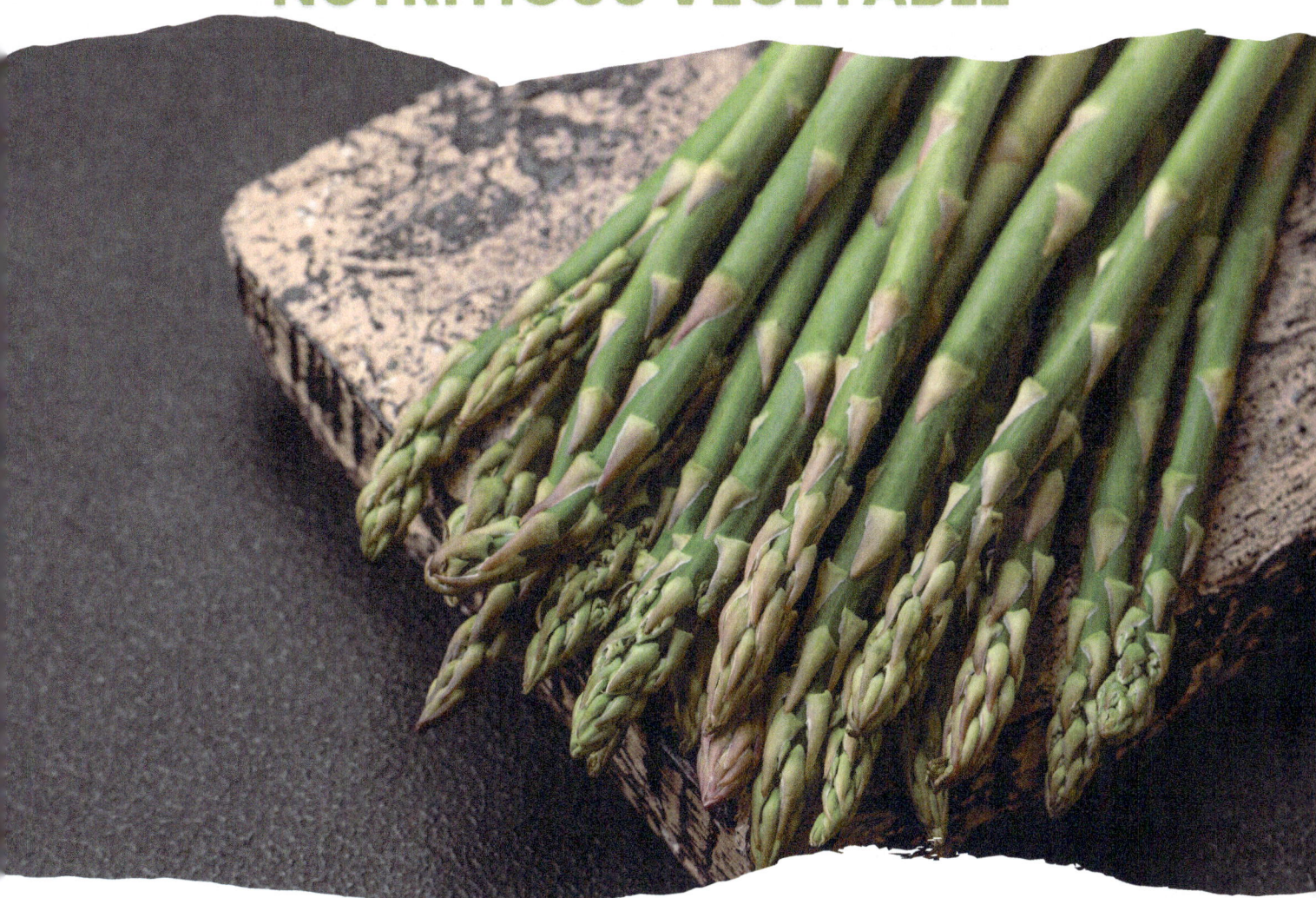

On Day 21, as we continue our Anti-Inflammatory Meal Plan, let's highlight asparagus, featured in our dinner. This slender, green vegetable is not just a side dish enhancer; it's a nutritional star, offering a host of health benefits, particularly in the realm of anti-inflammatory diets.

The Health Benefits of Asparagus

- Nutrient-Rich: Asparagus is loaded with essential nutrients, including vitamins A, C, E, K, and B vitamins, along with fiber, folate, and trace minerals like chromium.
- Anti-Inflammatory Properties: The array of antioxidants and anti-inflammatory compounds in asparagus, such as glutathione, help combat oxidative stress and may aid in reducing inflammation in the body.
- Digestive Health Support: High in fiber and a natural diuretic, asparagus promotes good digestive health and helps in detoxifying the body.

Incorporating Asparagus into Your Diet

- Versatile Cooking: Asparagus can be grilled, roasted, steamed, or sautéed. It's a perfect complement to a variety of dishes, including our baked chicken with quinoa tabbouleh.
- Enhancing Flavor and Nutrition: Its distinct, mildly earthy flavor enhances the overall taste of meals, while its nutrient content boosts their health benefits.

Asparagus's Role in a Balanced Diet

- Ideal for Weight Management: Low in calories yet high in water and fiber, asparagus is excellent for those focusing on weight management or general health maintenance.
- Promoting a Varied Vegetable Intake: Regularly including vegetables like asparagus in your diet ensures a diverse nutrient intake, essential for combating inflammation and maintaining overall health.

In conclusion, asparagus is a superb addition to an anti-inflammatory diet. Its rich nutrient profile, coupled with its versatility in cooking, makes it a delightful and healthful choice for enhancing meals. Enjoy asparagus in your culinary creations for both its flavor and the multitude of health benefits it brings to the table.

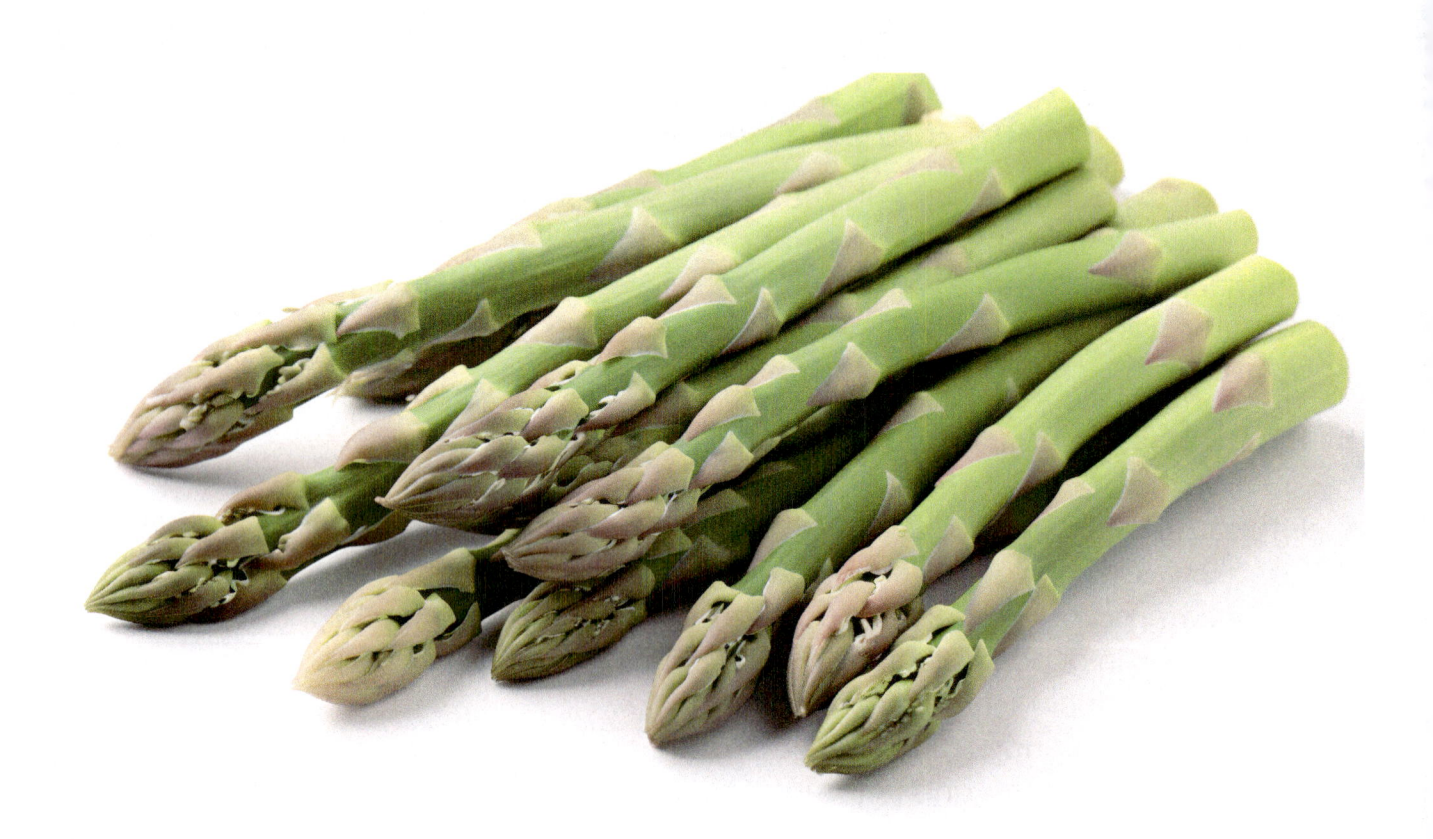

COMPLETION OF WEEK 3: A NOTE OF THANKS

Bravo on Completing Week 3!

You're now three-quarters through the Anti-Inflammatory Meal Plan. Your dedication to 'Mixing It Up' with creative and varied meals is commendable. Thank you for your continuous effort and for being an active participant in this health journey.

Celebrating Your Creativity and Progress

- Appreciation for Your Creativity: This week was all about creativity in the kitchen, and we're thankful for your willingness to experiment with new recipes and ideas.
- Acknowledging Your Journey: You're not just changing your diet; you're transforming your lifestyle. This takes courage and commitment, and we're so proud of the strides you've made.

Preparing for the Final Stretch

- Motivation for Week 4: As you move into Week 4, focus on sustainable swaps and long-term strategies. This is the perfect time to think about how you can continue these healthy habits beyond the meal plan.
- Recognizing Your Achievements: Every meal you've prepared and enjoyed is a testament to your dedication to better health. Keep this momentum going as you enter the final week of the plan.

As you reflect on Week 3, please use the Body Awareness Scale to assess the changes and benefits you've experienced. Your insights are valuable in tailoring the final week to your needs and preferences. Thank you for your incredible effort, and let's make Week 4 the best one yet!

WEEK 2 REFLECTION

After completing Week 3 of the Anti-Inflammatory Meal Plan, it's important to reflect on how your body has responded to the dietary changes. Use the following scale to rate your experiences in various aspects of your health and well-being. Rate each category from 1 to 10 (where 1 is 'no improvement' and 10 is 'significant improvement').

1. Digestive Comfort

- Question: How would you rate the overall comfort of your digestive system this week?
- Rating (1-10): _ _ _ _ _

2. Energy Levels

- Question: How do you feel about your energy levels after following the meal plan for a week?
- Rating (1-10): _ _ _ _ _

3. Sleep Quality

- Question: Have you noticed any changes in the quality of your sleep?
- Rating (1-10): _ _ _ _ _

4. Mood and Mental Clarity

- Question: How has your mood and mental clarity been affected by the dietary changes?
- Rating (1-10): _ _ _ _ _

5. Physical Comfort and Pain Levels

- Question: If you previously experienced any physical discomfort or pain, have you noticed any changes in its intensity or frequency?
- Rating (1-10): _ _ _ _ _

6. Skin Health

- Question: Have there been any noticeable changes in your skin health/appearance?
- Rating (1-10): _ _ _ _ _

7. Cravings and Appetite Control

- Question: How would you rate your control over cravings and appetite this week?
- Rating (1-10): _ _ _ _ _

8. Overall Well-being

- Question: Considering all factors, how would you rate your overall well-being after Week 1?
- Rating (1-10): _ _ _ _ _

Notes

Notes

- Daily Observations: Note any specific reactions or feelings on a day-to-day basis. This can include changes in mood, energy levels, digestive reactions, or any other physical or mental responses you notice.

- Dietary Adaptations: If you made any modifications to the meal plan, such as substituting ingredients or altering meal times, document these changes. This can help you understand how different foods or eating patterns affect you.

- Challenges and Successes: Reflect on any challenges you faced, such as cravings or difficulty in meal preparation, and how you addressed them. Also, celebrate successes, like resisting a particular craving or noticing positive changes in your health.

- Physical and Emotional Well-being: Expand on the ratings you provided by describing in more detail how you feel physically and emotionally. This could include noting any reduction in pain, improvements in skin health, or changes in mental clarity and mood.

- Future Adjustments: Based on your week's experience, jot down any thoughts on what you might want to try differently in the upcoming week. This could be trying new recipes, adjusting portion sizes, or incorporating more of a particular type of food.

- Questions and Research: If you have questions or areas of curiosity that arose during the week, such as the effects of certain foods or why you experienced specific reactions, note these down. You can then research these topics or discuss them with a healthcare professional.

- Overall Reflection: Conclude with a general reflection on how the week went, what you learned about your body's response to the diet, and how you feel about continuing with the meal plan.

DAY 22 MEAL PLAN

BREAKFAST: AVOCADO AND EGG SALAD ON WHOLE-GRAIN TOAST
LUNCH: GRILLED PORTOBELLO MUSHROOM BURGER WITH SWEET POTATO FRIES
DINNER: BAKED HADDOCK WITH LEMON-HERB DRESSING AND QUINOA ARUGULA SALAD
SNACK: CUCUMBER SLICES WITH BEETROOT HUMMUS
SNACK: MIXED NUTS
DRINK: NETTLE TEA

BREAKFAST: AVOCADO AND EGG SALAD ON WHOLE-GRAIN TOAST

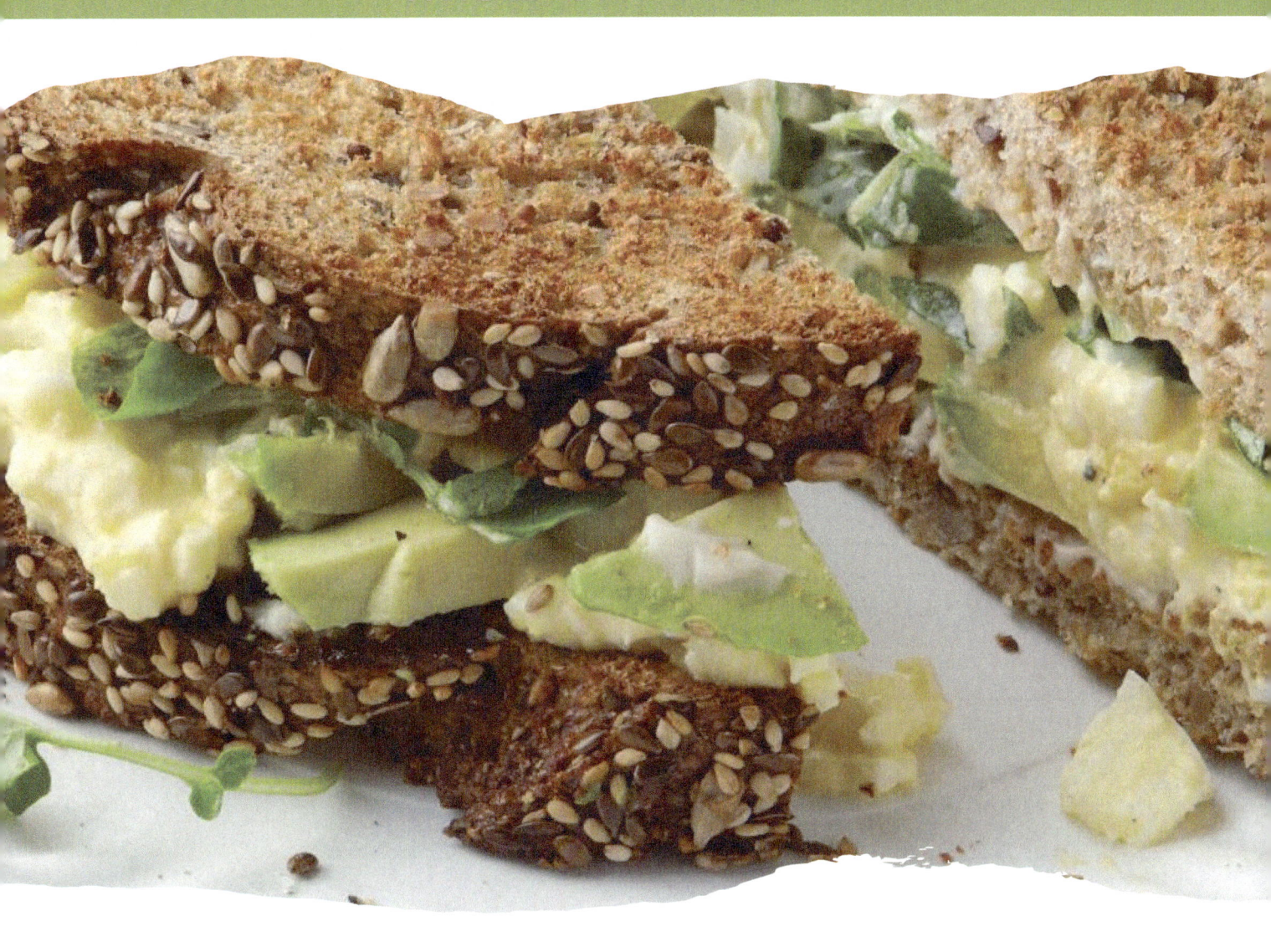

INGREDIENTS

- 2 eggs, hard-boiled and chopped
- 1 ripe avocado, mashed
- Whole-grain bread
- Salt, pepper, and lemon juice for seasoning

INSTRUCTIONS

- Prepare Egg Salad: Mix chopped eggs with mashed avocado. Season with salt, pepper, and a squeeze of lemon juice.
- Toast Bread: Toast whole-grain bread slices.
- Assemble: Spread egg salad on toast.

KITCHEN TOOLS NEEDED
- Knife and cutting board
- Bowl for mixing
- Toaster

LUNCH: GRILLED PORTOBELLO MUSHROOM BURGER WITH SWEET POTATO FRIES

INGREDIENTS

- Portobello mushrooms
- Whole-grain burger buns
- Lettuce, tomato, and other desired toppings
- Sweet potatoes, cut into fries
- Olive oil, salt, and spices for seasoning

INSTRUCTIONS

- Prepare and Grill Mushrooms: Clean portobello mushrooms, grill until tender.
- Bake Sweet Potato Fries: Toss sweet potato fries with olive oil and spices, bake until crispy.
- Assemble Burger: Place grilled mushrooms on buns with lettuce, tomato, and other toppings.
- Serve: Enjoy the burger with a side of sweet potato fries.

KITCHEN TOOLS NEEDED
- Grill or grill pan
- Oven for baking fries
- Knife and cutting board

DINNER: BAKED HADDOCK WITH LEMON-HERB DRESSING AND QUINOA ARUGULA SALAD

INGREDIENTS

- Haddock fillets
- Lemon juice, olive oil, herbs for dressing
- Quinoa
- Arugula
- Cherry tomatoes, cucumber, and other salad ingredients

INSTRUCTIONS

- Bake Haddock: Season haddock and bake with lemon-herb dressing.
- Cook Quinoa: Prepare quinoa as per package instructions.
- Prepare Salad: Toss arugula, cherry tomatoes, cucumber, and cooked quinoa.
- Serve: Plate the baked haddock with a side of quinoa and arugula salad.

KITCHEN TOOLS NEEDED
- Oven for baking haddock
- Pot for quinoa
- Mixing bowl

DRINK: NETTLE TEA

INGREDIENTS
- 1 nettle tea bag
- 1 cup boiling water

INSTRUCTIONS
- Boil Water: Heat the water.
- Steep Tea: Place the tea bag in a mug, pour hot water over it.

KITCHEN TOOLS NEEDED
- Kettle or pot for boiling water
- Mug

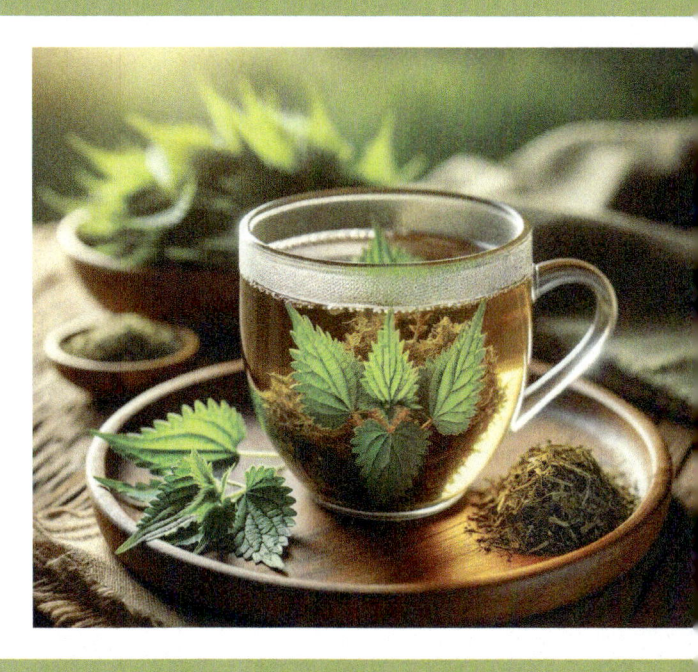

SNACK: CUCUMBER SLICES WITH BEETROOT HUMMUS

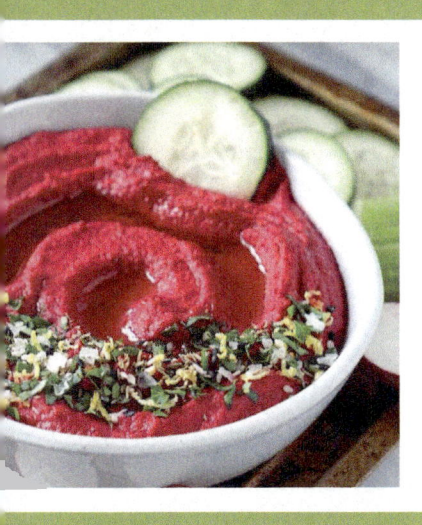

INGREDIENTS
- Cucumber, sliced
- Beetroot hummus

INSTRUCTIONS
- Prepare Snack: Slice cucumber and serve with a bowl of beetroot hummus for dipping.

KITCHEN TOOLS NEEDED
- Knife and cutting board

SNACK: MIXED NUTS

INGREDIENTS
- A small serving of mixed nuts (almonds, walnuts, cashews)

PREPARATION TIME: NONE, READY TO EAT.

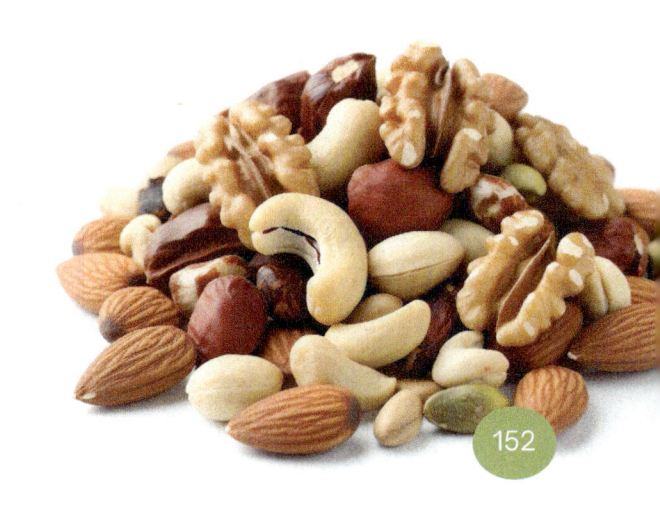

SWEET POTATO FRIES VS. REGULAR FRIES: A NUTRITIONAL COMPARISON

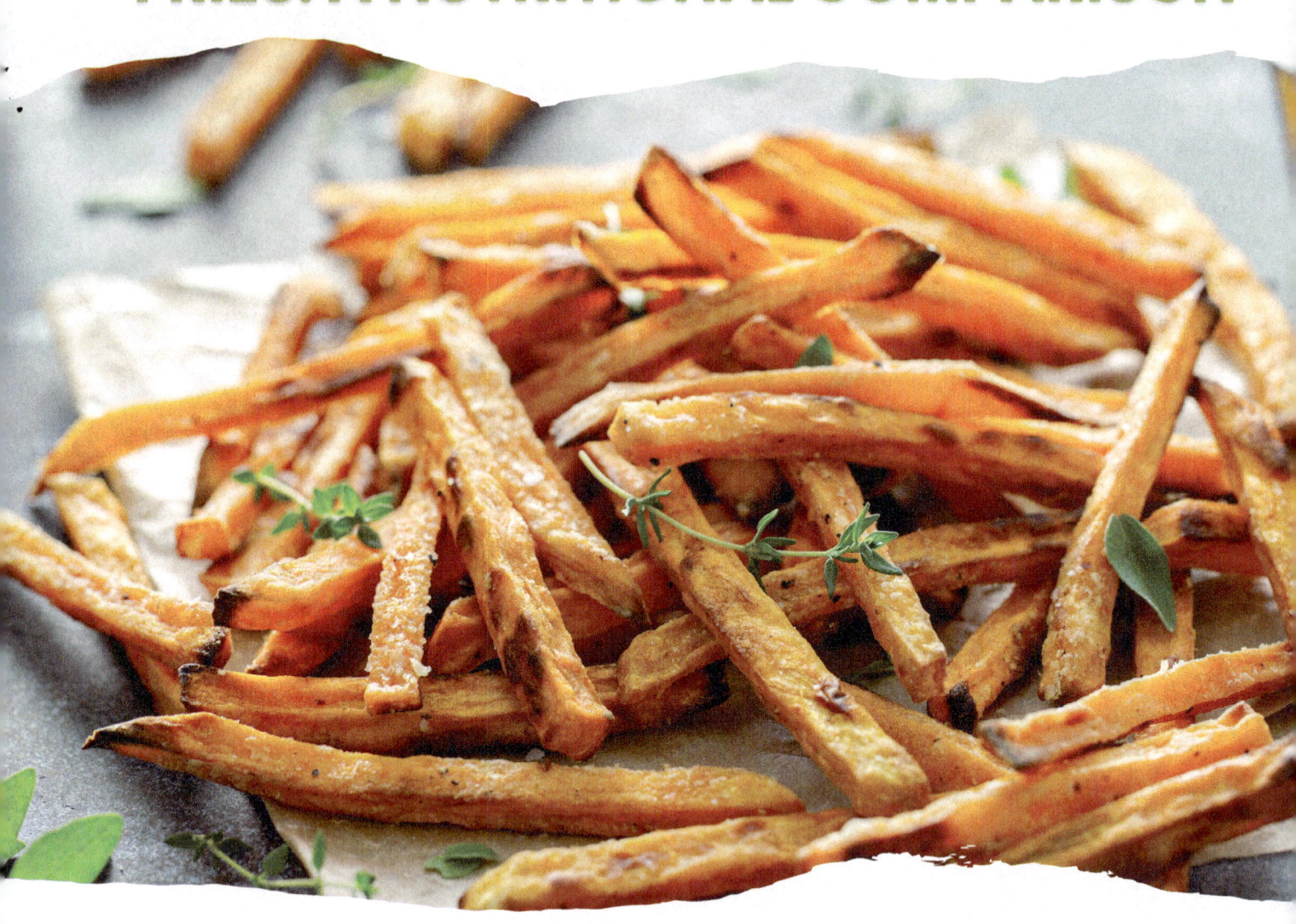

On Day 22 of our Anti-Inflammatory Meal Plan, we've chosen sweet potato fries as a side for lunch. This choice invites a comparison with regular fries, typically made from white potatoes. Both can be a delicious treat, but when it comes to nutritional value and health benefits, particularly in an anti-inflammatory diet, sweet potato fries have a distinct edge.

Nutritional Profile and Health Benefits

- Sweet Potato Fries:
    - Rich in Vitamins: Sweet potatoes are high in vitamins A and C, which are potent antioxidants. Vitamin A is crucial for eye health, immune function, and skin health.
    - Lower Glycemic Index: They have a lower glycemic index compared to white potatoes, meaning they cause a slower rise in blood sugar levels. This makes them a better choice for blood sugar management.
    - Dietary Fiber: Sweet potatoes are a good source of dietary fiber, which is beneficial for digestive health and can aid in weight management.

- Regular Fries:
    - Potassium Source: White potatoes provide potassium, which is essential for heart health and muscle function.
    - B Vitamins: They offer some B vitamins necessary for energy metabolism.
    - Higher Glycemic Index: Regular fries made from white potatoes have a higher glycemic index, which can lead to quicker spikes in blood sugar levels.

Preparation Method Matters

- Baked vs. Fried: How the fries are prepared can significantly impact their healthiness. Baking either type of fries, as we do with our sweet potato fries, is a healthier option than deep frying, reducing the calorie and fat content.

In the Context of an Anti-Inflammatory Diet

- Sweet Potato Fries as a Healthier Alternative: Given their nutrient richness, lower glycemic index, and high levels of antioxidants, sweet potato fries are a more favorable choice in an anti-inflammatory diet.
- Moderation is Key: Regardless of the type, fries should be consumed in moderation as part of a balanced diet.

In summary, while both sweet potato fries and regular fries can fit into a balanced diet, sweet potato fries offer greater nutritional benefits, particularly for those managing inflammation and blood sugar levels. Their rich flavor, coupled with health benefits, makes them a delightful and sensible choice for a meal accompaniment.

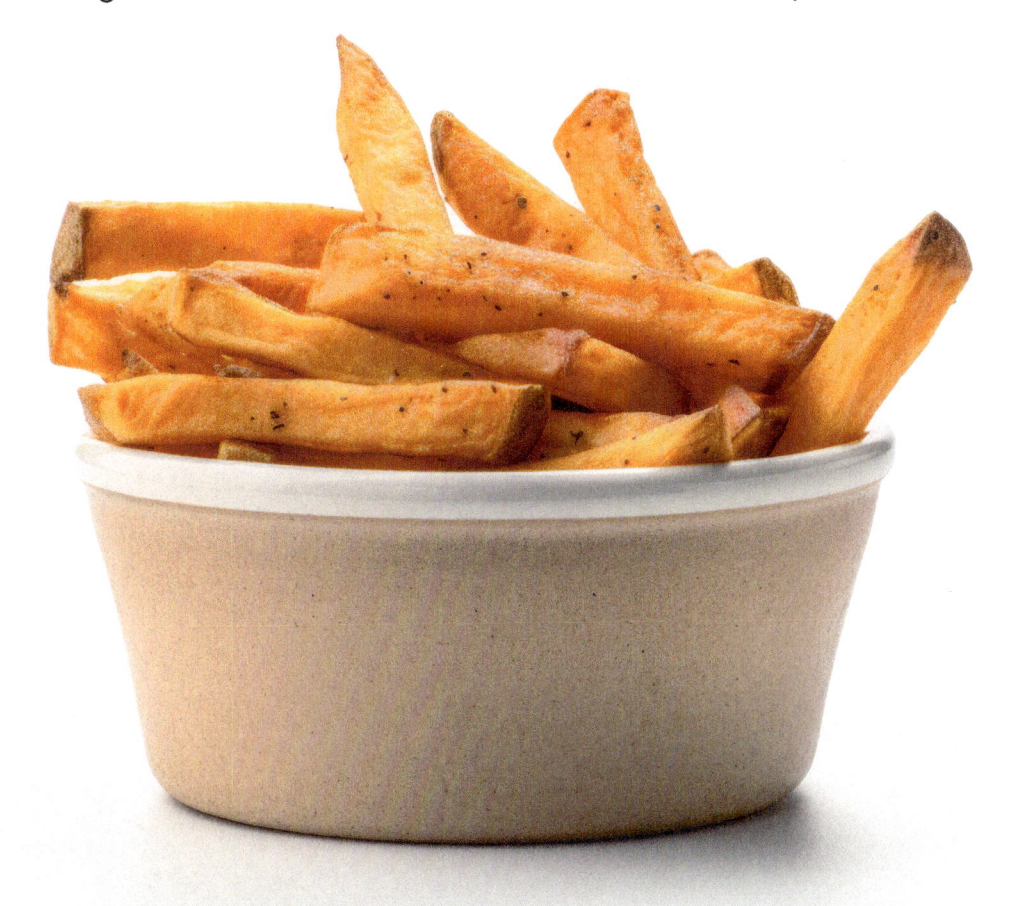

DAY 23 MEAL PLAN

BREAKFAST: PROTEIN SMOOTHIE WITH SPINACH, ALMOND BUTTER, AND COCONUT MILK
LUNCH: LENTIL AND VEGETABLE STEW
DINNER: GRILLED CHICKEN WITH ROASTED MEDITERRANEAN VEGETABLES AND FARRO
SNACK: A SMALL HANDFUL OF OLIVES
SNACK: A MEDIUM-SIZED PEAR
DRINK: ROOIBOS TEA

BREAKFAST: PROTEIN SMOOTHIE WITH SPINACH, ALMOND BUTTER, AND COCONUT MILK

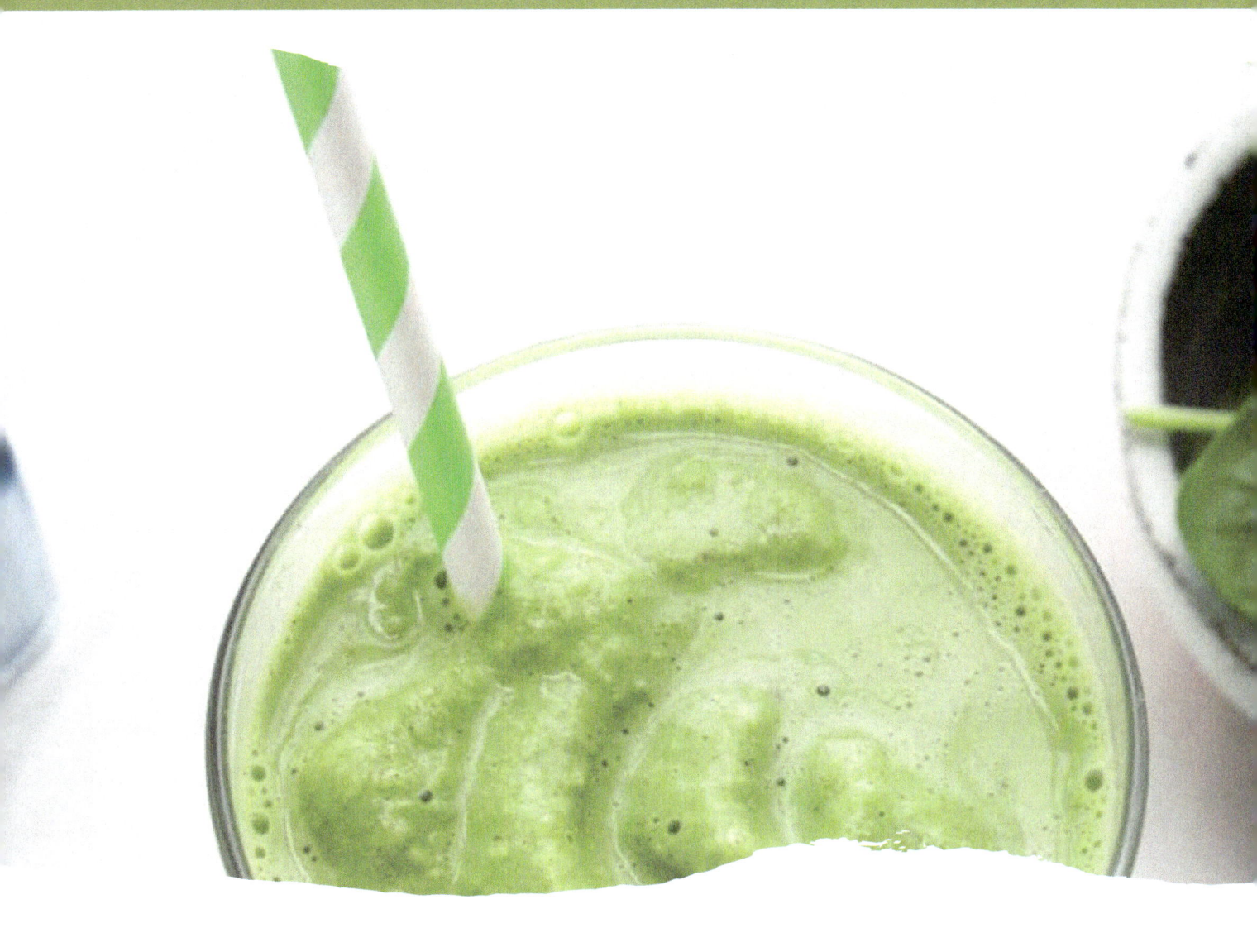

INGREDIENTS

- 1 cup spinach leaves
- 1 tablespoon almond butter
- 1 cup coconut milk
- Protein powder (optional)
- Ice cubes (optional)

INSTRUCTIONS

- Blend Ingredients: Combine spinach, almond butter, coconut milk, and protein powder in the blender.
- Add Ice: Add ice if you prefer a colder smoothie.
- Blend until Smooth: Blend until all ingredients are well combined.

KITCHEN TOOLS NEEDED

- Blender
- Measuring cups and spoons

LUNCH: LENTIL AND VEGETABLE STEW

INGREDIENTS

- 1 cup lentils
- Assorted vegetables (carrots, celery, onion, tomatoes)
- Vegetable broth or water
- Herbs and spices (such as thyme, bay leaf, garlic)

INSTRUCTIONS

- Cook Stew: Sauté vegetables, add lentils and broth, and simmer until lentils are tender.
- Season: Add herbs and spices for flavor.

KITCHEN TOOLS NEEDED

- Pot
- Knife and cutting board

DINNER: GRILLED CHICKEN WITH ROASTED MEDITERRANEAN VEGETABLES AND FARRO

INGREDIENTS

- Chicken breasts
- Mediterranean vegetables (zucchini, bell peppers, eggplant)
- Farro
- Olive oil, herbs, salt, and pepper for seasoning

INSTRUCTIONS

- Grill Chicken: Season chicken breasts and grill until cooked through.
- Roast Vegetables: Toss vegetables with olive oil and herbs, roast in the oven.
- Cook Farro: Prepare farro as per package instructions.
- Serve: Plate the grilled chicken with roasted vegetables and a side of farro.

KITCHEN TOOLS NEEDED

- Grill or grill pan
- Oven for roasting vegetables
- Pot for cooking farro
- Knife and cutting board

DRINK: ROOIBOS TEA

INGREDIENTS
- 1 rooibos tea bag
- 1 cup boiling water

INSTRUCTIONS
- Boil Water: Heat the water.
- Steep Tea: Place the tea bag in a mug, pour hot water over it.

KITCHEN TOOLS NEEDED
- Kettle or pot for boiling water
- Mug

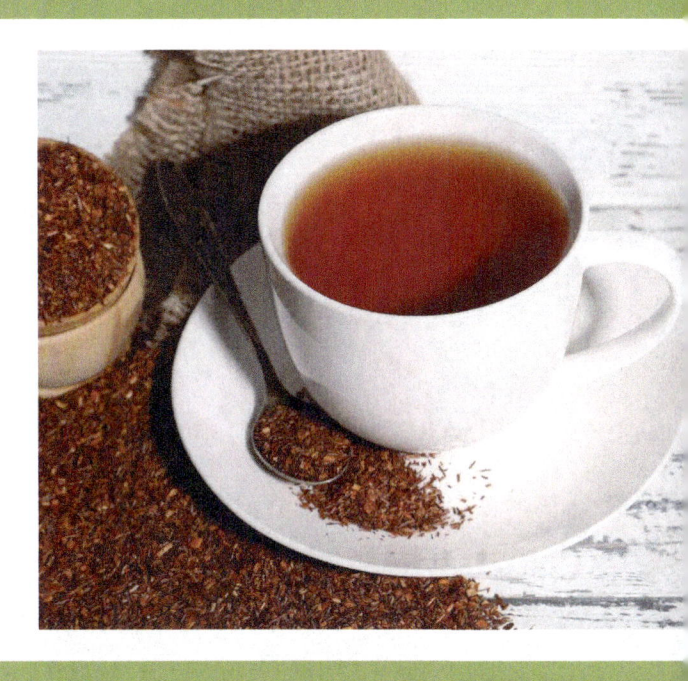

SNACK: A MEDIUM-SIZED PEAR

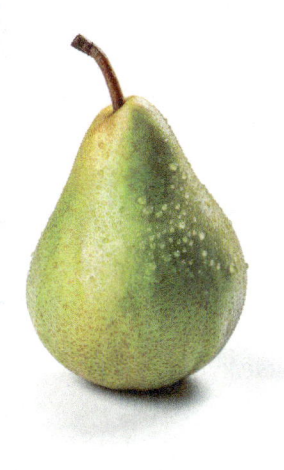

INGREDIENTS
- 1 medium-sized pear

PREPARATION TIME: NONE, READY TO EAT.

SNACK: A SMALL HANDFUL OF OLIVES

INGREDIENTS
- A small handful of olives (green or black)

PREPARATION TIME: NONE, READY TO EAT.

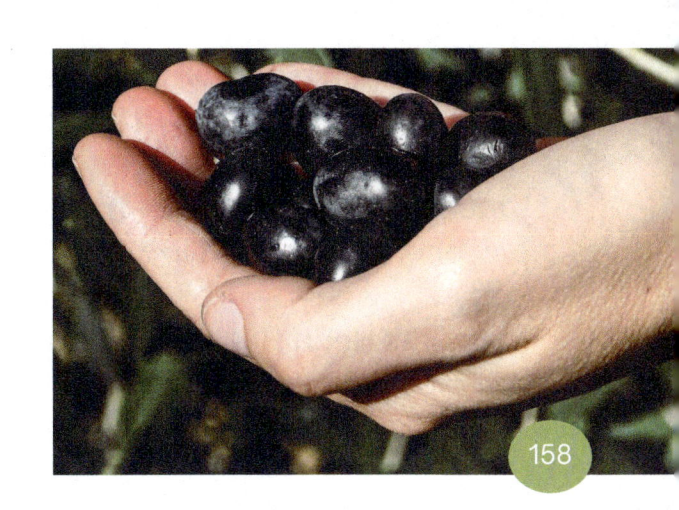

OLIVES - THE FLAVORFUL AND NUTRIENT-RICH FRUIT

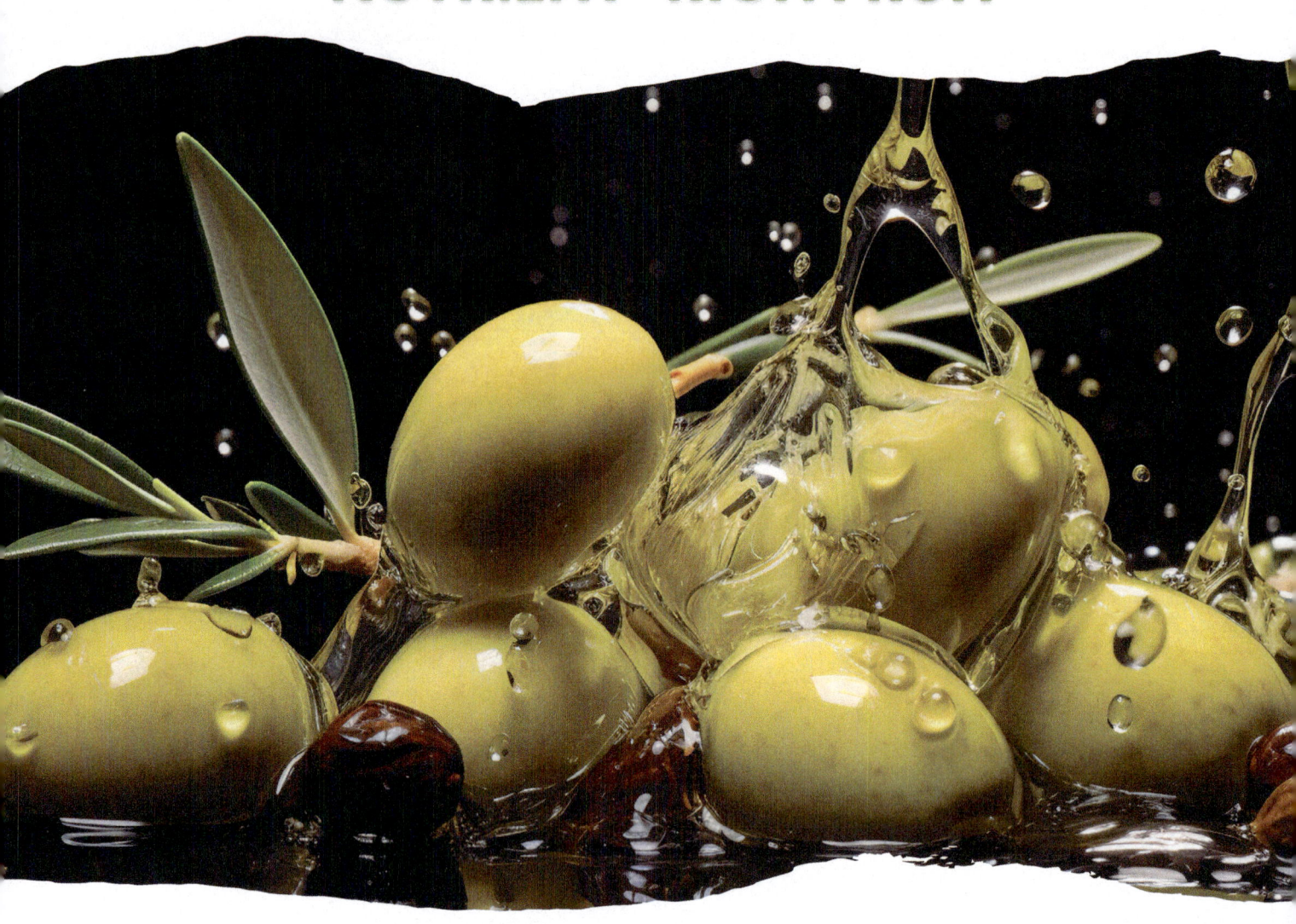

On Day 23 of our Anti-Inflammatory Meal Plan, we introduce olives as a snack. These small fruits are renowned not just for their unique flavor but also for their impressive array of health benefits, making them an excellent addition to an inflammation-conscious diet.

The Health Benefits of Olives

- Rich in Healthy Fats: Olives are a great source of monounsaturated fats, particularly oleic acid, which is known for its heart health benefits and anti-inflammatory properties.
- Loaded with Antioxidants: They are high in antioxidants, including vitamin E and polyphenols, which help combat oxidative stress and reduce inflammation in the body.
- Promotes Heart Health: The healthy fats in olives contribute to improved heart health by helping to regulate cholesterol levels and reducing the risk of heart disease.

Incorporating Olives into Your Diet

- Versatile in Use: Olives can be enjoyed as a snack on their own, added to salads, or used to enhance the flavor of various dishes, such as the roasted Mediterranean vegetables in our dinner recipe.
- A Flavor Booster: Their salty, tangy taste makes them a perfect flavor enhancer, adding depth to both savory and some sweet dishes.

Olives' Role in a Balanced Diet

- A Nutrient-Dense Snack Option: Olives provide essential nutrients without the high calorie count, making them an ideal snack for those mindful of their overall health and calorie intake.
- Encouraging Varied Healthy Fat Sources: Regularly including healthy fat sources like olives in your diet ensures a balanced intake of essential fatty acids, important for maintaining good health.

In conclusion, olives are a fantastic addition to an anti-inflammatory diet. Their combination of healthy fats, antioxidants, and unique flavor profile makes them a valuable food choice for enhancing overall health and adding zest to your meals. Enjoy olives in your daily diet to benefit from their nutritious and flavorful properties.

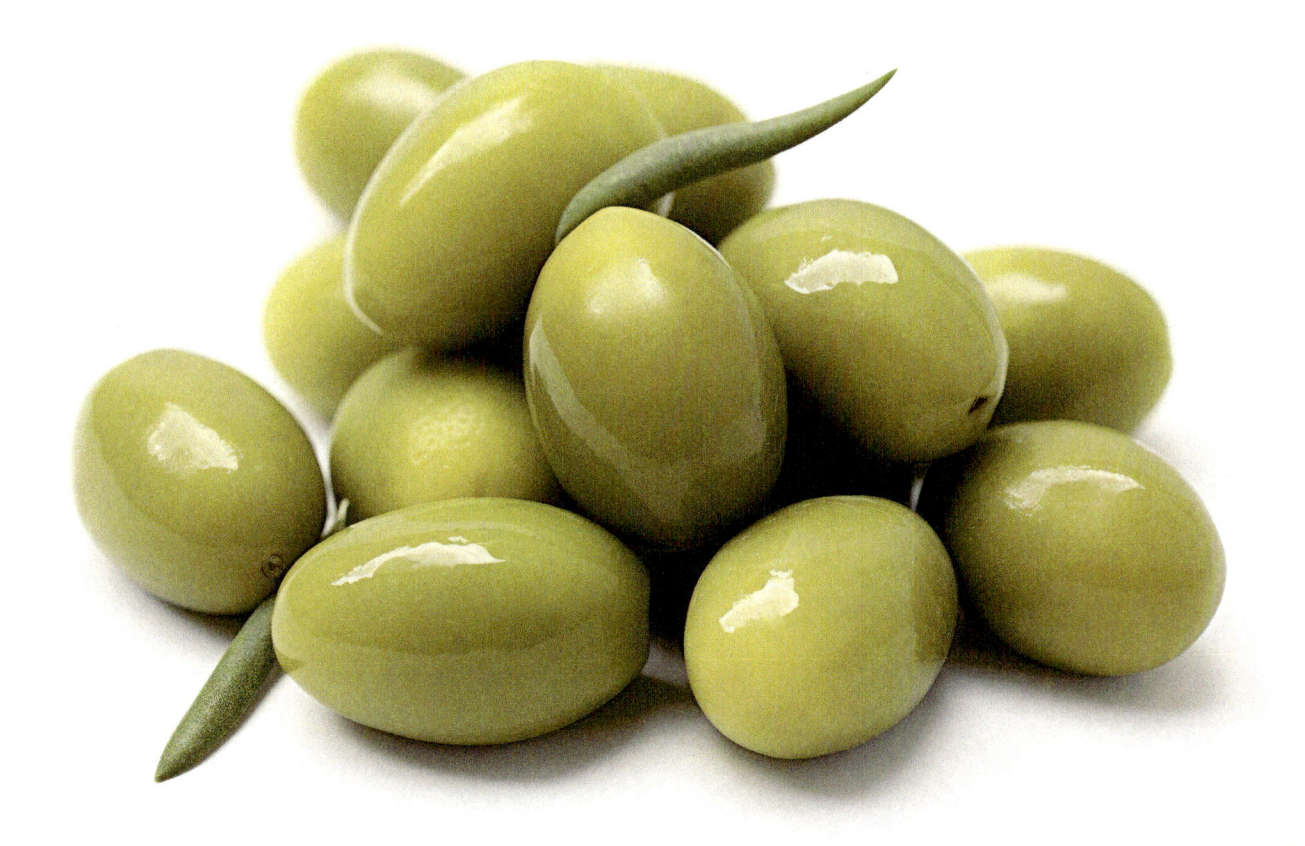

DAY 24 MEAL PLAN

BREAKFAST: BUCKWHEAT PORRIDGE WITH BERRIES AND CHIA SEEDS
LUNCH: RAINBOW SALAD
DINNER: VEGETABLE STIR-FRY WITH TOFU AND BROWN RICE
SNACK: APPLE SLICES WITH ALMOND BUTTER
SNACK: DARK CHOCOLATE
DRINK: CUCUMBER AND MINT INFUSED WATER

BREAKFAST: BUCKWHEAT PORRIDGE WITH BERRIES AND CHIA SEEDS

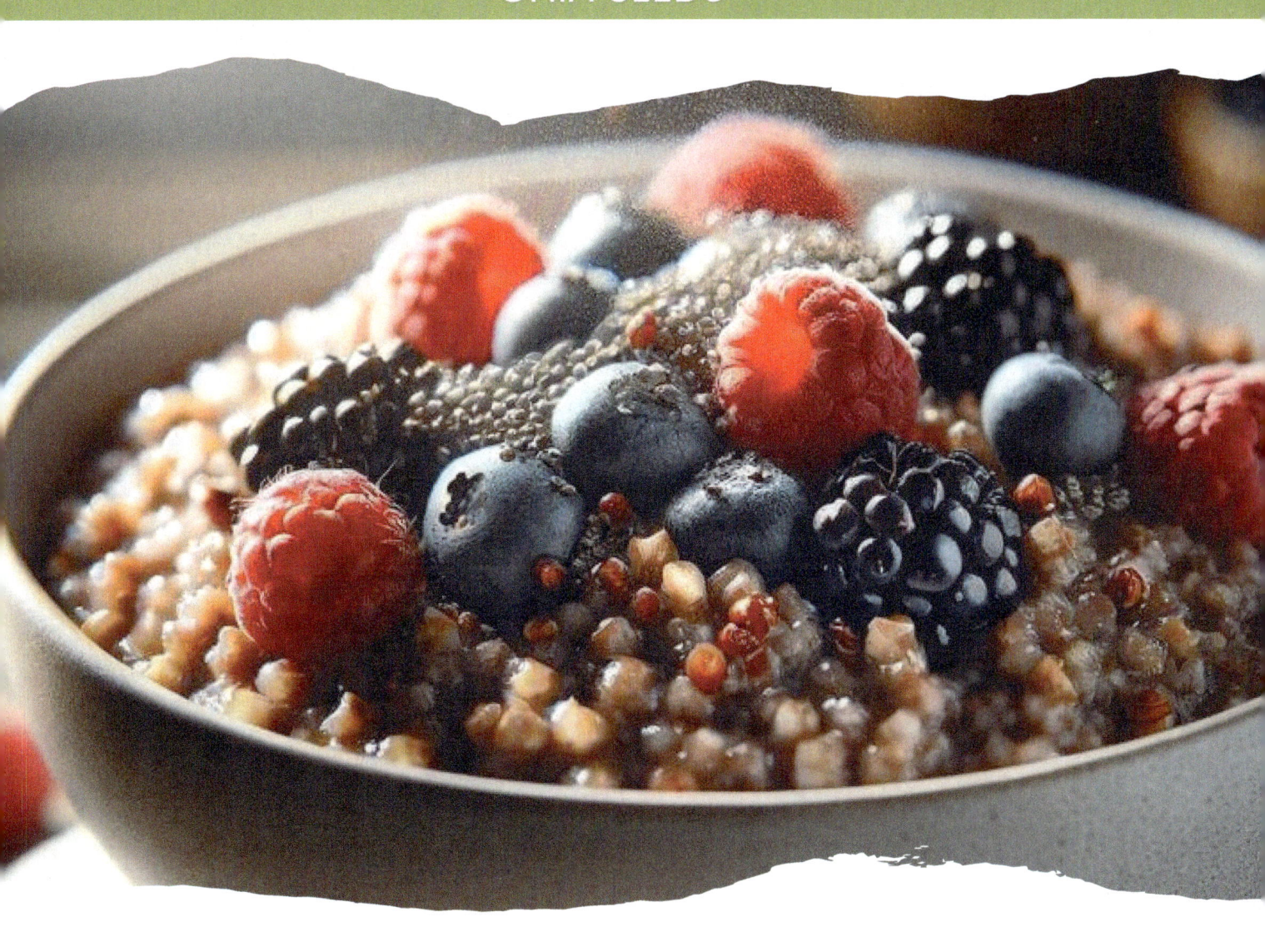

INGREDIENTS

- ½ cup buckwheat groats
- 1 cup water or milk (dairy or plant-based)
- Mixed berries (fresh or frozen)
- A sprinkle of chia seeds

INSTRUCTIONS

- Cook Buckwheat: Rinse buckwheat groats and cook in water or milk until soft.
- Serve: Top the porridge with berries and a sprinkle of chia seeds.

KITCHEN TOOLS NEEDED	- Pot - Bowl - Spoon

LUNCH: RAINBOW SALAD

INGREDIENTS

- Mixed greens (spinach, arugula, lettuce)
- Bell peppers, sliced
- Carrots, grated or sliced
- Vinaigrette dressing (olive oil, vinegar, mustard, honey)

INSTRUCTIONS

- Prepare Salad: Combine mixed greens, bell peppers, and carrots in a salad bowl.
- Dress Salad: Toss with vinaigrette dressing before serving.

KITCHEN TOOLS NEEDED
- Salad bowl
- Knife and cutting board

DINNER: VEGETABLE STIR-FRY WITH TOFU AND BROWN RICE

INGREDIENTS

- Assorted vegetables (broccoli, bell peppers, snap peas)
- Tofu, cubed
- Brown rice
- Stir-fry sauce (soy sauce, ginger, garlic, sesame oil)

INSTRUCTIONS

- Cook Rice: Prepare brown rice as per package instructions.
- Stir-Fry Vegetables and Tofu: Stir-fry tofu until golden, add vegetables and sauce, cook until veggies are tender.
- Serve: Serve the stir-fry over a bed of brown rice.

KITCHEN TOOLS NEEDED
- Wok or frying pan
- Pot for rice
- Knife and cutting board

DRINK: CUCUMBER AND MINT INFUSED WATER

INGREDIENTS

- Cucumber, thinly sliced
- Fresh mint leaves
- Water

INSTRUCTIONS

- Prepare Infused Water: Add cucumber slices and mint leaves to a pitcher of water.
- Infuse: Let it sit for an hour or more to infuse the flavors.

KITCHEN TOOLS NEEDED

- Pitcher or jar

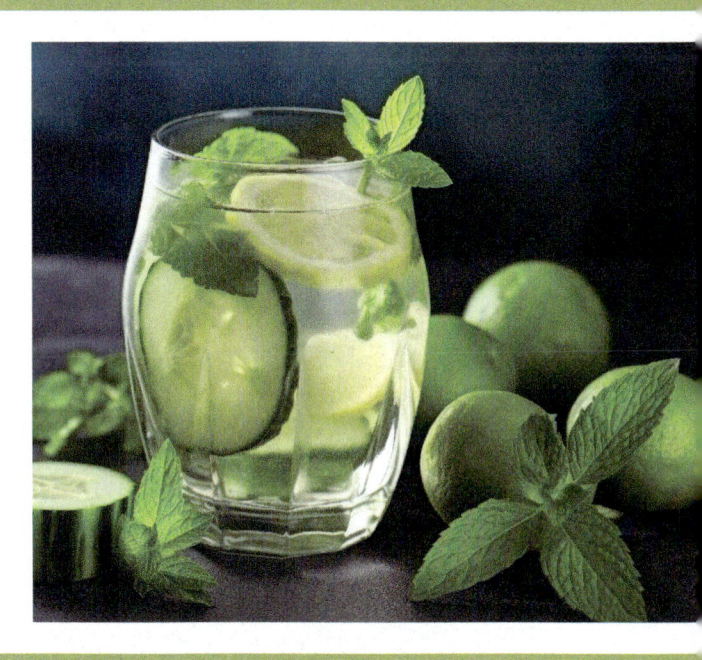

SNACK: APPLE SLICES WITH ALMOND BUTTER

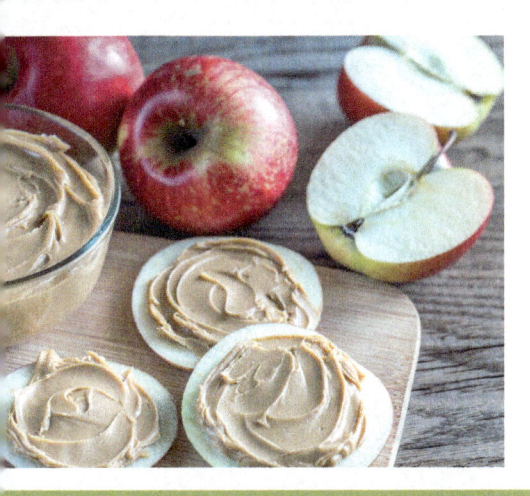

INGREDIENTS

- 1 apple, sliced
- Almond butter for dipping

INSTRUCTIONS

- Prepare Snack: Slice the apple and serve with a side of almond butter for dipping.

KITCHEN TOOLS NEEDED

- Knife and cutting board

SNACK: DARK CHOCOLATE

INGREDIENTS

- A few pieces of dark chocolate (70% cocoa or more)

PREPARATION TIME: NONE, READY TO EAT.

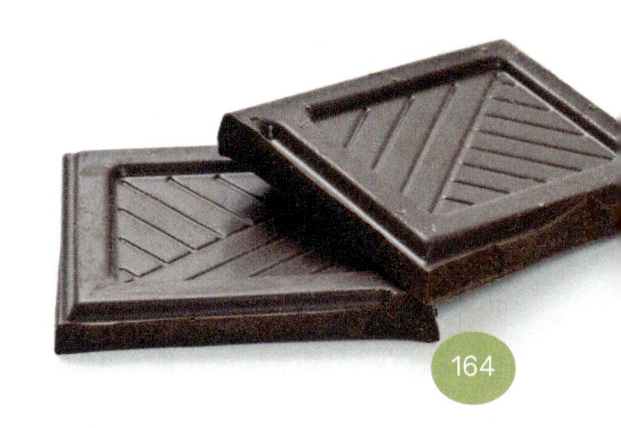

DARK CHOCOLATE – THE DELICIOUS ANTIOXIDANT TREAT

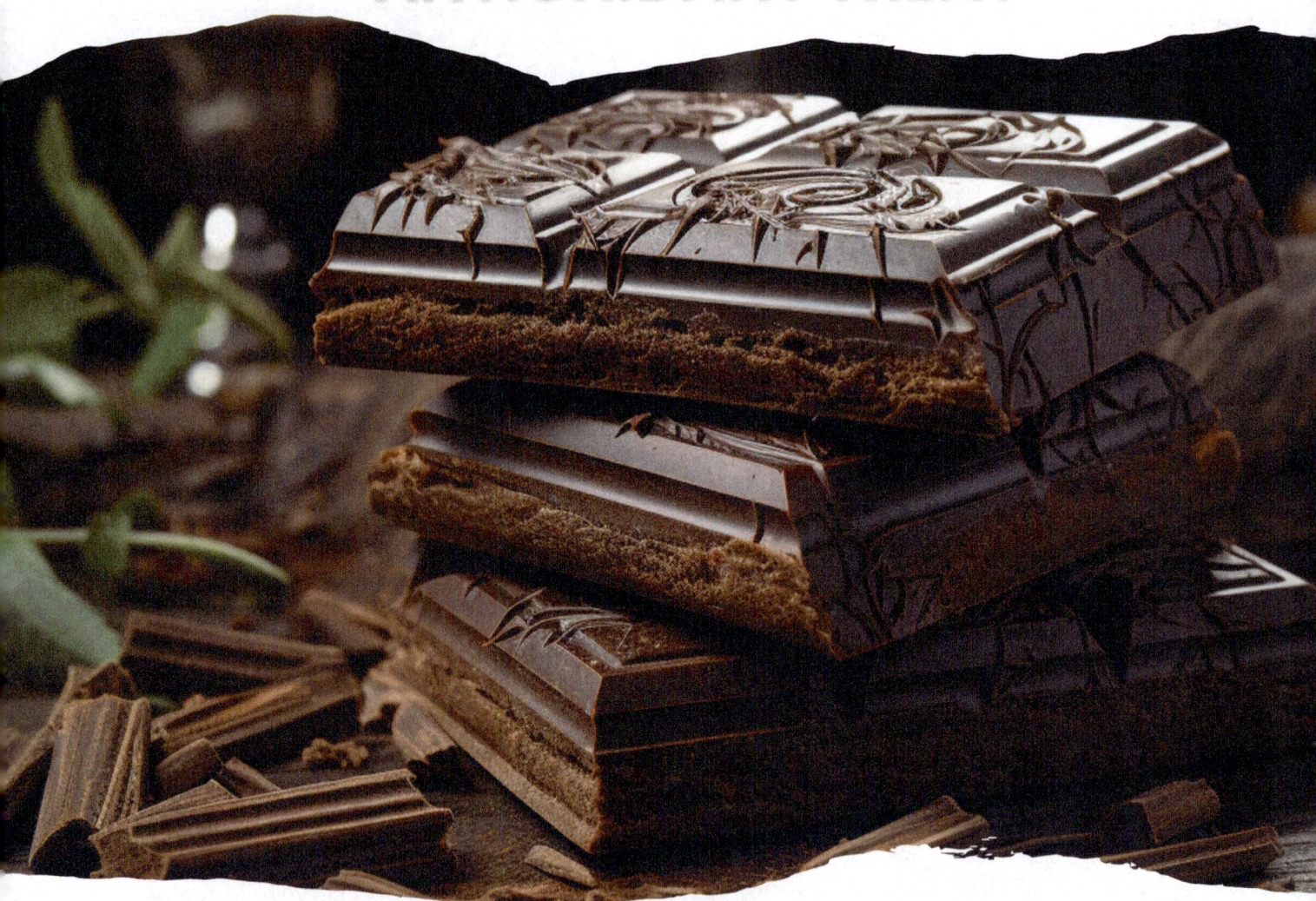

On Day 24 of our Anti-Inflammatory Meal Plan, we delight in a snack of dark chocolate. Beyond its rich and indulgent taste, dark chocolate is lauded for its health benefits, especially when it contains a high percentage of cocoa. It's a sweet treat that can actually be good for you, particularly in the context of an anti-inflammatory diet.

The Healthful Allure of Dark Chocolate

- Rich in Flavonoids: Dark chocolate with at least 70% cocoa is packed with flavonoids, a group of antioxidants known for their anti-inflammatory properties. These compounds can help reduce inflammation and have been linked to various health benefits.
- Heart Health: The antioxidants in dark chocolate contribute to improved heart health by enhancing blood flow, reducing blood pressure, and lowering the risk of heart disease.
- Mood Booster: Dark chocolate is known to stimulate the production of endorphins, the body's natural "feel-good" chemicals. It also contains serotonin, a neurotransmitter that acts as an anti-depressant.

Incorporating Dark Chocolate into Your Diet

- A Mindful Indulgence: Enjoying a few pieces of dark chocolate as a snack, as in our meal plan, can satisfy sweet cravings while still providing health benefits.
- Balance and Moderation: While dark chocolate is beneficial, it's also high in calories and can be rich in sugars, especially in lower cocoa percentages. It's best enjoyed in moderation.

Dark Chocolate's Role in a Balanced Diet

- Satisfying Sweetness with Benefits: Dark chocolate offers a way to indulge in something sweet without the negative effects often associated with sugary treats.
- A Versatile Ingredient: Besides being a snack, dark chocolate can be used in baking, added to oatmeal or yogurt, or melted and drizzled over fruits for a delicious and healthful dessert.

In conclusion, dark chocolate is a delightful addition to an anti-inflammatory diet. Its rich flavor and antioxidant content make it not just a treat for the taste buds but also a contributor to overall health. Enjoy dark chocolate in moderation as part of your diverse and nutritious diet.

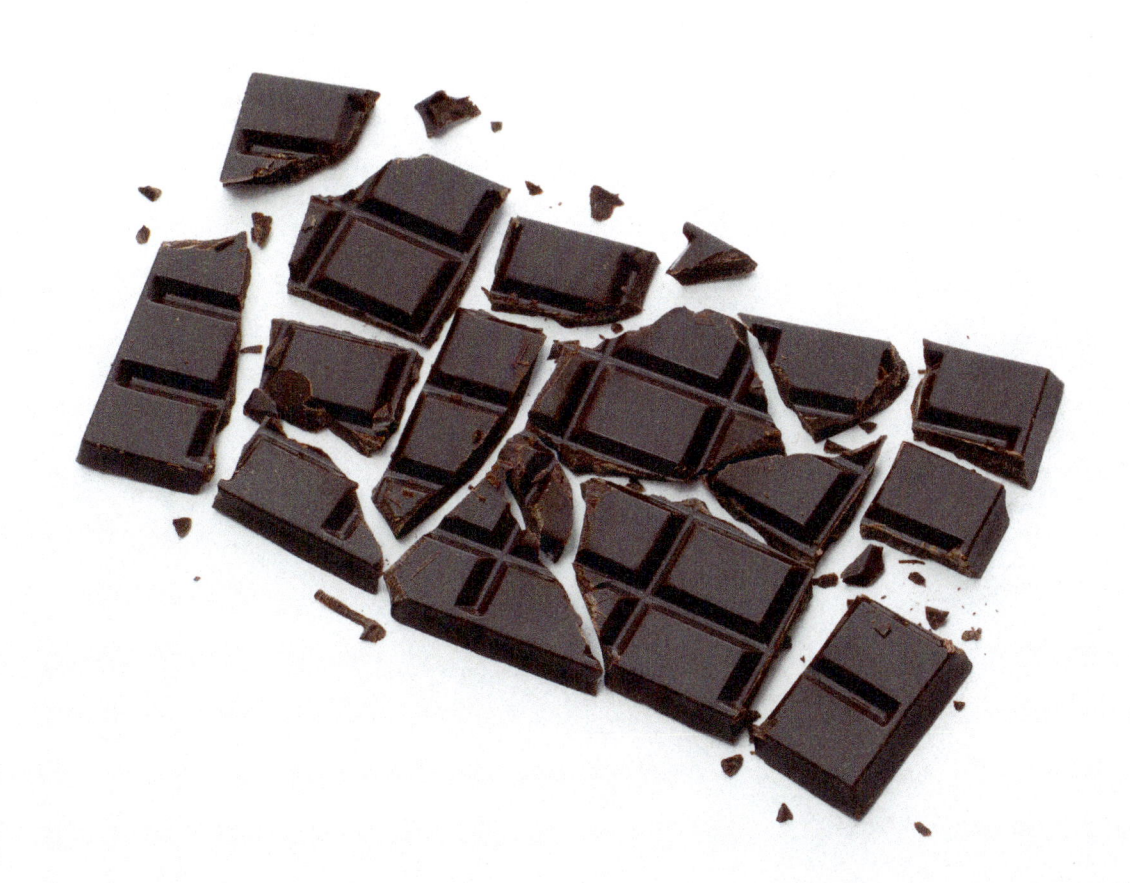

DAY 25 MEAL PLAN

BREAKFAST: GREEK YOGURT WITH GRANOLA AND MAPLE SYRUP
LUNCH: TURKEY AND AVOCADO WRAP
DINNER: GRILLED SALMON WITH DILL SAUCE AND STEAMED ASPARAGUS
SNACK: FRESH PINEAPPLE
SNACK: A SMALL BANANA
DRINK: GINGER AND LEMON TEA

BREAKFAST: GREEK YOGURT WITH GRANOLA AND MAPLE SYRUP

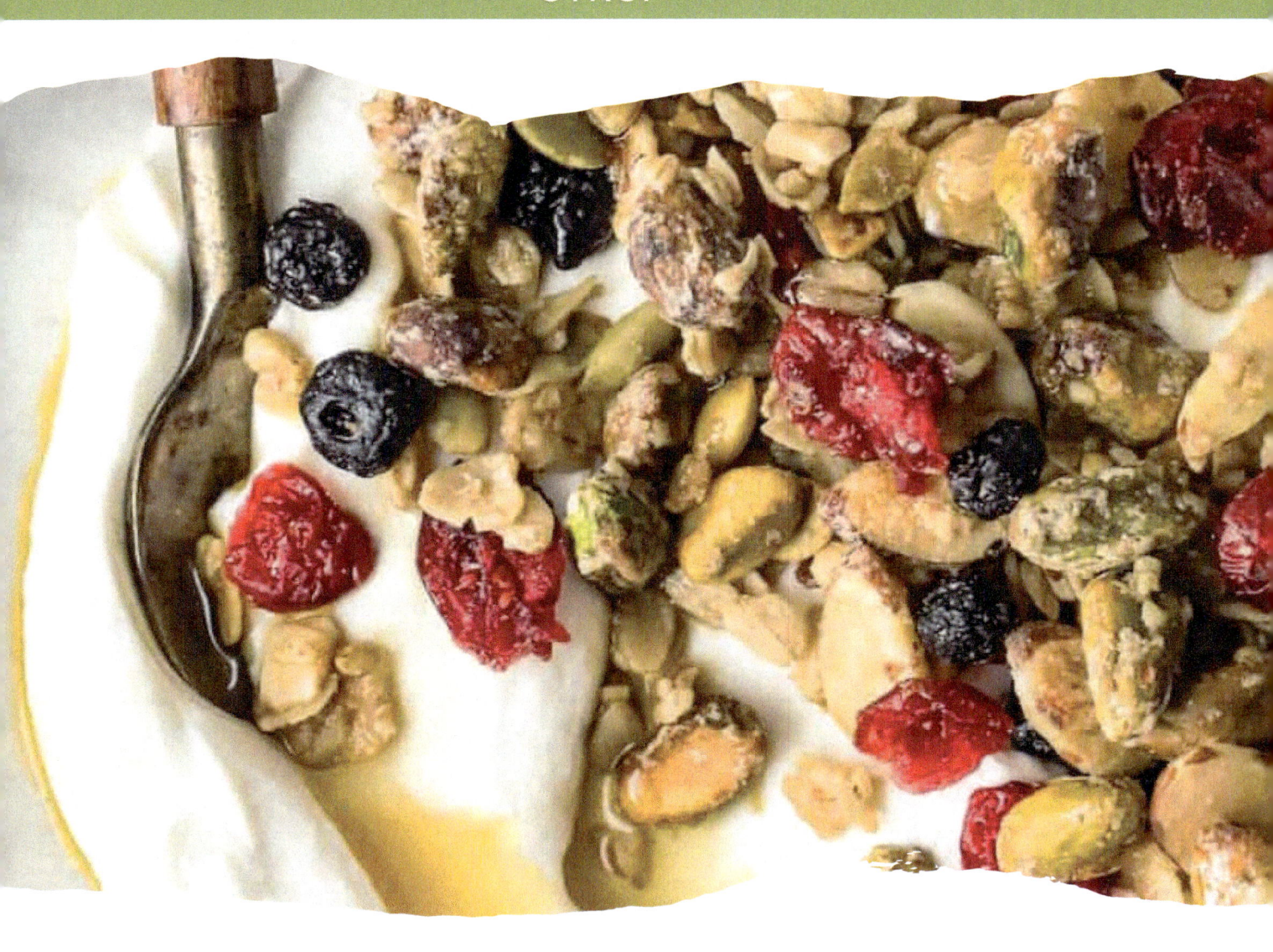

INGREDIENTS

- 1 cup Greek yogurt (plain or unsweetened)
- ½ cup granola
- Maple syrup for drizzling

INSTRUCTIONS

- Serve Yogurt: Scoop Greek yogurt into a bowl.
- Add Granola: Sprinkle granola on top.
- Drizzle Maple Syrup: Finish with a drizzle of maple syrup.

KITCHEN TOOLS NEEDED

- Bowl
- Spoon

LUNCH: TURKEY AND AVOCADO WRAP

INGREDIENTS

- Whole-grain tortilla
- Sliced turkey breast
- Sliced avocado
- Lettuce or spinach leaves
- Mustard or hummus for spreading (optional)

INSTRUCTIONS

- Assemble Wrap: Spread mustard or hummus on the tortilla, layer with turkey, avocado, and lettuce/spinach.
- Roll and Serve: Roll up the tortilla tightly, cut in half if desired.

KITCHEN TOOLS NEEDED

- Knife and cutting board

DINNER: GRILLED SALMON WITH DILL SAUCE AND STEAMED ASPARAGUS

INGREDIENTS

- Salmon fillets
- Fresh dill, lemon juice, and yogurt or mayo for the sauce
- Asparagus spears

INSTRUCTIONS

- Grill Salmon: Season salmon fillets and grill until cooked through.
- Prepare Dill Sauce: Mix chopped dill, lemon juice, and yogurt/mayo to create a sauce.
- Steam Asparagus: Steam asparagus spears until tender-crisp.
- Serve: Plate the grilled salmon with dill sauce and a side of steamed asparagus.

KITCHEN TOOLS NEEDED

- Grill or grill pan
- Steamer or pot for asparagus
- Bowl for sauce

DRINK: GINGER AND LEMON TEA

INGREDIENTS
- Fresh ginger, sliced
- Lemon juice
- 1 cup boiling water

INSTRUCTIONS
- Prepare Tea: Add ginger slices and lemon juice to a mug.
- Steep: Pour boiling water over them and let steep for several minutes.

KITCHEN TOOLS NEEDED
- Kettle or pot for boiling water
- Mug

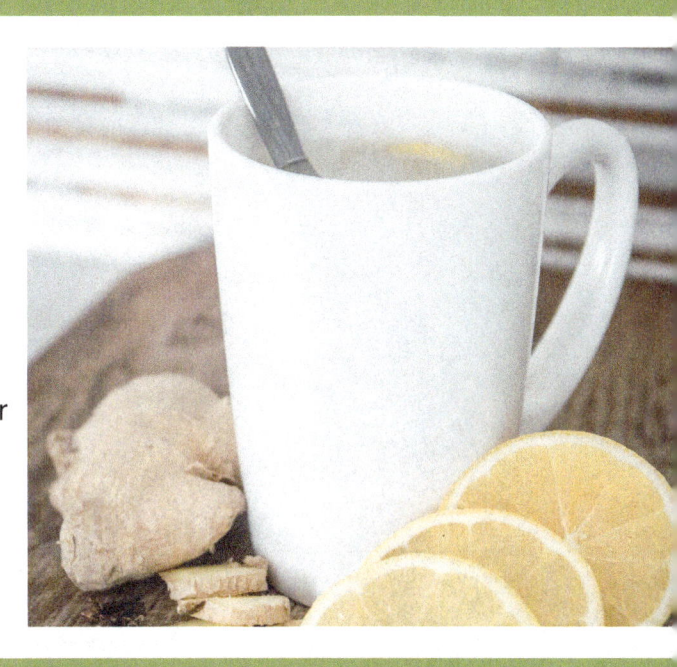

SNACK: FRESH PINEAPPLE

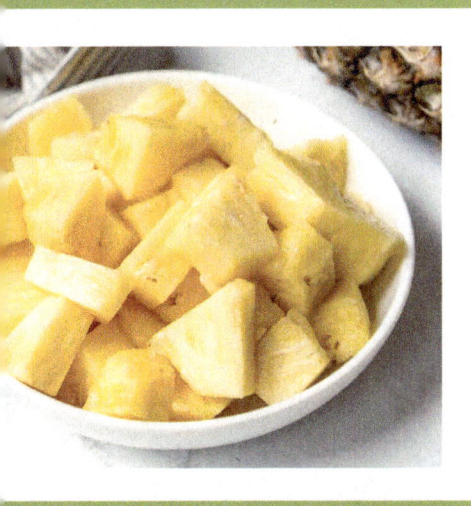

INGREDIENTS
- A small bowl of fresh pineapple, cut into chunks

INSTRUCTIONS
- Prepare Pineapple: Peel and cut the pineapple into bite-sized pieces.

KITCHEN TOOLS NEEDED
- Knife and cutting board

SNACK: A SMALL BANANA

INGREDIENTS
- 1 small banana

PREPARATION TIME: NONE, READY TO EAT.

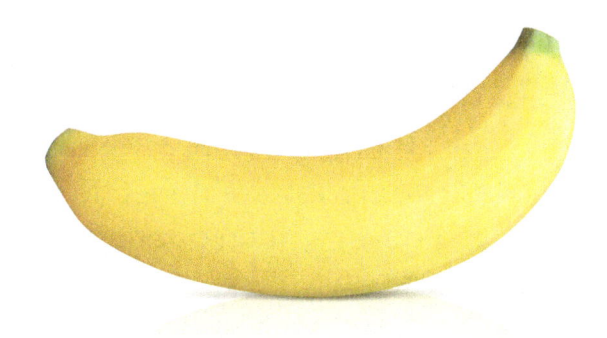

GRANOLA - THE CRUNCHY, WHOLESOME STAPLE

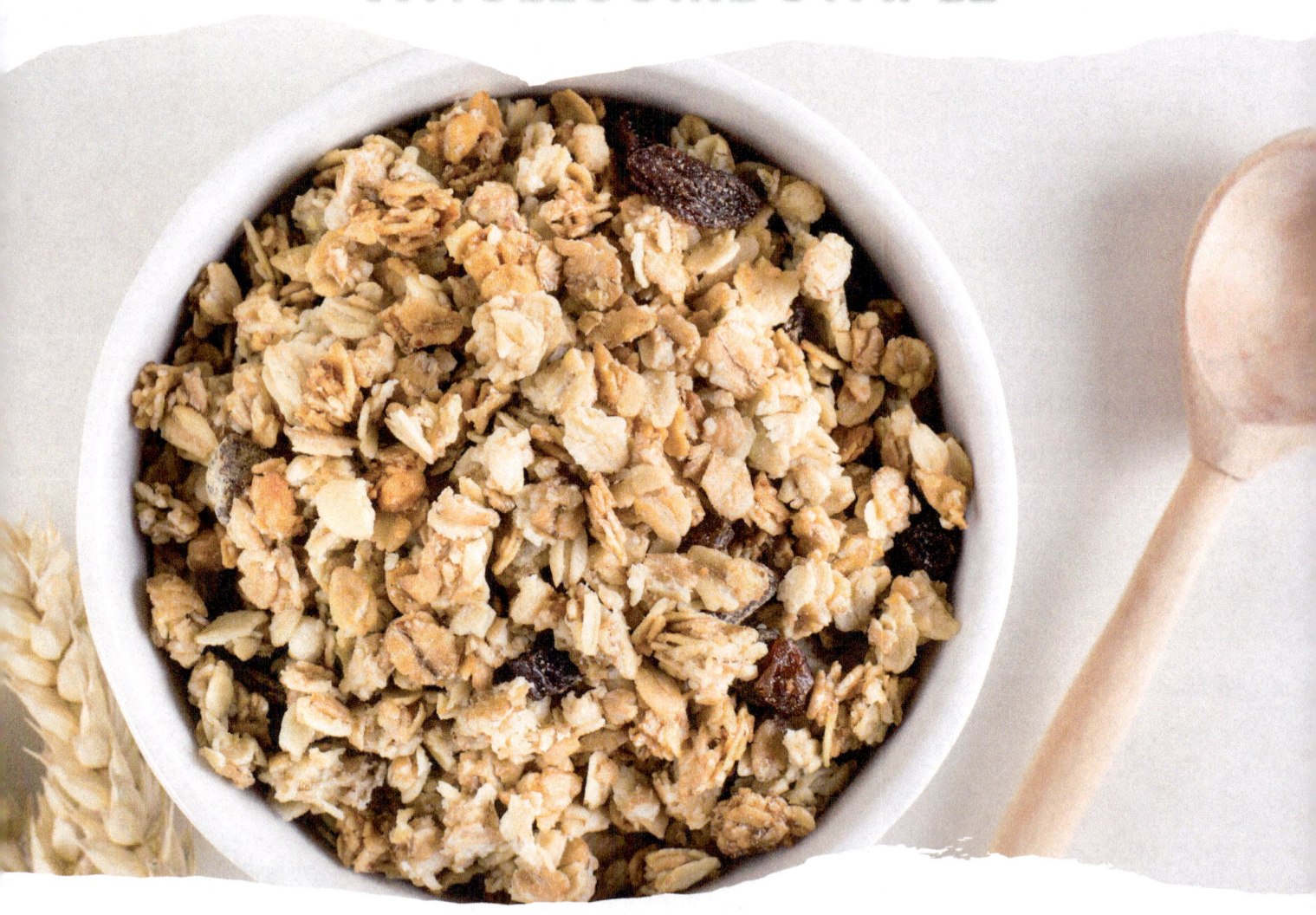

On Day 25 of our Anti-Inflammatory Meal Plan, granola takes a spotlight in our breakfast. This popular, crunchy food is more than just a breakfast staple; it's a versatile mix that can be nutrient-dense, making it a valuable part of a diet aimed at reducing inflammation.

The Nutritious Profile of Granola

- Rich in Fiber and Whole Grains: Many granola blends include whole grains such as oats, which are high in dietary fiber. This fiber is beneficial for digestive health and can help to regulate blood sugar levels.
- Loaded with Healthy Fats: When granola includes nuts and seeds, it provides healthy fats that are essential for heart health and can help to reduce inflammation.
- Customizable for Added Nutrients: Granola can be fortified with a variety of ingredients, such as dried fruits, nuts, seeds, and spices, which enhance its nutritional value.

Incorporating Granola into Your Diet

- Versatile and Convenient: Granola can be enjoyed in many ways - as a topping for yogurt, mixed into smoothies, or simply with a splash of milk. Its crunchy texture and sweet flavor make it a delightful addition to various dishes.
- Energy-Boosting Meal Option: The combination of granola with Greek yogurt and a touch of maple syrup, as in our breakfast, offers a balanced meal of protein, carbohydrates, and healthy fats, ideal for starting the day with sustained energy.

Choosing the Right Granola

- Mindful of Added Sugars and Fats: It's important to choose granola that is low in added sugars and unhealthy fats. Homemade granola or brands with simple, natural ingredients are often the healthiest choices.
- Enhancing Nutrient Intake: Including granola in your diet can be a delicious way to consume more fiber, vitamins, and minerals, contributing to a balanced and anti-inflammatory diet.

In conclusion, granola is a valuable addition to an anti-inflammatory diet when chosen wisely and consumed in moderation. Its versatility, combined with its potential for high nutritional value, makes it an excellent choice for a wholesome and satisfying meal or snack. Enjoy granola as part of your varied and nutritious diet for both its health benefits and delicious taste.

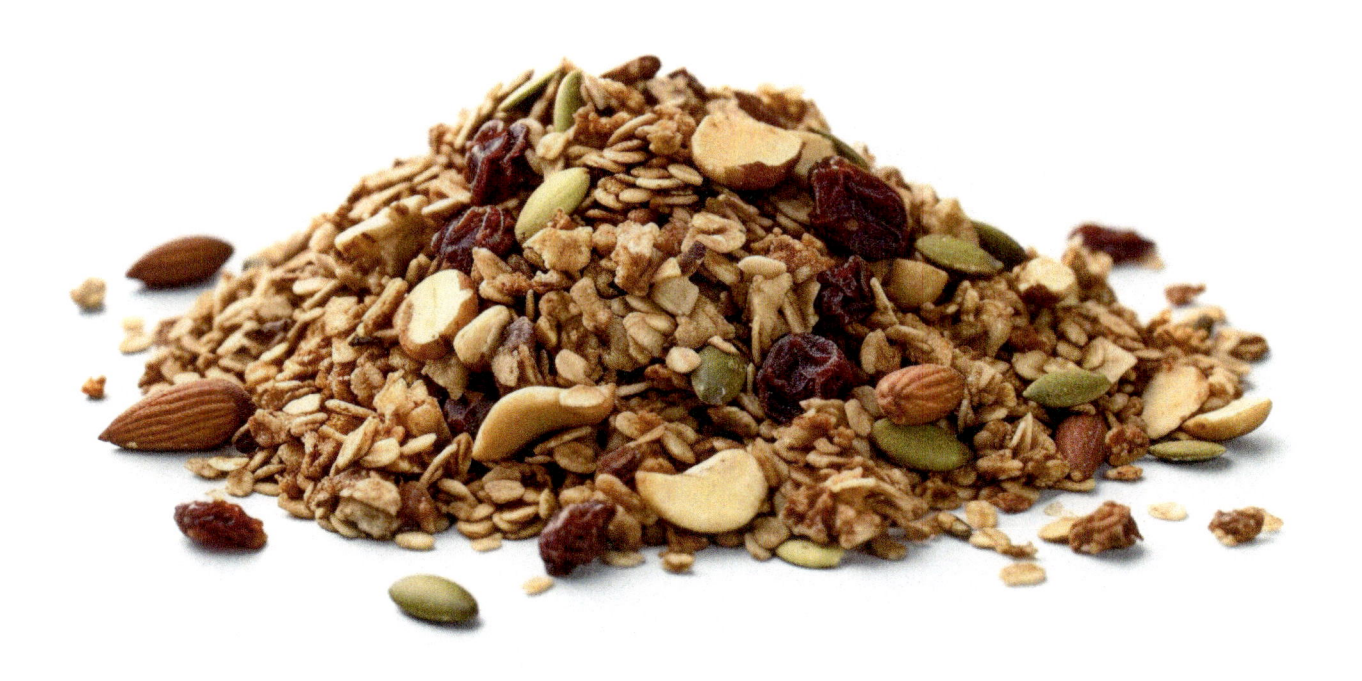

DAY 26 MEAL PLAN

BREAKFAST: SCRAMBLED TOFU WITH TURMERIC, KALE, AND TOMATOES
LUNCH: QUINOA SALAD WITH BLACK BEANS, CORN, AND CILANTRO-LIME DRESSING
DINNER: SLOW-COOKED LAMB SHANK WITH ROOT VEGETABLES
SNACK: A MEDIUM-SIZED ORANGE
SNACK: HANDFUL OF SEED MIX
DRINK: HERBAL SLEEP TEA

BREAKFAST: SCRAMBLED TOFU WITH TURMERIC, KALE, AND TOMATOES

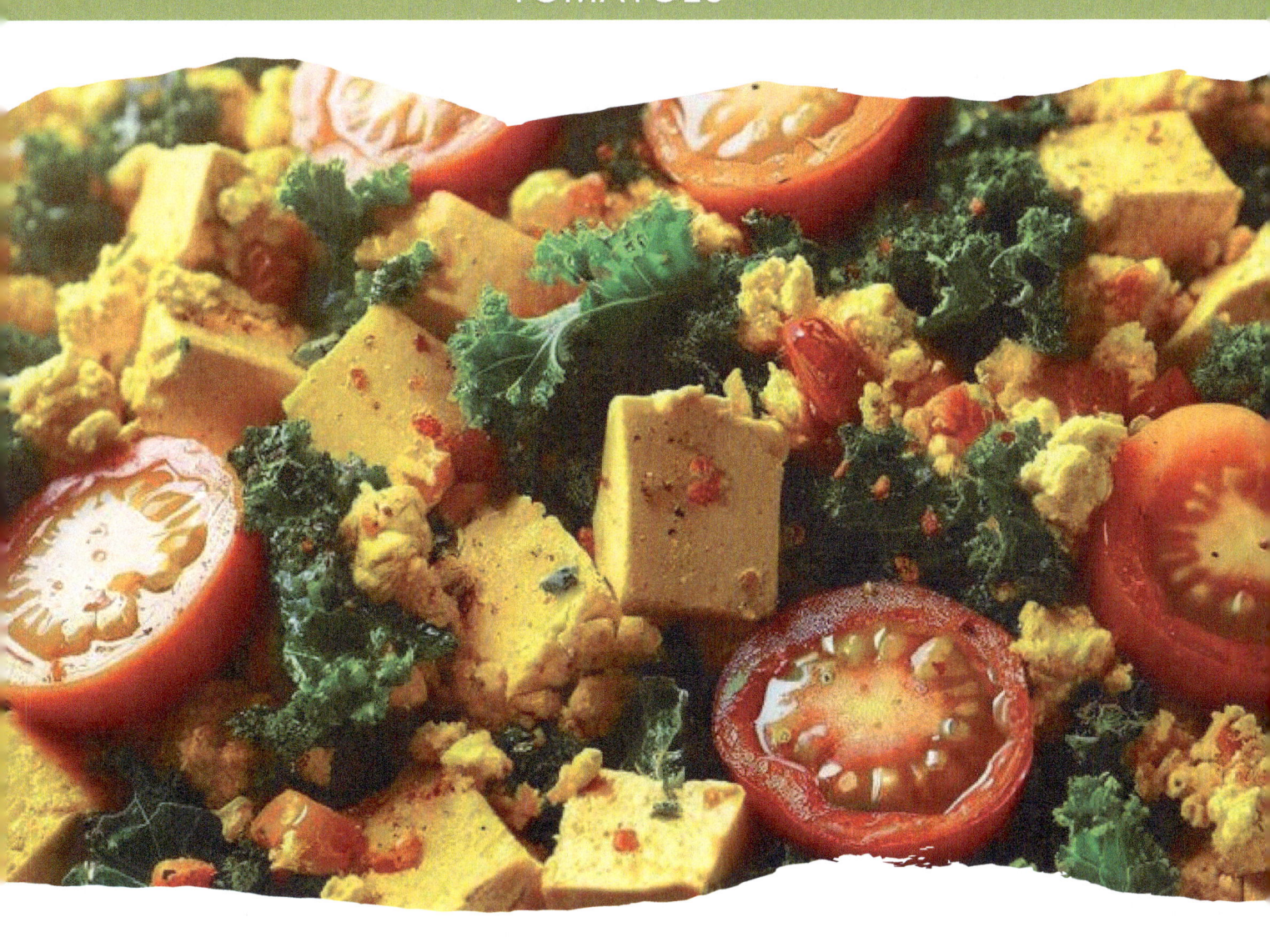

INGREDIENTS

- 1 block of firm tofu, crumbled
- ½ teaspoon turmeric
- 1 cup kale, chopped
- 1 tomato, diced
- Salt and pepper to taste
- Olive oil for cooking

INSTRUCTIONS

- Cook Tofu: Heat olive oil in a pan, add crumbled tofu and turmeric, cook until slightly browned.
- Add Vegetables: Mix in kale and tomatoes, cook until vegetables are tender.
- Season: Add salt and pepper to taste.

KITCHEN TOOLS NEEDED

- Frying pan
- Knife and cutting board

LUNCH: QUINOA SALAD WITH BLACK BEANS, CORN, AND CILANTRO-LIME DRESSING

INGREDIENTS

- 1 cup cooked quinoa
- ½ cup black beans
- ½ cup corn
- Cilantro, chopped
- Lime juice and olive oil for dressing

INSTRUCTIONS

- Prepare Salad: Combine quinoa, black beans, and corn in a bowl.
- Add Dressing: Mix in chopped cilantro, lime juice, olive oil, salt, and pepper.

KITCHEN TOOLS NEEDED

- Mixing bowl

DINNER: SLOW-COOKED LAMB SHANK WITH ROOT VEGETABLES

INGREDIENTS

- Lamb shanks
- Assorted root vegetables (carrots, parsnips, potatoes)
- Herbs and spices for seasoning (rosemary, thyme, garlic)
- Broth or water

INSTRUCTIONS

- Prepare Lamb and Vegetables: Season lamb shanks and chop root vegetables.
- Slow Cook: Place lamb and vegetables in the slow cooker, add broth or water, and cook until the lamb is tender.

KITCHEN TOOLS NEEDED

- Slow cooker or large pot
- Knife and cutting board

DRINK: HERBAL SLEEP TEA

INGREDIENTS

- A bag of herbal tea blend for sleep (such as chamomile or valerian root)
- 1 cup boiling water

INSTRUCTIONS

- Boil Water: Heat the water.
- Steep Tea: Place the tea bag in a mug, pour hot water over it.

KITCHEN TOOLS NEEDED

- Kettle or pot for boiling water
- Mug

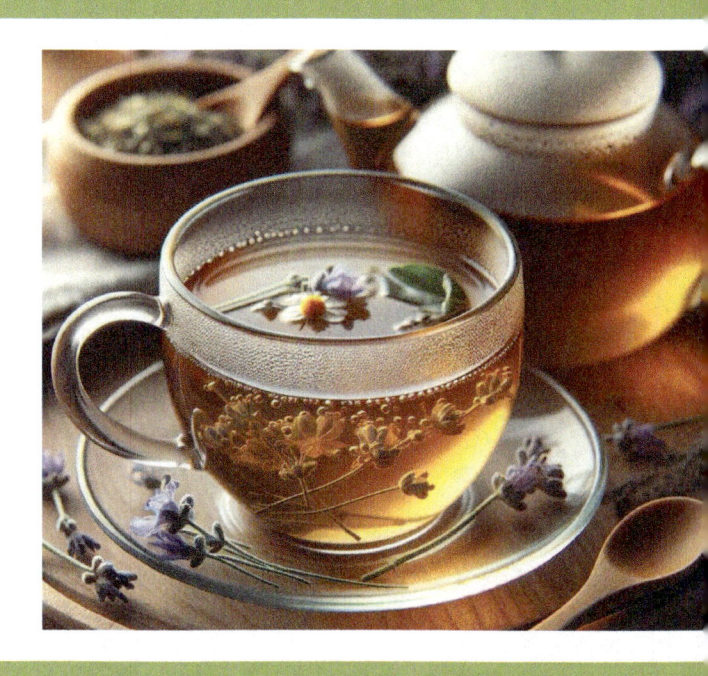

SNACK: HANDFUL OF SEED MIX

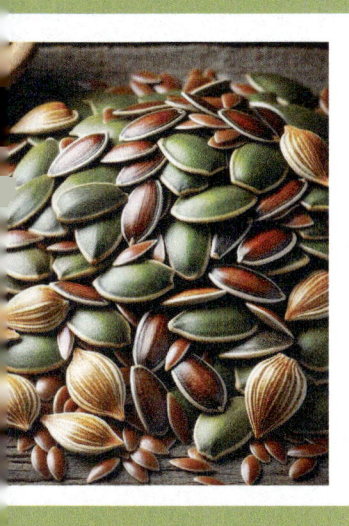

INGREDIENTS

- A mix of seeds (pumpkin seeds, sunflower seeds, flaxseeds)

PREPARATION TIME: NONE, READY TO EAT.

SNACK: A MEDIUM-SIZED ORANGE

INGREDIENTS

- 1 medium-sized orange

PREPARATION TIME: NONE, READY TO EAT.

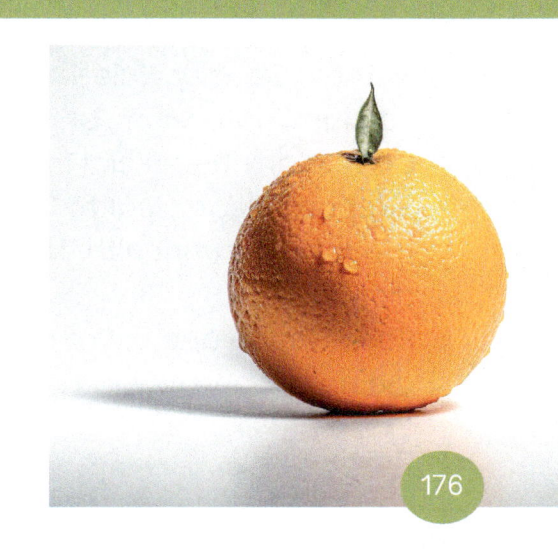

KALE - THE LEAFY GREEN SUPERFOOD

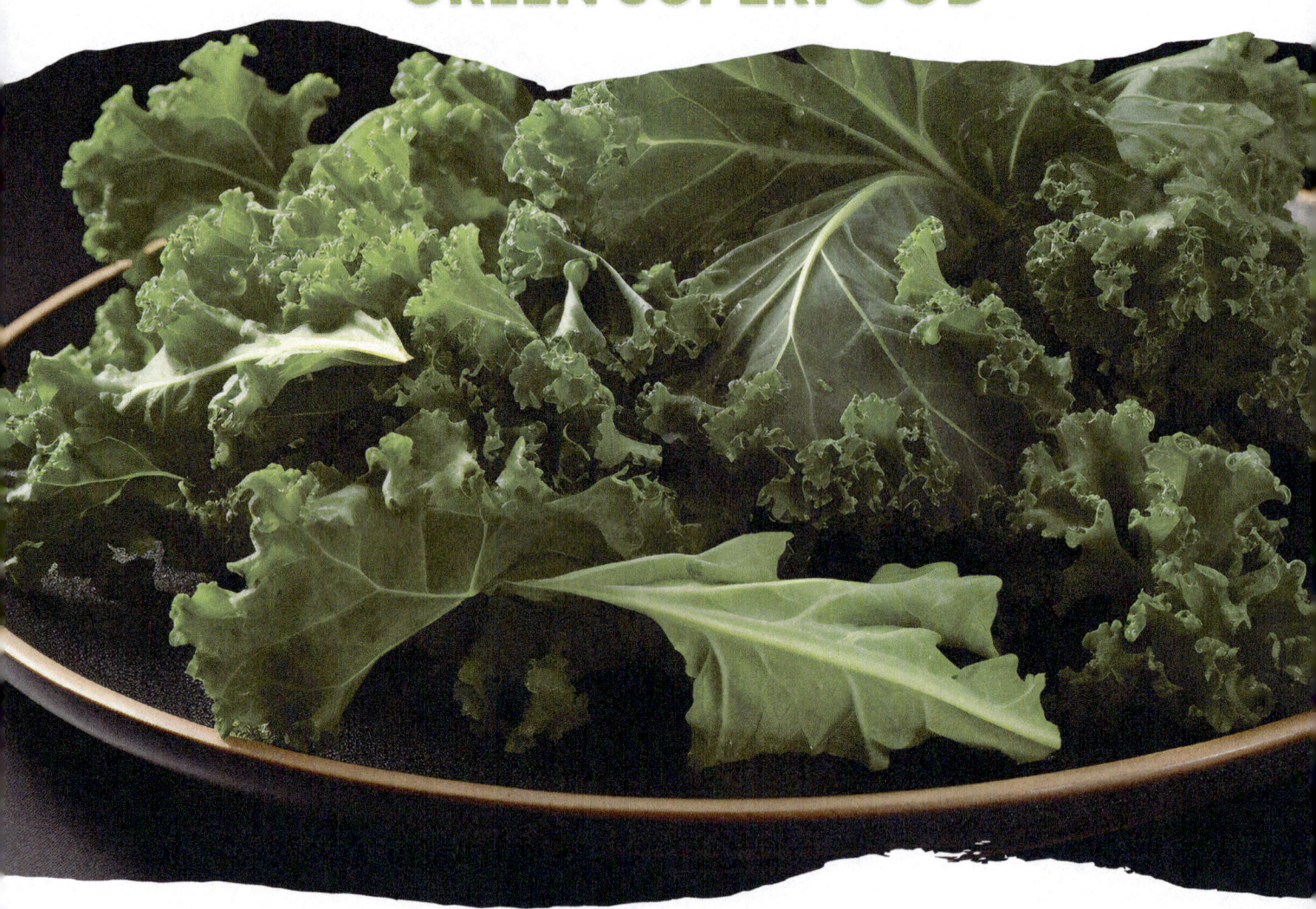

On Day 26 of our Anti-Inflammatory Meal Plan, kale plays a starring role in our breakfast. This leafy green is much more than just a trendy ingredient; it's a nutrient powerhouse, renowned for its health benefits and particularly effective in an anti-inflammatory diet.

The Exceptional Benefits of Kale

- Nutrient Density: Kale is incredibly rich in vitamins A, C, and K, along with minerals like calcium, potassium, and magnesium. These nutrients are vital for overall health and particularly beneficial for their anti-inflammatory and antioxidant properties.
- Supports Heart Health: The fiber, antioxidants, and omega-3 fatty acids in kale are great for heart health. They help lower cholesterol levels and reduce the risk of heart disease.
- Bone Health and Beyond: The high vitamin K content in kale is crucial for bone health, aiding in bone formation and reducing the risk of osteoporosis.

Incorporating Kale into Your Diet

- Versatility in Cooking: Kale can be added to a variety of dishes. It's excellent in salads, smoothies, stir-fries, and as a side dish. In our breakfast recipe, it adds both color and nutrients to the scrambled tofu.
- A Flavorful Addition: Kale's slightly peppery and earthy taste enhances the overall flavor of meals, making it a popular choice for both health-conscious and flavor-seeking individuals.

Embracing Kale for Holistic Health

- Ideal for Weight Management: Kale is low in calories but high in fiber, making it an ideal food for those focusing on weight management without sacrificing nutrient intake.
- Promoting a Varied Vegetable Intake: Including a variety of vegetables like kale in your diet ensures a broad nutrient intake and is key to a balanced and anti-inflammatory diet.

In summary, kale is an outstanding addition to an anti-inflammatory diet. Its rich nutritional profile, combined with its versatility in cooking, makes it a valuable ingredient for enhancing meals and promoting overall health. Enjoy kale in your daily diet to reap its multitude of health benefits and add delicious variety to your meals.

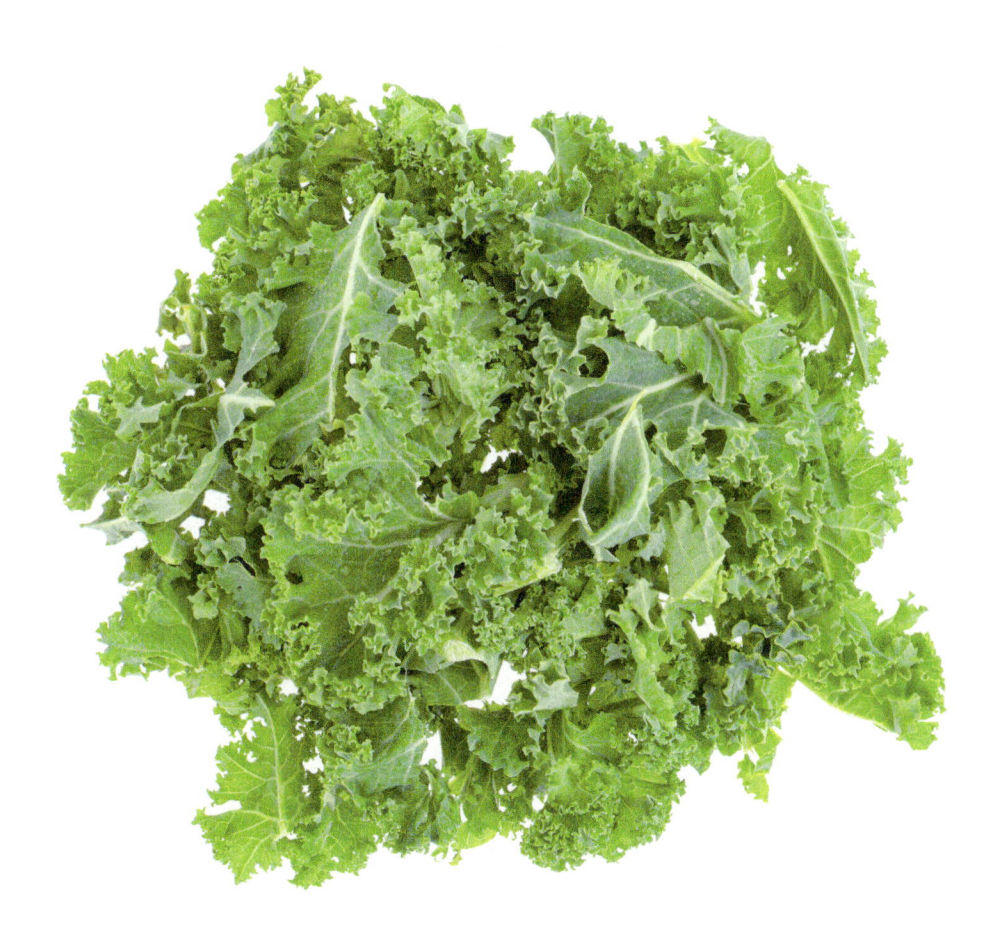

DAY 27 MEAL PLAN

BREAKFAST: CHIA AND ALMOND MILK PUDDING WITH FRESH MANGO
LUNCH: CHICKEN CAESAR SALAD WITH YOGURT-BASED DRESSING
DINNER: SPAGHETTI SQUASH WITH HOMEMADE TOMATO SAUCE AND LEAN GROUND BEEF
SNACK: WALNUT HALVES
SNACK: CARROT STICKS WITH TAHINI DIP
DRINK: CHAMOMILE AND LAVENDER TEA

BREAKFAST: CHIA AND ALMOND MILK PUDDING WITH FRESH MANGO

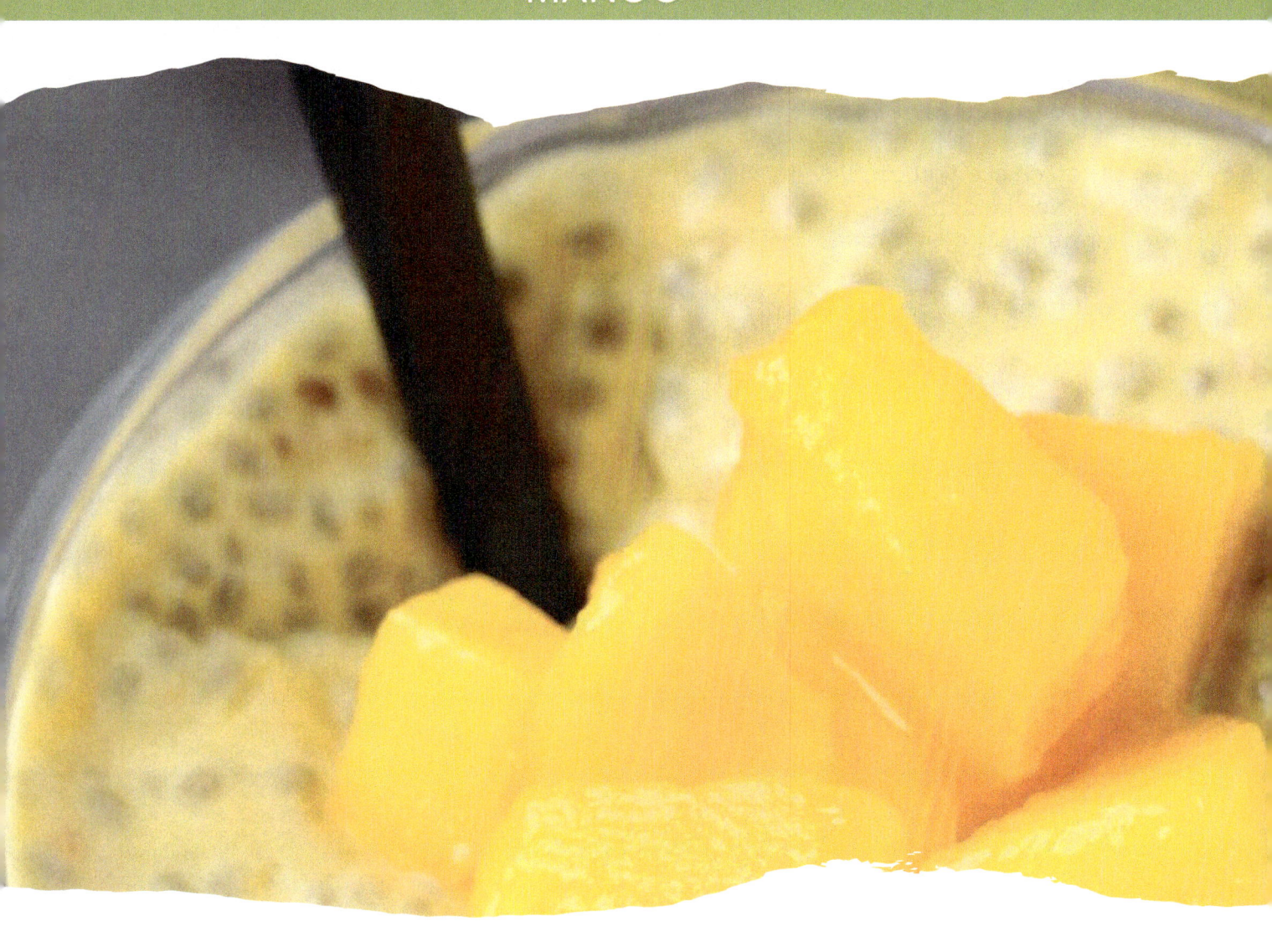

INGREDIENTS

- ¼ cup chia seeds
- 1 cup almond milk
- 1 mango, diced

INSTRUCTIONS

- Prepare Pudding: Mix chia seeds with almond milk and let sit overnight or at least a few hours until it forms a pudding-like consistency.
- Top with Mango: Add fresh diced mango on top before serving.

KITCHEN TOOLS NEEDED
- Bowl
- Spoon

LUNCH: CHICKEN CAESAR SALAD WITH YOGURT-BASED DRESSING

INGREDIENTS

- Grilled chicken breast, sliced
- Romaine lettuce
- Parmesan cheese, grated
- Croutons (optional)
- Yogurt-based Caesar dressing

INSTRUCTIONS

- Assemble Salad: Toss lettuce with grilled chicken, parmesan, and croutons.
- Add Dressing: Drizzle with yogurt-based Caesar dressing.

KITCHEN TOOLS NEEDED

- Mixing bowl
- Knife and cutting board

DINNER: SPAGHETTI SQUASH WITH HOMEMADE TOMATO SAUCE AND LEAN GROUND BEEF

INGREDIENTS

- 1 spaghetti squash
- Lean ground beef
- Tomato sauce ingredients (tomatoes, garlic, onion, herbs)

INSTRUCTIONS

- Roast Spaghetti Squash: Halve the squash, remove seeds, and roast until tender.
- Prepare Tomato Sauce: Cook tomatoes with garlic, onion, and herbs.
- Cook Beef: Brown the ground beef in a pan.
- Combine: Mix the cooked beef with tomato sauce, serve over spaghetti squash strands.

KITCHEN TOOLS NEEDED

- Oven for roasting squash
- Frying pan for beef
- Pot for tomato sauce
- Knife and cutting board

DRINK: CHAMOMILE AND LAVENDER TEA

INGREDIENTS
- 1 chamomile and lavender tea bag
- 1 cup boiling water

INSTRUCTIONS
- Boil Water: Heat the water.
- Steep Tea: Place the tea bag in a mug, pour hot water over it.

KITCHEN TOOLS NEEDED
- Kettle or pot for boiling water
- Mug

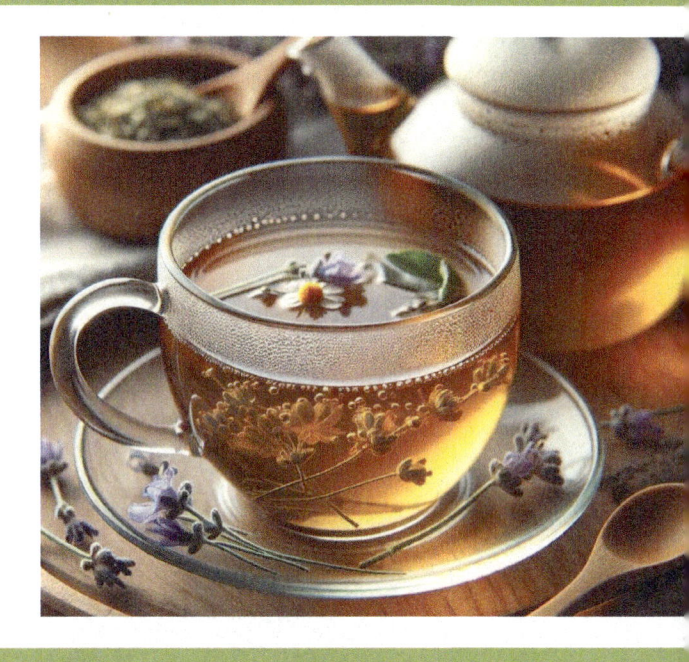

SNACK: CARROT STICKS WITH TAHINI DIP

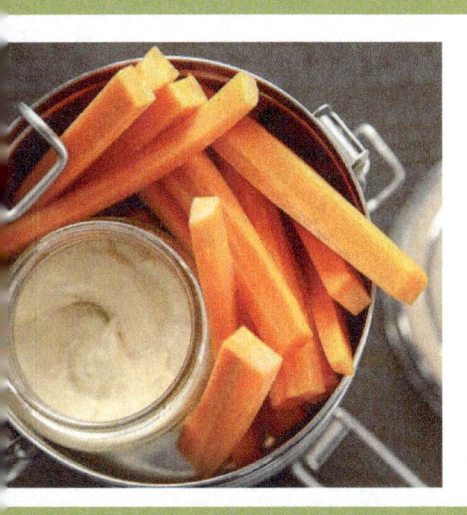

INGREDIENTS
- Carrots, cut into sticks
- Tahini for dipping

INSTRUCTIONS
- Prepare Snack: Serve carrot sticks with a side of tahini dip.

KITCHEN TOOLS NEEDED
- Knife and cutting board

SNACK: WALNUT HALVES

INGREDIENTS
- A few walnut halves

PREPARATION TIME: NONE, READY TO EAT.

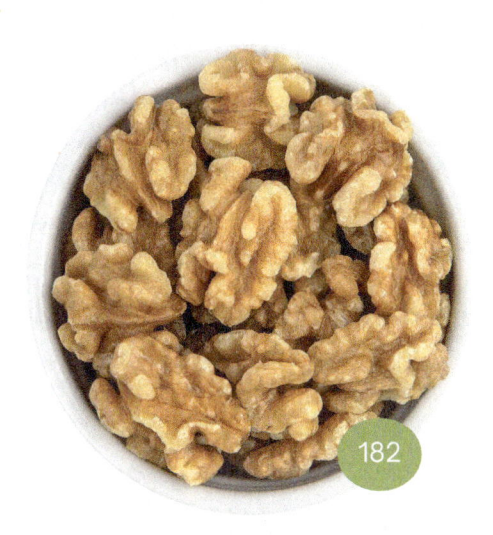

MANGO – THE TROPICAL NUTRIENT TREASURE

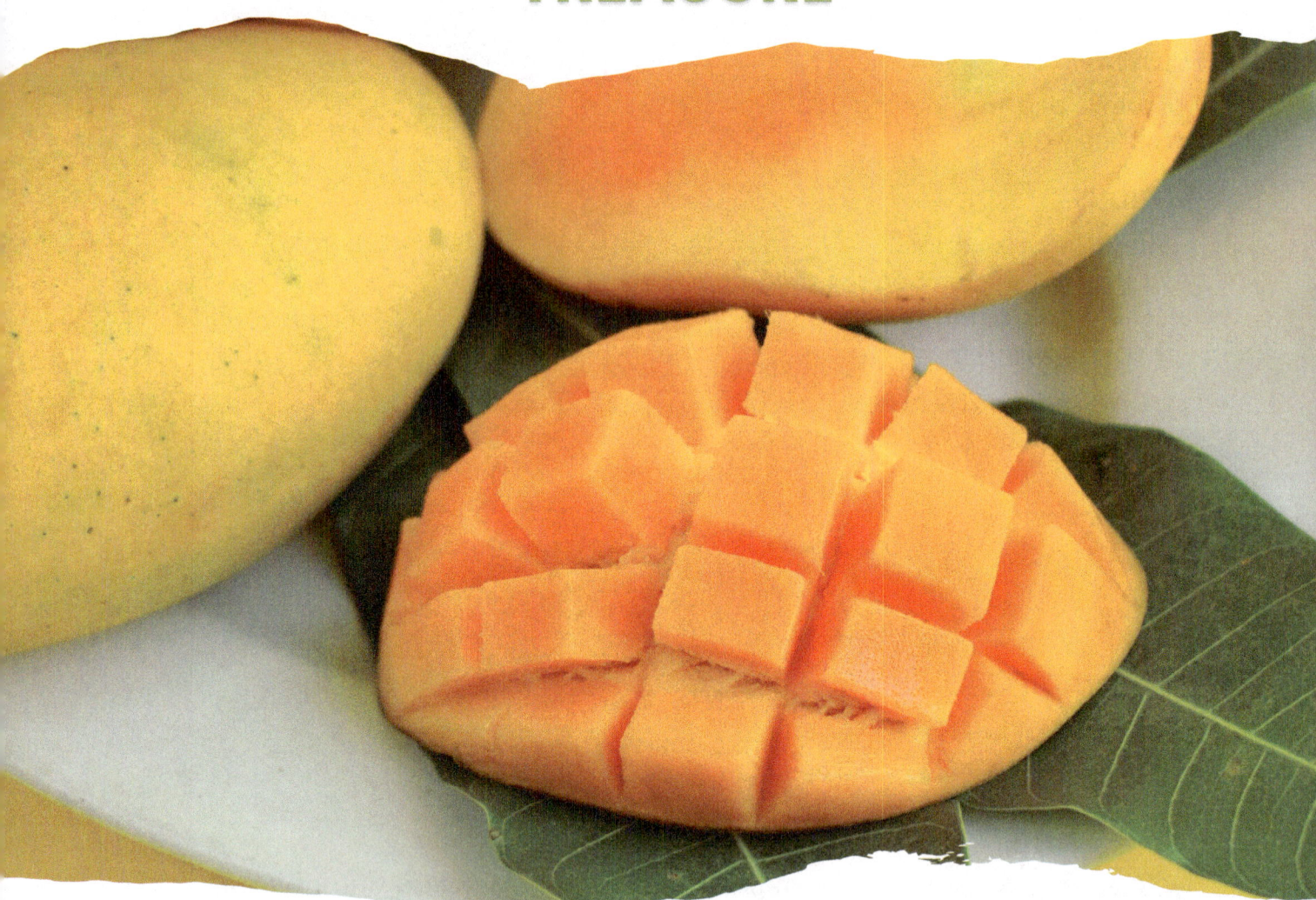

On Day 27 of our Anti-Inflammatory Meal Plan, we introduce mango as a delightful topping for our breakfast. Mangoes are not only celebrated for their sweet, tropical flavor but also for their impressive array of nutrients and health benefits, making them an excellent addition to an anti-inflammatory diet.

The Health Benefits of Mango

- Rich in Vitamins and Antioxidants: Mangoes are a fantastic source of vitamins C and A, both powerful antioxidants. Vitamin C boosts immune function and skin health, while Vitamin A is essential for eye health and immune defense.
- Digestive Health Support: Mangoes contain enzymes that aid in digestion and are high in dietary fiber, which promotes gut health and regularity.
- Anti-Inflammatory Properties: The unique combination of polyphenols and antioxidants in mangoes helps in reducing inflammation and combating oxidative stress.

Incorporating Mango into Your Diet

- Versatile and Flavorful: Fresh mango can be enjoyed on its own, added to smoothies, salads, desserts, or as a sweet topping for breakfast dishes like chia pudding.
- A Sweet Addition to Diverse Meals: Its natural sweetness and rich texture enhance the flavor profile of a variety of dishes, adding both nutritional value and a burst of tropical taste.

Embracing Mango for Well-Rounded Nutrition

- Ideal for a Balanced Diet: Mangoes are not only delicious but also nutrient-dense, making them an excellent choice for a balanced diet focused on reducing inflammation.
- Promoting Varied Fruit Intake: Including a variety of fruits like mangoes in your diet ensures a broad intake of nutrients and antioxidants, which is key to maintaining overall health and wellness.

In conclusion, mangoes are a superb addition to an anti-inflammatory diet. Their rich flavor and nutritional profile make them an ideal choice for enhancing the taste and health benefits of your meals. Enjoy mangoes in your daily diet for a delicious, nutrient-packed tropical twist.

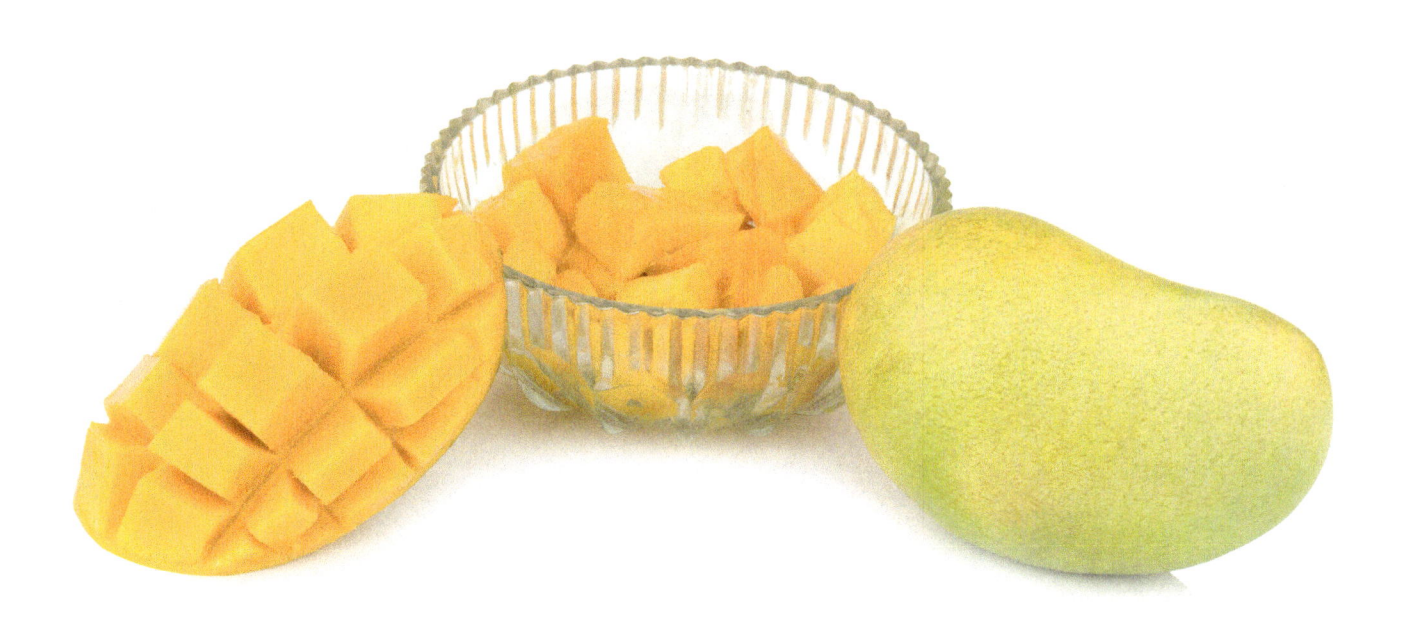

DAY 28 MEAL PLAN

BREAKFAST: SMOOTHIE BOWL WITH MIXED BERRIES, COCONUT FLAKES, AND PUMPKIN SEEDS
LUNCH: GRILLED SHRIMP OVER MIXED GREENS WITH AVOCADO DRESSING
DINNER: RATATOUILLE WITH BROWN RICE
SNACK: CUCUMBER SLICES WITH HUMMUS
SNACK: BLUEBERRIES
DRINK: HERBAL DETOX TEA

BREAKFAST: SMOOTHIE BOWL WITH MIXED BERRIES, COCONUT FLAKES, AND PUMPKIN SEEDS

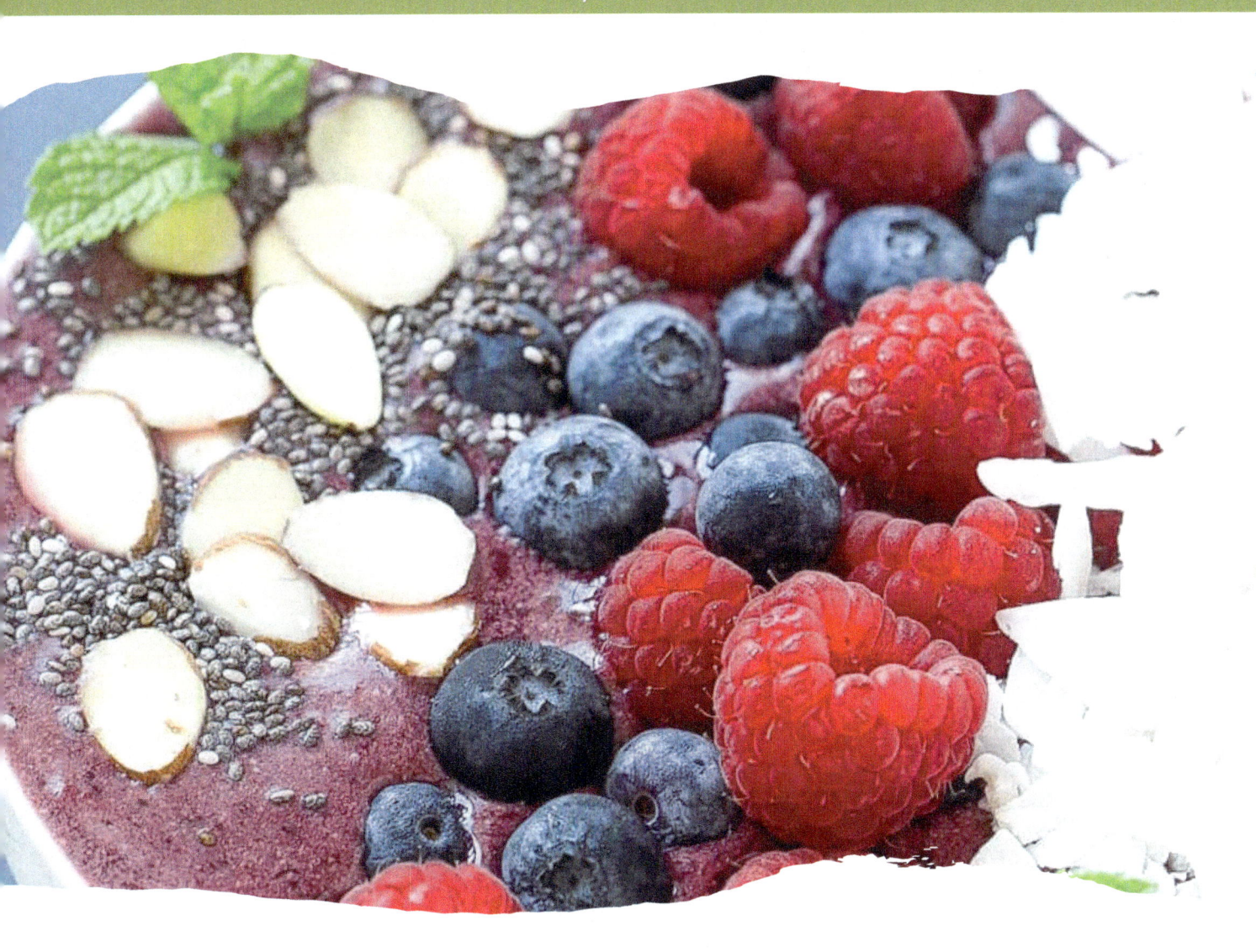

INGREDIENTS

- Mixed berries (strawberries, blueberries, raspberries)
- Coconut flakes
- Pumpkin seeds
- Base smoothie mix (banana, almond milk or yogurt)

INSTRUCTIONS

- Blend Smoothie: Blend a base of banana with almond milk or yogurt.
- Create Bowl: Pour the smoothie into a bowl.
- Add Toppings: Top with mixed berries, coconut flakes, and pumpkin seeds.

KITCHEN TOOLS NEEDED
- Blender
- Bowl
- Spoon

LUNCH: GRILLED SHRIMP OVER MIXED GREENS WITH AVOCADO DRESSING

INGREDIENTS

- Shrimp, peeled and deveined
- Mixed greens (lettuce, spinach, arugula)
- Avocado, lemon juice, olive oil for dressing

INSTRUCTIONS

- Grill Shrimp: Season shrimp and grill until cooked through.
- Prepare Salad: Arrange mixed greens on a plate.
- Make Dressing: Blend avocado with lemon juice and olive oil for a creamy dressing.
- Assemble: Top salad with grilled shrimp and avocado dressing.

KITCHEN TOOLS NEEDED
- Grill or grill pan
- Salad bowl

DINNER: RATATOUILLE WITH BROWN RICE

INGREDIENTS

- Assorted vegetables for ratatouille (eggplant, zucchini, bell peppers, tomatoes)
- Herbs (basil, thyme)
- Olive oil
- 1 cup brown rice

INSTRUCTIONS

- Cook Ratatouille: Sauté chopped vegetables with herbs and olive oil until tender.
- Cook Rice: Prepare brown rice as per package instructions.
- Serve: Dish the ratatouille over a bed of brown rice.

KITCHEN TOOLS NEEDED
- Pot for ratatouille
- Pot for rice
- Knife and cutting board

DRINK: HERBAL DETOX TEA

INGREDIENTS

- 1 bag of herbal detox tea (ingredients like dandelion, nettle, ginger)
- 1 cup boiling water

INSTRUCTIONS

- Boil Water: Heat the water.
- Steep Tea: Place the tea bag in a mug, pour hot water over it.

KITCHEN TOOLS NEEDED

- Kettle or pot for boiling water
- Mug

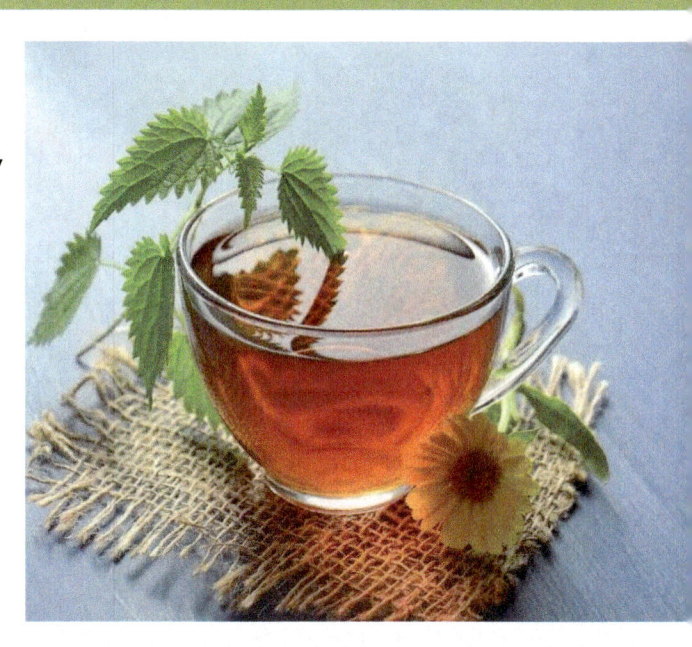

SNACK: CUCUMBER SLICES WITH HUMMUS

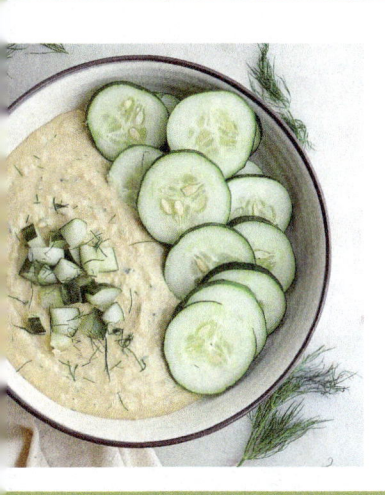

INGREDIENTS

- Cucumber, sliced
- Hummus for dipping

INSTRUCTIONS

- Prepare Snack: Serve cucumber slices with a side of hummus for dipping.

KITCHEN TOOLS NEEDED

- Knife and cutting board

SNACK: BLUEBERRIES

INGREDIENTS

A small serving of blueberries

PREPARATION TIME: NONE, READY TO EAT.

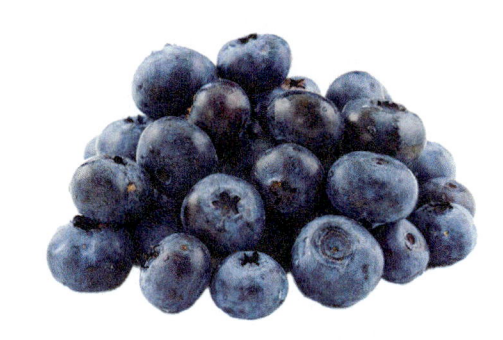

PUMPKIN SEEDS – THE NUTRIENT-PACKED POWER HOUSE

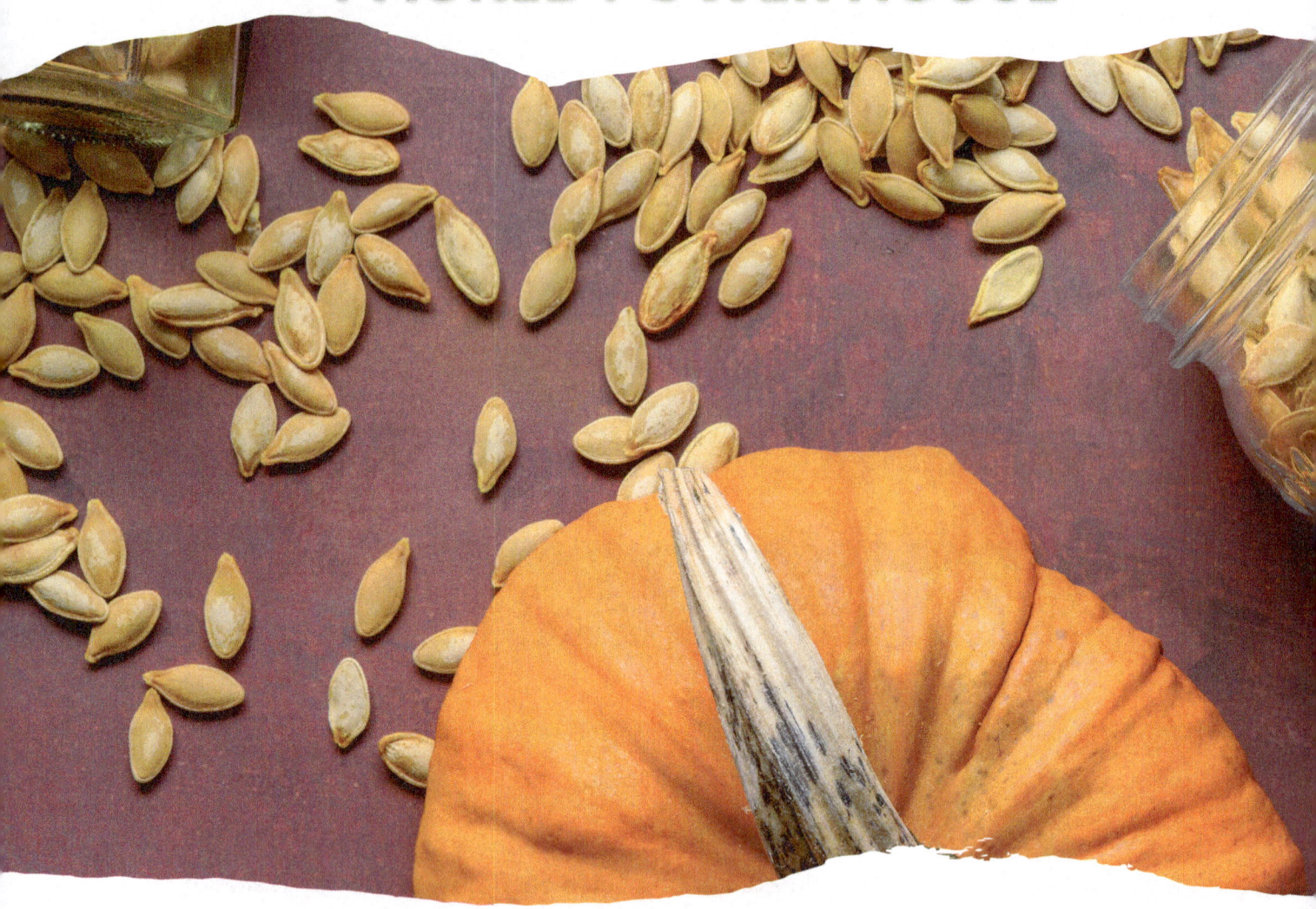

On Day 28, the final day of our Anti-Inflammatory Meal Plan, we highlight pumpkin seeds, featured in our breakfast smoothie bowl. These small but mighty seeds are not just a crunchy add-on; they're packed with nutrients and health benefits, making them an excellent choice for anyone looking to enhance their diet, particularly in reducing inflammation.

The Impressive Benefits of Pumpkin Seeds

- Rich in Magnesium: Pumpkin seeds are a great source of magnesium, a mineral essential for various bodily functions, including muscle and nerve function, blood sugar control, and blood pressure regulation.
- High in Omega-3 Fatty Acids: Like other seeds and nuts, they contain omega-3 fatty acids, known for their anti-inflammatory properties.
- Antioxidant-Rich: They're also rich in antioxidants, which help to reduce oxidative stress and inflammation in the body.

Incorporating Pumpkin Seeds into Your Diet

- Versatile Addition to Meals: Pumpkin seeds can be sprinkled over salads, smoothie bowls, or yogurt, and can also be added to baked goods or eaten as a standalone snack.
- Enhancing Breakfast and Snacks: Adding them to your morning smoothie bowl, as in our breakfast recipe, provides a nutritious start to your day with added crunch and flavor.

Pumpkin Seeds' Role in a Healthy Diet

- Great for Heart Health and More: Regular consumption of pumpkin seeds is beneficial for heart health and can aid in improving sleep quality, thanks to their magnesium and tryptophan content.
- Promoting Diverse Nutrient Intake: Their inclusion in our meal plan is a reminder of the importance of incorporating a variety of seeds and nuts for their unique nutritional benefits and flavors.

In conclusion, pumpkin seeds are a valuable addition to an anti-inflammatory diet. Their combination of essential nutrients, heart-healthy fats, and antioxidants make them a smart choice for anyone looking to improve their health through diet. Enjoy pumpkin seeds in your meals or as a snack to benefit from their numerous health properties and add a satisfying crunch to your diet.

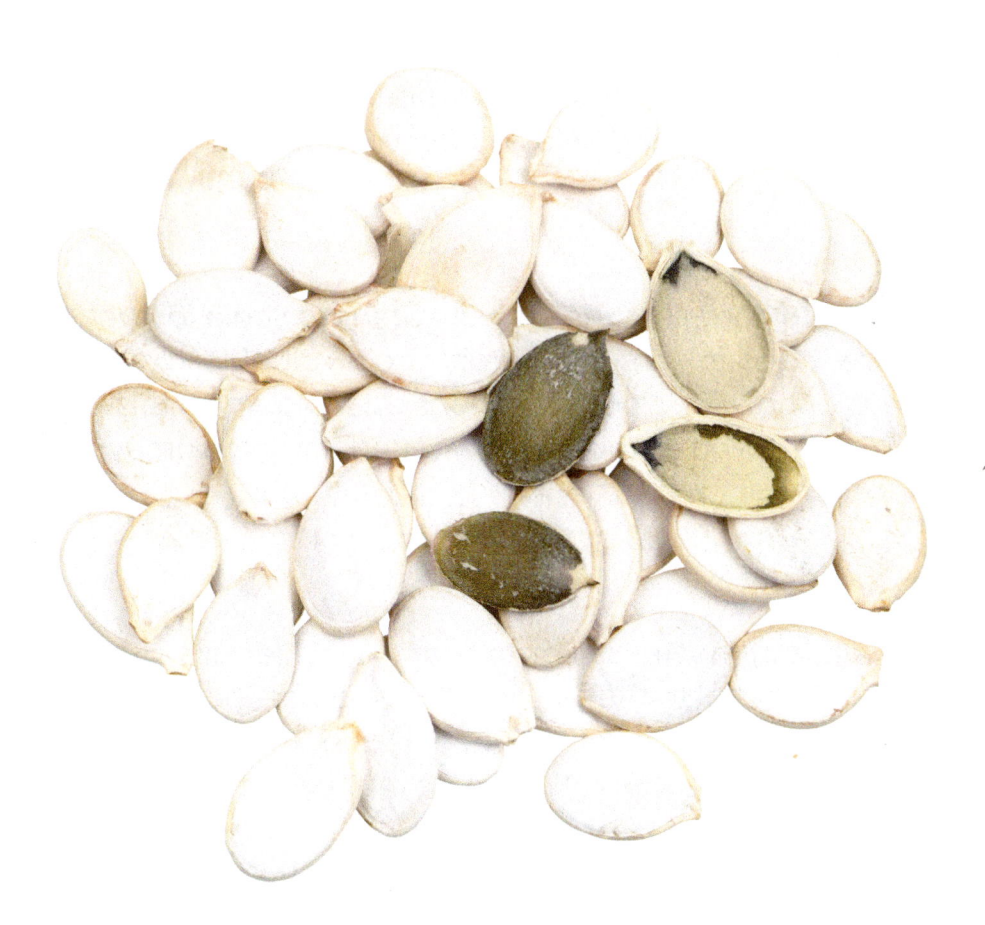

COMPLETION OF WEEK 4: A MESSAGE OF CONGRATULATIONS

You Did It! Completing the 28-Day Plan

Congratulations on completing the 28-Day Anti-Inflammatory Meal Plan! Your commitment to following through Week 4's sustainable swaps and strategies is truly inspiring. Thank you for being with us on this transformative journey.

Acknowledging Your Dedication and Learning

- Gratitude for Your Journey: It has been a pleasure to see you grow and adapt throughout these four weeks. Your dedication to learning and implementing these dietary changes is commendable.
- Celebrating Your Achievements: You've not only completed the plan but also laid the groundwork for a healthier, anti-inflammatory lifestyle. This is a significant achievement worth celebrating.

Embracing the Future with New Habits

- Looking Ahead: As you move beyond this meal plan, remember the lessons learned and the habits formed. These will be your tools in maintaining a healthful, anti-inflammatory diet in your daily life.
- Continued Support: Remember, the journey doesn't end here. We encourage you to continue exploring, learning, and enjoying the vast world of anti-inflammatory foods and recipes.

Please take a moment to complete the Body Awareness Scale for Week 4. Your reflections on this week and the entire program are invaluable in understanding the impact of your dietary changes. Congratulations once again on this remarkable achievement, and we wish you all the best in your continued journey to wellness!

WEEK 4 REFLECTION

After completing Week 4 of the Anti-Inflammatory Meal Plan, it's important to reflect on how your body has responded to the dietary changes. Use the following scale to rate your experiences in various aspects of your health and well-being. Rate each category from 1 to 10 (where 1 is 'no improvement' and 10 is 'significant improvement').

1. Digestive Comfort

- Question: How would you rate the overall comfort of your digestive system this week?
- Rating (1-10): _____

2. Energy Levels

- Question: How do you feel about your energy levels after following the meal plan for a week?
- Rating (1-10): _____

3. Sleep Quality

- Question: Have you noticed any changes in the quality of your sleep?
- Rating (1-10): _____

4. Mood and Mental Clarity

- Question: How has your mood and mental clarity been affected by the dietary changes?
- Rating (1-10): _____

5. Physical Comfort and Pain Levels

- Question: If you previously experienced any physical discomfort or pain, have you noticed any changes in its intensity or frequency?
- Rating (1-10): _____

6. Skin Health

- Question: Have there been any noticeable changes in your skin health/appearance?
- Rating (1-10): _____

7. Cravings and Appetite Control

- Question: How would you rate your control over cravings and appetite this week?
- Rating (1-10): _____

8. Overall Well-being

- Question: Considering all factors, how would you rate your overall well-being after Week 1?
- Rating (1-10): _____

Notes

Notes

- Daily Observations: Note any specific reactions or feelings on a day-to-day basis. This can include changes in mood, energy levels, digestive reactions, or any other physical or mental responses you notice.

- Dietary Adaptations: If you made any modifications to the meal plan, such as substituting ingredients or altering meal times, document these changes. This can help you understand how different foods or eating patterns affect you.

- Challenges and Successes: Reflect on any challenges you faced, such as cravings or difficulty in meal preparation, and how you addressed them. Also, celebrate successes, like resisting a particular craving or noticing positive changes in your health.

- Physical and Emotional Well-being: Expand on the ratings you provided by describing in more detail how you feel physically and emotionally. This could include noting any reduction in pain, improvements in skin health, or changes in mental clarity and mood.

- Future Adjustments: Based on your week's experience, jot down any thoughts on what you might want to try differently in the upcoming week. This could be trying new recipes, adjusting portion sizes, or incorporating more of a particular type of food.

- Questions and Research: If you have questions or areas of curiosity that arose during the week, such as the effects of certain foods or why you experienced specific reactions, note these down. You can then research these topics or discuss them with a healthcare professional.

- Overall Reflection: Conclude with a general reflection on how the week went, what you learned about your body's response to the diet, and how you feel about continuing with the meal plan.

WEEK 1

DIGESTIVE COMFORT	1	2	3	4	5	6	7	8	9	10
ENERGY LEVELS	1	2	3	4	5	6	7	8	9	10
SLEEP QUALITY	1	2	3	4	5	6	7	8	9	10
MOOD & MENTAL CLARITY	1	2	3	4	5	6	7	8	9	10
PHYSICAL COMFORT	1	2	3	4	5	6	7	8	9	10
SKIN HEALTH	1	2	3	4	5	6	7	8	9	10
CRAVINGS CONTROL	1	2	3	4	5	6	7	8	9	10
OVERALL WELL-BEING	1	2	3	4	5	6	7	8	9	10

Notes

WEEK 2

DIGESTIVE COMFORT	1	2	3	4	5	6	7	8	9	10
ENERGY LEVELS	1	2	3	4	5	6	7	8	9	10
SLEEP QUALITY	1	2	3	4	5	6	7	8	9	10
MOOD & MENTAL CLARITY	1	2	3	4	5	6	7	8	9	10
PHYSICAL COMFORT	1	2	3	4	5	6	7	8	9	10
SKIN HEALTH	1	2	3	4	5	6	7	8	9	10
CRAVINGS CONTROL	1	2	3	4	5	6	7	8	9	10
OVERALL WELL-BEING	1	2	3	4	5	6	7	8	9	10

Notes

WEEK 3

Category	Rating
DIGESTIVE COMFORT	1 2 3 4 5 6 7 8 9 10
ENERGY LEVELS	1 2 3 4 5 6 7 8 9 10
SLEEP QUALITY	1 2 3 4 5 6 7 8 9 10
MOOD & MENTAL CLARITY	1 2 3 4 5 6 7 8 9 10
PHYSICAL COMFORT	1 2 3 4 5 6 7 8 9 10
SKIN HEALTH	1 2 3 4 5 6 7 8 9 10
CRAVINGS CONTROL	1 2 3 4 5 6 7 8 9 10
OVERALL WELL-BEING	1 2 3 4 5 6 7 8 9 10

Notes

WEEK 4

DIGESTIVE COMFORT	1	2	3	4	5	6	7	8	9	10
ENERGY LEVELS	1	2	3	4	5	6	7	8	9	10
SLEEP QUALITY	1	2	3	4	5	6	7	8	9	10
MOOD & MENTAL CLARITY	1	2	3	4	5	6	7	8	9	10
PHYSICAL COMFORT	1	2	3	4	5	6	7	8	9	10
SKIN HEALTH	1	2	3	4	5	6	7	8	9	10
CRAVINGS CONTROL	1	2	3	4	5	6	7	8	9	10
OVERALL WELL-BEING	1	2	3	4	5	6	7	8	9	10

Notes

HOW TO INTERPRET YOUR PROGRESS

Score Improvements:

- Incremental Benefits: A gradual increase in scores week over week suggests that the anti-inflammatory diet is positively impacting your health. This can manifest in various ways, from enhanced energy levels to improved digestive comfort.
- Understanding Your Body's Responses: Consistently high scores in certain areas may indicate aspects of your health that particularly benefit from the diet. Conversely, areas with lower scores might need more attention or a different approach.

Identifying Patterns:

- Connecting Diet and Well-being: Regularly high or low scores in certain categories can reveal how specific dietary changes influence different facets of your health, such as mood swings, sleep quality, or physical discomfort.
- Holistic View: Look beyond individual scores to see the broader pattern of how your body responds to the diet. This can help you tailor future dietary choices more effectively.

Considering Limitations:

- Contextual Factors: Understand that these scores are subjective and influenced by various external factors. Stress levels, life changes, physical activity, and even weather can affect how you feel and, consequently, your scores.
- Scores as a Guideline: Treat these scores as guidelines rather than definitive measures of health. They are tools to help you reflect on your experiences and are most effective when considered alongside other aspects of your lifestyle.

Reflecting on Your Journey

- Holistic Reflection: At the end of the 28 days, take time to review your overall progress. Consider not just the scores, but also qualitative aspects like how you felt emotionally and physically during the plan.
- Lessons Learned: Use this reflection period to identify what worked well for you and what didn't. This can guide you in maintaining or adjusting your dietary habits post-plan.
- Future Focus: Consider areas where you might want to continue making changes or where you've seen the most significant benefits. This could be in terms of specific foods, meal timings, or even the balance of nutrients in your diet.

BEYOND THE 28 DAYS: SUSTAINING AN ANTI-INFLAMMATORY LIFESTYLE

1. Strategies for Maintaining an Anti-Inflammatory Diet Long-Term

- Diversify Your Diet: Incorporate a wide range of anti-inflammatory foods to prevent dietary boredom. Experiment with different fruits, vegetables, whole grains, lean proteins, and healthy fats.
- Plan Your Meals: Regular meal planning can help you stay on track. Prepare a weekly menu and grocery list to ensure you have the right ingredients on hand.
- Mindful Eating Habits: Pay attention to portion sizes, eat slowly, and savor your food. This practice helps with better digestion and maintaining a healthy weight.

2. Reintegrating or Continuing to Avoid Certain Foods

- Listen to Your Body: Gradually reintroduce foods that were eliminated and notice how your body reacts. This can help identify any food sensitivities or triggers.
- Keep Inflammatory Foods Limited: If you choose to reintegrate certain items like dairy or gluten, do so in moderation and balance them with anti-inflammatory foods.
- Stay Informed: Keep up-to-date with nutritional research and be open to adjusting your diet as new information becomes available.

3. Building a Sustainable and Enjoyable Anti-Inflammatory Lifestyle

- Cook at Home More Often: Preparing your own meals gives you complete control over ingredients and cooking methods. Explore new recipes and cooking techniques.
- Balance is Key: It's okay to indulge occasionally. The goal is to create a balanced approach to eating that can be maintained long-term.
- Incorporate Physical Activity: Regular exercise complements an anti-inflammatory diet and boosts overall health. Find activities you enjoy and make them a part of your routine.
- Mindfulness and Stress Reduction: Chronic stress can contribute to inflammation. Incorporate stress-reduction techniques like meditation, yoga, or deep breathing into your daily life.
- Stay Hydrated: Drink plenty of water throughout the day. Proper hydration is crucial for all bodily functions and helps reduce inflammation.
- Community and Support: Share your journey with friends or online communities. Having support can make maintaining this lifestyle more manageable and enjoyable.
- Regular Health Check-ups: Keep up with regular medical check-ups and discuss your dietary approach with healthcare professionals to ensure it aligns with your health needs.

ENHANCING YOUR ANTI-INFLAMMATORY JOURNEY THROUGH MINDFUL PRACTICES

Welcome to a crucial part of your anti-inflammatory journey, as mentioned in week 2 - understanding and implementing mindful eating and stress reduction techniques. This section of the book is dedicated to helping you cultivate practices that not only complement your dietary efforts but also enrich your overall well-being.

Mindful Eating Techniques

- Mindful eating is the practice of fully focusing on the experience of eating and savoring each bite.
- Benefits include improved digestion, better control over eating habits, and a deeper connection between food and body wellness.
- Mindful eating has been linked to reduced inflammation by promoting a balanced approach to food, reducing overeating, and improving gut health.

Chewing Slowly

- Why It's Important: Chewing slowly and thoroughly is a fundamental aspect of mindful eating. It aids in breaking down food more effectively, making it easier to digest. This process allows for better absorption of nutrients and can reduce digestive issues like bloating and indigestion.
- Benefits: By chewing slowly, you give your body time to recognize when it's full, which helps in portion control and prevents overeating. It also enhances the enjoyment of the flavors and textures of your food.
- Practical Tips:
    - Try to chew each bite around 20-30 times before swallowing.
    - Place your utensils down between bites to encourage slower eating.
    - Example: When eating an apple, notice the crisp texture and the sweetness that emerges as you chew slowly, enhancing the sensory experience.

2. Eliminating Distractions

- Why It's Important: Eating without distractions allows you to fully concentrate on your meal. Distractions like TV, phones, or computers can lead to mindless eating, where you may consume more than necessary without truly enjoying the meal.
- Benefits: Focused eating helps in recognizing hunger and fullness cues more accurately. It fosters a healthier relationship with food, as you're more aware of what and how much you're eating.

- **Practical Tips:**
    - Make mealtime an 'electronic-free zone.'
    - Use meals as a time to relax and enjoy your food without the rush.
    - Example: During lunch, instead of scrolling through social media, focus on the aroma, taste, and texture of your meal, such as the crunchiness of a salad or the warmth of a soup.

3. Journaling Food Experiences

- Why It's Important: Keeping a food journal helps in tracking not only what you eat but also your emotional responses to food. It can be a powerful tool in identifying triggers for overeating or choosing unhealthy foods.
- Benefits: Journaling can reveal patterns in eating habits and emotional eating. It helps in identifying foods that might cause discomfort or inflammation, leading to more mindful food choices.
- Practical Tips:
    - Note down details like time, place, mood, and physical sensations during and after each meal.
    - Don't just focus on the food; include thoughts and feelings associated with eating.
    - Example: If you notice discomfort after eating dairy, you might record this in your journal, helping you make more informed choices in the future.

Interactive Exercises:

- Guided Mindful Eating Practices: Follow along with exercises that help you eat more slowly and deliberately.
- Reflection Questions: Regularly ask yourself how certain foods make you feel and how your mood influences your eating choices.

Stress Reduction Techniques

The Link Between Stress and Inflammation:
- Chronic stress triggers the release of pro-inflammatory cytokines, exacerbating inflammation.
- Understanding how stress affects your body can help in developing strategies to manage it.

Practical Stress Management Strategies:

- Deep Breathing and Meditation: Regularly practice deep breathing or meditation to reduce stress levels.
- Physical Activity: Incorporate activities like yoga or walking, which have dual benefits of exercise and stress reduction.
- Effective Time Management: Develop techniques to manage your time better, reducing the stress that comes from feeling overwhelmed.

Creating a Personalized Stress Reduction Plan:

- Identify Stressors: Recognize what causes you stress and develop coping mechanisms.
- Daily Routine: Include relaxation and self-care in your daily schedule.

Additional Resources

Books:
- "The Mindful Diet" by Ruth Wolever and Beth Reardon
- "Full Catastrophe Living" by Jon Kabat-Zinn

Documentaries:
- "In Search of Balance"
- "The Connection: Mind Your Body"

YouTube Channels/Podcasts:
- "The Mindful Kind" (podcast by Rachael Kable)
- "Yoga With Adriene" (YouTube channel for accessible yoga practices)

These resources offer further insight into mindful eating and stress management, complementing the information and exercises provided in this program. They will guide you in creating a more balanced lifestyle, reducing inflammation, and promoting overall health and well-being.

Food to Avoid or minimize
- Refined Sugars (Score: 5)
  - Identification: Look for terms like 'sucrose', 'high-fructose corn syrup', or 'dextrose' on labels. Common in soft drinks, candies, and baked goods.
  - Why to Avoid: Causes blood sugar and insulin spikes, leading to increased inflammation.
  - Other Effects: Weight gain, diabetes risk, and energy fluctuations.
- **Trans Fats (Score: 5)**
  - Identification: Often listed as 'partially hydrogenated oils'. Found in many fast-food items, such as certain products from McDonald's, and in packaged snacks.
  - Why to Avoid: Triggers systemic inflammation.
  - Other Effects: Raises bad cholesterol, increasing heart disease risk.
- **Red and Processed Meats (Score: 4)**
  - Identification: Includes products like bacon, sausages, and deli meats. Check labels for 'processed' or 'cured' meats.
  - Why to Avoid: Linked to increased inflammation, particularly in processed forms.
  - Other Effects: Higher risk of heart disease and certain cancers.
- **Refined Carbohydrates (Score: 4)**
  - Identification: White bread, pastries, and other foods made with white flour. Check for 'refined wheat flour' on labels.
  - Why to Avoid: High glycemic index, causing blood sugar spikes.
  - Other Effects: Weight gain and type 2 diabetes risk.
- **Artificial Additives (Score: 3)**
  - Identification: Look for names like 'monosodium glutamate (MSG)', 'aspartame', or 'acesulfame potassium' on packaged foods.
  - Why to Avoid: Can trigger inflammatory responses.
  - Other Effects: Headaches, allergic reactions.
- **Dairy Products (Score: 2)**
  - Identification: Includes milk, cheese, and some yogurts. Be aware of dairy in baked goods and processed foods.
  - Why to Minimize: Inflammatory for those with lactose intolerance or sensitivities.
  - Other Effects: Digestive discomfort, acne.
- **Gluten (Score: 2)**
  - Identification: Found in wheat, barley, and rye. Look for 'gluten-free' alternatives if sensitive.
  - Why to Minimize: Can cause inflammation in individuals with celiac disease or sensitivities.
  - Other Effects: Gastrointestinal discomfort, autoimmune disease exacerbation.

- **Fried Foods (Score: 4)**
  - Identification: Common in fast food and restaurants; includes items like fries, fried chicken, and doughnuts.
  - Why to Avoid: High in unhealthy fats and trans fats.
  - Other Effects: Obesity and heart disease risk.
- **Sodium-Heavy Foods (Score: 3)**
  - Identification: Common in canned soups, snacks, and some frozen meals. Check sodium content on nutrition labels.
  - Why to Minimize: Can lead to inflammation and high blood pressure.
  - Other Effects: Increased risk of heart disease and stroke.

In addition to the previously listed foods, it's crucial to consider other substances like nicotine or alcohol, which can have indirect effects on diet and inflammation.

Alcohol (Score: 3)

Identification:
- Alcohol is found in a variety of beverages, including beers, wines, spirits, and mixed drinks. Excessive consumption, particularly of high-alcohol content drinks, can be problematic.

Why to Avoid:
- Disruption of Gut and Liver Function: Alcohol can significantly disrupt the balance of the gut microbiome and liver function. This disruption can contribute to systemic inflammation, affecting overall health.
- Direct Inflammatory Response: Alcohol can trigger an immediate inflammatory response in the body. Chronic consumption can lead to a persistent inflammatory state, aggravating conditions like gastritis and liver disease.

Other Effects:
- Risk of Liver Disease: Chronic alcohol consumption is a well-known risk factor for liver diseases, including fatty liver, hepatitis, and cirrhosis, all of which are linked to increased inflammation.
- Exacerbation of Health Issues: Excessive alcohol intake can worsen existing health conditions, particularly those associated with inflammation, such as heart disease.

Impact on Diet and Lifestyle:
- Appetite and Digestion: Alcohol can initially stimulate appetite but later disrupt normal digestion, leading to poor nutrient absorption and gastrointestinal issues.
- Impaired Judgment: Alcohol can impair judgment, leading to poor dietary choices, such as high consumption of fatty, salty, or sugary foods often associated with drinking.

Implementing Avoidance and Moderation Strategies:

- Moderation is Key: For those who choose to drink, moderation is crucial. Guidelines often suggest limiting intake to one drink per day for women and two for men.
- Healthier Choices: Opt for lower-alcohol beverages and avoid high-calorie mixers. Choosing a glass of red wine, known for its antioxidants, over hard liquors can be a healthier option.
- Support for Cessation: If alcohol consumption is a concern, seeking professional help or support groups can be essential for cessation and managing its impact on health.
- Mindful Drinking: Pay attention to the reasons behind alcohol consumption and its effects on your body. This awareness can help in making more conscious decisions regarding alcohol intake.

Nicotine (Score: 4)

- Identification: Nicotine is primarily consumed through smoking tobacco products, including cigarettes and e-cigarettes.
- Why to Avoid: Nicotine can indirectly affect eating habits and inflammation. While it's not a food, its impact on the body can exacerbate inflammatory responses.

- **Impact on Appetite and Eating Habits:**

  - Appetite Suppression: Nicotine initially acts as an appetite suppressant, which might lead to irregular eating patterns.
  - Increased Consumption Later: Once the effect wears off, there can be a tendency to overeat or crave unhealthy foods, contributing to poor dietary choices.
  - Metabolic Impact: Nicotine affects metabolism and can disrupt normal digestive processes, potentially leading to gastrointestinal inflammation.
- Other Effects: Aside from its well-known risks such as lung cancer, heart disease, and respiratory problems, nicotine can also contribute to stress and anxiety, further exacerbating inflammation.

Implementing Avoidance Strategies

- Seeking Alternatives: For those struggling with nicotine addiction, seeking professional help for cessation is crucial. There are various support systems and programs available to aid in quitting.
- Mindful Eating Post-Cessation: After quitting nicotine, it's important to be mindful of changes in appetite and eating patterns. Focusing on a balanced, anti-inflammatory diet can help manage weight and maintain overall health.
- Regular Physical Activity: Incorporating regular exercise can help regulate appetite, reduce stress, and lower the risk of weight gain post-cessation.

F*** ULTRA PROCESSED FOOD

The Health Risks

- Chronic Inflammation: These foods can trigger and exacerbate inflammation, contributing to a range of chronic diseases such as obesity, diabetes, heart disease, and even certain cancers.
- Impact on Gut Health: Ultra-processed foods can disrupt the balance of gut bacteria, leading to poor digestive health and further inflammation.
- Addictive Qualities: The high sugar and fat content in these foods can have addictive properties, making it challenging to moderate consumption.

But you already probably know this !

But how did we get here ?

The Evolution of Eating Habits in a Fast-Paced World

In our journey to understand modern diets, it's crucial to recognize the significant shift towards ultra-processed food consumption, a trend deeply rooted in cultural and industrial changes.

A Quick History Lesson: The American Machine and Its Global Impact
- Post-World War II Changes: The landscape of food production and consumption underwent a dramatic transformation post-World War II, particularly in America. The era marked the advent of mass-produced, easily accessible processed foods, driven by advancements in food technology and manufacturing.
- The Convenience Revolution: The rise of fast-food chains and the introduction of TV dinners in the 1950s epitomized America's growing appetite for convenience. These changes catered to the bustling lifestyle of the post-war era, offering quick, ready-to-eat meal solutions.
- Global Proliferation: This trend quickly spread across Europe and other parts of the world. The allure of convenience, coupled with aggressive marketing strategies, made ultra-processed foods a global phenomenon.
- Cultural Shifts: Over the decades, these foods became ingrained in cultural practices, influencing eating habits and preferences. The idea of quick, easy meals became synonymous with modern living.

Impact Across America, Europe, and Beyond

- Dietary Changes: The dominance of ultra-processed foods led to significant changes in traditional diets worldwide. Countries with rich culinary histories saw a surge in the consumption of ready-to-eat products, altering traditional eating patterns.
- Health Implications: This shift has had profound health implications. Regions that embraced these dietary changes witnessed rising rates of obesity, diabetes, and other diet-related health issues.
- Economic and Social Factors: Economic growth, urbanization, and lifestyle changes further fueled the demand for ultra-processed foods. Time constraints and the search for cost-effective meal options made these foods a staple in many households.

Understanding the history and widespread impact of ultra-processed foods sheds light on how deeply they are embedded in our society. It highlights the challenge of navigating a dietary landscape where convenience often overshadows nutritional value, underscoring the need for a more mindful and informed approach to eating in the modern world.

INTEGRATING ANTI-INFLAMMATORY CHOICES IN A FAST-PACED WORLD

Navigating Modern Lifestyle Demands with a Focus on Anti-Inflammatory Eating
In a world where ultra-processed foods are often the default due to work demands, social dynamics, and lifestyle constraints, incorporating anti-inflammatory choices requires both awareness and strategy.

The Intersection of Convenience and Nutrition

- Choosing Wisely: Even in the realm of convenience, there are options that can align with anti-inflammatory principles. For instance, many stores offer mixed nuts and seeds, which, despite being processed, can be a healthy choice.
- Understanding Labels: Not all processed foods are created equal. Some mixed nuts, for instance, may be heavily salted or sweetened. Opting for unsalted, raw or dry-roasted versions without added oils or sugars can provide the benefits of nuts and seeds without the inflammatory downsides.

Meal Planning and Preparation with an Anti-Inflammatory Twist

- Efficient and Healthy Cooking: When meal prepping, focus on recipes that are both time-efficient and rich in anti-inflammatory ingredients. For example, a quinoa salad with mixed vegetables, olive oil, and lemon dressing can be a quick yet healthy choice.
- Batch Cooking: Prepare anti-inflammatory meals in bulk, like stews or casseroles with lean proteins, whole grains, and vegetables. These can be refrigerated or frozen for convenience.

Balancing Convenience with Anti-Inflammatory Choices

- Healthiest Available Options: In situations where you have to rely on convenience foods, choose the options that align most closely with anti-inflammatory principles. Salads, grilled proteins, and vegetable-based dishes are often available in fast-food settings.
- Smart Snacking: Instead of reaching for chips or sugary snacks, keep a stash of anti-inflammatory snacks like mixed nuts, fresh fruits, or carrot sticks with hummus.

Adapting to Social and Lifestyle Realities

- Social Eating: When attending social events, try to opt for dishes that are closer to the anti-inflammatory spectrum. If you're bringing a dish, make it something that aligns with your dietary goals.
- Lifestyle Integration: Incorporate anti-inflammatory foods into your lifestyle in a way that feels natural and sustainable. This might mean having a go-to list of restaurants that offer healthier options or carrying healthy snacks during travel.

ACKNOWLEDGMENTS AND FURTHER LEARNING RESOURCES

First and foremost, thank you sincerely for taking the time to explore and embrace the principles outlined in this Anti-Inflammatory Meal Plan. Your commitment to enhancing your health and well-being is truly commendable. As you continue on this journey, expanding your knowledge and finding inspiration is key to maintaining a sustainable and enjoyable anti-inflammatory lifestyle. Below is a curated list of resources, including books, documentaries, websites, and YouTube channels, that can provide further insights and encouragement:

Websites

Harvard Health Blog

- What It Is: An online resource provided by Harvard Medical School offering articles and insights on various health topics.
- Benefits: You'll find up-to-date, research-backed information on a range of health subjects, including the latest trends in anti-inflammatory eating. This site is ideal for keeping abreast of evolving nutritional science and health advice.

NutritionFacts.org

- What It Is: A non-profit, science-based public service providing free updates on the latest in nutrition research via bite-sized videos.
- Benefits: Offers evidence-based information on nutrition and health, helping you make informed dietary choices. It's particularly beneficial for understanding the scientific rationale behind different foods and their impact on health.

The Whole30 Program

- What It Is: A 30-day dietary program designed to reset eating habits and help identify food sensitivities.
- Benefits: Although it's not specifically anti-inflammatory, it encourages the elimination and gradual reintroduction of certain foods, which can be helpful in identifying triggers for inflammation and other health issues.

YouTube Channels

Mind Over Munch

- What It Is: A YouTube channel focusing on making healthy eating both easy and fun.
- Benefits: Provides practical, accessible advice on creating sustainable and healthy eating habits. It's great for finding inspiration for meal prep and learning how to make healthier versions of your favorite foods.

Dr. Mike Hansen

- What It Is: A channel run by a physician, offering insights into various medical topics, including diet and its impact on health.
- Benefits: Dr. Hansen breaks down complex medical information into understandable content. This channel is useful for gaining medical perspectives on how diet affects overall health, including the role of anti-inflammatory eating.

Documentaries

"The Game Changers"

- What It Is: A documentary that explores the benefits of plant-based eating, particularly for athletes.
- Benefits: Provides compelling arguments and evidence for the impact of a plant-based diet on physical performance and health. It's inspiring for anyone considering more plant-centric eating habits, highlighting the benefits beyond just anti-inflammatory effects.

Books

The Longevity Diet" by Valter Longo

- What It Is: A book by a biochemist and gerontologist offering insights into how diet affects longevity and health.
- Benefits: It explores the relationship between nutrition and longevity, providing guidance on how to eat for a long and healthy life. The principles in this book can complement an anti-inflammatory diet, emphasizing foods that support healthy aging and disease prevention.

Each of these resources offers unique insights and practical advice, aiding in expanding your understanding of nutrition and health, particularly regarding anti-inflammatory eating and overall well-being. They can be invaluable tools as you continue to cultivate a lifestyle that supports health, longevity, and vitality.

BNW
PUBLISH

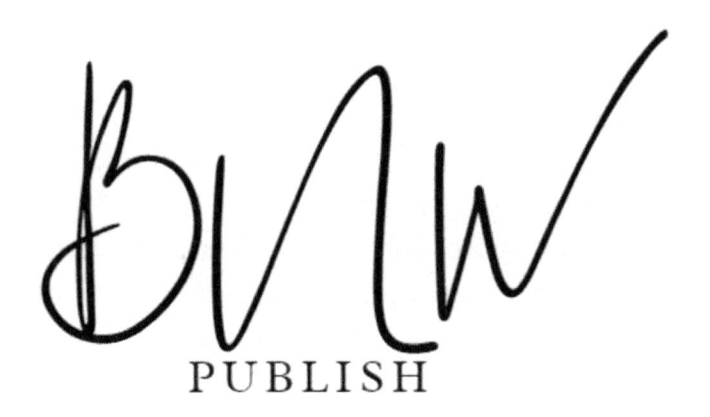

Join us on your favourite platform, Scan the QR code on your phone or tablet

Thank you

Please review on Amazon

★★★★★

B N William

Printed in Great Britain
by Amazon